ACCEPTANCE-BASED BEHAVIORAL THERAPY

Also Available

FOR GENERAL READERS

The Mindful Way through Anxiety:
Break Free from Chronic Worry and Reclaim Your Life
Susan M. Orsillo and Lizabeth Roemer

Worry Less, Live More:
The Mindful Way through Anxiety Workbook
Susan M. Orsillo and Lizabeth Roemer

Acceptance-Based Behavioral Therapy

TREATING ANXIETY AND RELATED CHALLENGES

Lizabeth Roemer
Susan M. Orsillo

THE GUILFORD PRESS
New York   London

See page 318 for terms of use for audio files.

The authors have checked with sources believed to be reliable in their efforts to provide
information that is complete and generally in accord with the standards of practice that are
accepted at the time of publication. However, in view of the possibility of human error or
changes in behavioral, mental health, or medical sciences, neither the authors, nor the editors
and publisher, nor any other party who has been involved in the preparation or publication
of this work warrants that the information contained herein is in every respect accurate or
complete, and they are not responsible for any errors or omissions or the results obtained from
the use of such information. Readers are encouraged to confirm the information contained in
this book with other sources.

Library of Congress Cataloging-in-Publication data

Names: Roemer, Lizabeth, 1967– author. | Orsillo, Susan M., 1964– author.
Title: Acceptance-based behavioral therapy : treating anxiety and related challenges /
    Lizabeth Roemer, Susan M. Orsillo.
Description: New York : The Guilford Press, [2020] | Includes bibliographical references
    and index. |
Identifiers: LCCN 2020022641 | ISBN 9781462544875 (paperback) |
    ISBN 9781462543946 (hardcover)
Subjects: LCSH: Acceptance and commitment therapy. | Anxiety disorders—Treatment. |
    Anxiety—Treatment.
Classification: LCC RC489.C62 R635 2020 | DDC 616.89/1425—dc23
LC record available at https://lccn.loc.gov/2020022641

About the Authors

Lizabeth Roemer, PhD, is Professor of Psychology at the University of Massachusetts Boston, where she is actively involved in research and clinical training of doctoral students in clinical psychology. Dr. Roemer's research examines how people understand, react to, and cope with intense emotional reactions, most often in the contexts of anxiety disorders and posttraumatic functioning. She also supports her students in examining the relevance of cultural and contextual factors in these phenomena, with an emphasis on helping people thrive in the face of discrimination and racism. Her research team has a recent focus on dissemination, health promotion, and identifying and addressing barriers to care. Dr. Roemer has published over 120 journal articles and book chapters. She is coauthor, with Susan M. Orsillo, of *The Mindful Way through Anxiety* and *Worry Less, Live More* (for general readers). Their website is *www.mindfulwaythroughanxiety.com*.

Susan M. Orsillo, PhD, is Professor of Psychology at Suffolk University in Boston, where she is actively involved in the education, training, and professional development of undergraduates and doctoral students in clinical psychology. Dr. Orsillo studies how acceptance-based behavioral therapy-informed strategies can help buffer against contextual stressors, build resilience, improve psychosocial functioning, and enhance quality of life. Her research team also has a focus on improving widespread access to evidence-based care. Dr. Orsillo has published over 120 journal articles and book chapters. Her books with Lizabeth Roemer include *The Mindful Way through Anxiety* and *Worry Less, Live More*. Their website is *www.mindfulwaythroughanxiety.com*.

Preface

Our initial intention was to briefly revise our 2009 book into a second edition. However, as we revisited the initial text and began the process of revision, we realized that the last 10 years of research, supervision, clinical trainings, consultation, and scholarly developments in the field had generated a lot of new material, leading to this new volume that rests on the foundation of the previous one. The basic tenets of our clinical approach haven't changed radically; however, we have learned so much from clients, trainees, therapists, and colleagues over the years about the importance of acknowledging and working with the complexities and contextual factors that impact our clients' lives, the aspects of acceptance-based behavioral therapy (ABBT) that are most central to therapeutic success, and the most effective methods of presenting our ideas (to both clinicians and clients) that this resulting work is largely new. The process of writing two self-help books in the interim (and feedback we've received on them) also taught us a great deal about how to clarify and get to the heart of key concepts, while also allowing for individual variability and flexibility in clients' presenting concerns, lived experiences, and individualized goals for therapy. We think those who have read our first therapist book will find a lot of new material here that we hope you will find useful. Specifically, this volume includes:

- More detailed, step-by-step guidance on how to conduct a detailed assessment and develop a case formulation to guide flexible application of these strategies.
- A more extensive description of the therapeutic relationship we aim to develop with clients when working from an acceptance-based behavioral orientation and the intentional ways we cultivate and use this relationship to support and create client change.
- Considerably more scaffolding and guidance in how to effectively and flexibly use strategies such as identifying and working with clear and muddy emotions and helping clients to clarify and affirm values that promote mindful engagement in life-fulfilling activities.

- A more refined description of how to seamlessly integrate and flexibly adapt formal and informal mindfulness practices with behavioral change strategies to help clients with their specific presenting concerns and to support their achievement of individualized therapy goals.
- A deeper focus on methods used to cultivate self-compassion within this approach.
- More discussion of how to recognize and address barriers that can arise at all of the different points of treatment, particularly within values-based living.
- An integration of considerations of context, cultural factors, and systemic oppression across all aspects of treatment.
- Guidelines for conducting therapy when time is limited to facilitate adaptation of this approach in different contexts of care.
- Updated forms and handouts to use with clients and activities that therapists can try to deepen their experiential understanding of the material.

As with the previous book, *Mindfulness- and Acceptance-Based Behavioral Therapies in Practice*, our hope is to provide clinicians and clinicians-in-training with a helpful framework and guidelines for conducting psychotherapy that uses mindfulness- and acceptance-based behavioral approaches with clients with diverse clinical presentations. This book differs from typical treatment protocol books in that we do not present a standardized protocol, nor do we focus on a single type of ABBT. Instead, this clinical guide is grounded in our two decades of collaborative work that was initially focused on developing an ABBT for clients with a principal diagnosis of generalized anxiety disorder (GAD) along with a range of comorbid disorders (Roemer & Orsillo, 2002, 2014) and evolved into a flexible, conceptualization-driven acceptance-based behavioral approach to a range of clinical presentations and health promotion efforts. When we initially developed our manualized treatment, we integrated material from a variety of evidence-based interventions that emphasize acceptance and mindfulness (e.g., acceptance and commitment therapy [ACT]: Hayes, Strosahl, & Wilson, 1999; dialectical behavior therapy [DBT]: Linehan, 1993; mindfulness-based cognitive therapy [MBCT]: Segal, Williams, & Teasdale, 2002), along with other behavioral and cognitive interventions that have received extensive empirical support (e.g., Barlow, 2014; Borkovec & Sharples, 2004). Over time we have continued to learn from these and other clinicians and researchers and to integrate material from a broad range of interventions under the acceptance, mindfulness, and behavioral umbrellas. In this way, we see our work as similar to that of cognitive-behavioral clinicians and researchers who draw from a range of empirically supported treatments to inform case conceptualizations and treatment plans that meet individualized needs of a particular client.

DEFINING THE APPROACH

In our work, we use the term *acceptance-based behavioral therapies* (ABBTs; or sometimes *mindfulness- and acceptance-based behavioral therapies)* to define an overarching approach that explicitly emphasizes altering the way clients relate to their internal experiences (reducing reactivity and avoidance, while promoting decentering and acceptance) as a central mechanism of therapeutic change, coupled with an emphasis on the central role of learning and behavior change in therapy. Approaches that fall under this umbrella term have also been called "third-wave" behavioral and cognitive therapies (Hayes, 2016) or contextual cognitive-behavioral therapies (CBTs) (Hayes, Villatte, Levin, & Hildebrandt, 2011), and a subset are often called mindfulness-based interventions or therapies (e.g., Khoury et al., 2013). Still another subset of (self) compassion-focused treatments have been developed that share a number of principles and strategies (e.g., Gilbert, 2009; Kolts, 2016; Neff & Germer, 2018). At the same time, it's important to note that similar mechanisms and processes are often identified as underlying what are sometimes called "traditional" behavioral therapies or CBTs (for in-depth reviews, see Arch & Craske, 2008; Orsillo, Roemer, Lerner, & Tull, 2004; Roemer, Arbid, Martinez, & Orsillo, 2017). Moreover, behavioral and cognitive-behavioral models continue to evolve in ways that more explicitly incorporate acceptance of internal experiences, which was often an implicit focus in these approaches (e.g., Barlow et al., 2017). Emotion regulation therapies (e.g., Mennin & Fresco, 2014) similarly posit overlapping targets and mechanisms of change. Further, nonbehavioral traditions also highlight a central role of acceptance (e.g., Rogers, 1961). We do not intend ABBT to refer to another specific protocol or to be a model in opposition to these other approaches. In fact, we are inspired and informed by the commonalities across treatment approaches and are particularly excited when therapists attending our workshops share that something we are talking about feels connected to another tradition or approach they've been trained in. When theories overlap, they are likely to be converging on some meaningful aspect of the human condition.

That said, we do find a coherent model of clinical challenges and intervention strategies that can guide case conceptualization and inform treatment planning to be an important part of collaboratively engaging clients in meaningful change. In this book, we share the specific ideas and strategies falling under this umbrella of acceptance-based behavioral therapies that we have found most helpful. We use the term ABBT to describe the approach for ease of communication; we intend it the same way one might use CBT: we are referring to a broad approach to understanding and treating clinical problems, not a narrow protocol. And we conceptualize ABBTs as falling within the broader scope of CBTs in that both rest on the foundation of learning theory. We incorporate a wide range of traditional CBT strategies in our work (e.g., self-monitoring, psychoeducation, adapted relaxation strategies, behavioral activation, and exposure [tied to valued action]), using them all in the service of targeting ABBT-related processes. Throughout the book we highlight the ways that an ABBT approach relates to and can be consistent with other CBT strategies such as relaxation therapy, cognitive restructuring, and emotion regulation. We hope readers will find information here that they can integrate effectively into their clinical approach.

THE EVIDENCE BASE FOR ABBT APPROACHES

The evidence base for ABBTs, and the cognitive-behavioral strategies incorporated in them, is too expansive and rapidly expanding to be effectively summarized here (see Hofmann & Asmundson, 2017, for overviews of evidence for specific approaches). Efficacy has been demonstrated for a range of ABBT approaches across a range of clinical presentations (e.g., Goldberg et al., 2018; A-Tjak et al., 2015), with effects generally comparable to CBT. Empirically supported protocols developed for specific clinical presentations typically incorporate evidence-based strategies (e.g., ACT for mixed anxiety disorders incorporating behavioral exposures; Arch, Eifert, Davies, Vilardaga, Rose, & Craske, 2012). We encourage readers to explore the literature regarding specific clinical presenting problems and contexts for the clients you're working with and to incorporate evidence-based strategies consistent with these evidence-based principles.

Our own collaborative research with colleagues and doctoral students focused first on developing an ABBT protocol for treating clients with GAD and comorbid presenting problems. This treatment leads to significant reductions in symptoms of anxiety and depression, improvements in quality of life that are comparable to those found with applied relaxation (e.g., Roemer, Orsillo, & Salters-Pedneault, 2008; Hayes-Skelton, Roemer, & Orsillo, 2013), as well as improvements in interpersonal functioning (Millstein, Orsillo, Hayes-Skelton, & Roemer, 2015) and clinically significant increases in self-reported engagement in valued action (Michelson, Lee, Orsillo, & Roemer, 2011). Both ABBT and applied relaxation (AR) targeted experiential avoidance and decentering, and these changes predicted clinical outcomes (Eustis, Hayes-Skelton, Roemer, & Orsillo, 2016; Hayes-Skelton, Calloway, Roemer, & Orsillo, 2015), with decentering changing prior to anxiety symptoms. Clients from marginalized backgrounds reported that values clarification/action and flexibility helped with the cultural responsiveness of the therapy (Fuchs et al., 2016). Abbreviated health promotion programs developed on the basis of these principles also significantly reduced anxiety and depressive symptoms through programs delivered in person (Danitz & Orsillo, 2014; Danitz, Suvak, & Orsillo, 2016; Eustis, Krill Williston, Morgan, Graham, Hayes-Skelton, & Roemer, 2017) and online (Eustis, Hayes-Skelton, Orsillo, & Roemer, 2018; Sagon, Danitz, Suvak, & Orsillo, 2018). We also have preliminary data suggesting that individuals in the community with generalized anxiety who used ABBT materials as self-help resources experienced significant decreases in worry, anxiety, depression, and functional impairment and increases in acceptance (Serowik, Roemer, Suvak, Liverant, & Orsillo, 2019). Correlational and experimental pilot studies have also begun to illustrate the ways that mindfulness and valued action may be beneficial in response to racist experiences (Graham, West, & Roemer, 2013, 2015; Miller & Orsillo, 2020; West, Graham, & Roemer, 2013).

We draw from our experience conducting these studies in our application of these principles here. As such, the context of these studies is relevant—our clinical trials involved a 16-session individual protocol therapy, while the health promotion studies involved single or multiple brief session general interventions. However, we have supervised ABBTs administered in more flexible structures, and we advocate the use of group contexts when possible for skills building and values-based action accountability support. In this book, we provide guidelines for flexible use of these principles and strategies.

HOW TO USE THIS BOOK

Rather than providing a prescriptive protocol for conducting ABBT, in this book we provide an in-depth description of how to use a range of clinical methods to target the factors presumed to contribute to and maintain client problems from an ABBT perspective. We hope this will allow clinicians to flexibly deliver ABBT, integrating it with other treatment approaches when indicated, adapting it to fit a range of treatment settings, and tailoring it to meet the individualized needs of specific clients. We explicitly describe the conceptual basis for choosing and applying each intervention to inform clinicians' choices and adaptations and provide a basis for troubleshooting challenges. Given the complexity of humans and the range of settings clinicians work in, we provide numerous case examples and a range of possible strategies, so that therapists can pick and choose and still have resources left to look at if some strategies seem to fit less well with a given client. These are meant to support flexible application of the treatment approach, not as an exhaustive list that therapists should follow. We encourage therapists to be creative in developing their own ways of presenting concepts and delivering the treatment in ways that meet clients' needs while monitoring progress and making data-driven choices about what is most relevant and effective.

Tips for Making the Best Use of This Book

- We recommend reading the whole book before applying the treatment to your work with a client. Assessing a client and developing a comprehensive case conceptualization require full understanding of the theory and course of therapy, which is reflected in the principles and methods described throughout the entire book.

- The divisions into assessment, strategies, and valued action are somewhat arbitrary—concepts overlap across these chapters. We provide cross-references to other parts of the book to draw these connections. It may be helpful to follow these cross-references when you see them in order to develop a deeper understanding of a given concept, or to come back to this part of the book once you've read a later description.

- This book is focused on targeting mechanisms that underlie a wide range of clinical presentations. Resources focused on addressing specific clinical presentations will be an important supplement. Given our research focus on generalized anxiety and comorbid disorders, we provide more details for these clinical presentations, but we also draw connections to other clinical presentations.

- We encourage you to create personalized handouts and mindfulness recordings for your clients and to supplement the handouts and recordings (available on the Guilford website; see the box at the end of the table of contents) we provide, so that you can more precisely reflect their own experiences and fit material to their needs.

- We encourage you to engage in the experiential exercises in the "Try This" boxes; this will allow you to bring your observations of your own experience to your work with clients.

- We have reprinted some material from our workbook *Worry Less, Live More: The Mindful Way through Anxiety Workbook*, but many more practical guides and exercises for clients appear in that book. Readers may find that it's helpful to supplement treatment with that self-help guide with clients who are experiencing anxiety and worry, particularly when time is limited.

We use the gender-neutral singular pronoun "they" in case examples to capture the range of gender identities of clients.

Acknowledgments

This book is a culmination of our collaborative work over the past two decades, and we are grateful to all the people who have inspired, encouraged, supported, and facilitated that work over all these years. Our work stands on the shoulders of countless clinical psychologists and Buddhist writers and teachers whose contributions helped us to identify effective ways to help people engage more fully and meaningfully in their lives. Although we can't possibly name all of these influences, we wish to specifically acknowledge the work of Dave Barlow, Tom Borkovec, Andrew Christensen, Kelly Koerner, Shelly Harrell, Steven Hayes, Richard Heimberg, Neil Jacobson, Marsha Linehan, Brett Litz, Alan Marlatt, Doug Mennin, Zindel Segal, John Teasdale, Mark Williams, and Kelly Wilson, as well as Toni Bernhard, Pema Chodron, Paul Gilbert, Les Greenberg, Jon Kabat-Zinn, Rhonda Magee, Jeremy Safran, Sharon Salzberg, Paul Wachtel, and Angel Kyodo Williams. We are most grateful to the clients who have continually taught and inspired us with their willingness to open up to their pain and their courage to make changes in order to experience more meaningful lives. We thank them for all they have taught us as psychologists and as human beings. We also thank all the therapists we have supervised over the years; their insights too are reflected in these pages. In particular, we thank our collaborator Sarah Hayes-Skelton, who has held, nurtured, nourished, and enhanced our work for the past 12 years. We also thank the National Institute of Mental Health for supporting our work and this book and everyone at The Guilford Press for supporting our books over the years.

In addition, I (LR) want to thank Sue, first and foremost, although there are no words to sufficiently capture my gratitude. Sue's wisdom, kindness, conscientiousness, perceptiveness, and care create and enrich our shared work and continually inspire me. Her steadfast, far-reaching support enables me to engage my life fully in ways that matter to me. I am also eternally grateful to my graduate school mentor, Tom Borkovec, for all of his teachings and for the model he provided of integrating science and practice, to which I continue to aspire. I have had the great privilege of working with many graduate students over the years whose wisdom, insights, commitment to social justice, and kindness continually teach, enrich, and motivate me; there are too many to list, but they know who they are and how much I appreciate them. They, along with my friends and colleagues Karen Suyemoto and Roxanne Donovan, influenced this volume immensely. Thanks also to my father and mother, who always took my writing and my ideas seriously. And last, but far from least, I thank my partner, Josh Bartok, whose discernments (and editorial skill) infuse this book, and whose love, care, and wisdom help me to be the person I want to be.

I (SMO) am deeply indebted to Liz, my coauthor, collaborator, and friend. What a gift it's been to have shared this journey with her. From the time our training paths crossed at the Boston VA, her generosity and compassion have challenged, inspired, and sustained me. I also want to thank the graduate students I've worked with across the years. The countless hours we shared together reading (and rereading) the literature, wrestling with challenging questions, reflecting on our clients' experiences, and exploring our own biases and blind spots have made me a better scholar, teacher, clinician, and human. I am grateful to my parents for surrounding me with books as a child, encouraging my love of learning, and supporting me in my journey from first-generation college student to faculty scholar. I thank my children, Sarah and Sam, for their love, support, and understanding, particularly during the many times that my writing encroached on family time. The joy and meaning they bring to my life are immeasurable. And finally, my deepest gratitude to my partner, Paul, for more than 30 years of friendship, unwavering support, and love.

Contents

PART I

Setting the Stage for Change

An essential component of successful therapy is developing a clear, shared understanding of a client's presenting challenges that is paired to a reasonable, acceptable plan for creating meaningful change. In these chapters, we present a general conceptualization of human challenges that forms the overarching basis for our clinical work, guidelines for assessing central concepts in this conceptualization, and a description of how to develop an individualized case conceptualization and share it with a client. This work forms the foundation for the more explicit interventions that follow in Parts II and III; those interventions are less likely to be effective when this foundation isn't clearly established. This shared understanding also provides a foundation to return to when challenges arise in treatment (described more fully in Chapter 11).

Although these early chapters focus specifically on assessing and conceptualizing clients at the beginning of therapy, the process of assessment and conceptualization is iterative across the course of treatment. Therefore, many of the suggestions we include here may be relevant later in treatment as well, when ongoing monitoring and observation (by both client and therapist) refine and expand the shared understanding of how clients came to be struggling in specific ways and how best to help them make meaningful changes. Similarly, initial sessions include important aspects of intervention as well (and this is particularly true when conducting brief interventions). We encourage therapists to apply principles from Chapter 4 describing the use of the therapeutic relationship as a context and mechanism for change when conducting assessments and sharing their case conceptualization.

Because acceptance-based behavioral therapy (ABBT) emphasizes cultivating a more expansive, clear awareness of responses as they unfold, therapeutic interventions like monitoring and mindfulness (described in Chapters 5 and 6) will naturally enhance clients' (and therapists') understanding of their experiences, and potential targets for learning new ways of responding. Therefore, Parts II and III include more in-depth, complex descriptions of central concepts in the model—reading the book all the way through will enhance your ability to skillfully and flexibly notice and clarify patterns of responding throughout treatment.

CHAPTER 1

Overview of an Acceptance-Based Behavioral Model of Clinical Problems

Although acceptance-based behavioral approaches to treatment, like all cognitive-behavioral approaches, are grounded in an idiographic case conceptualization of the client, they draw from an overarching evidence-based model of common factors that underlie clinical problems. This model integrates many theoretical orientations and is firmly grounded in behavioral theory. As such, it is an easy model for clinicians to learn and incorporate into their clinical thinking.

What you will learn

- An evidence-based understanding of clinical problems that can guide flexible application of acceptance-based behavioral, and other, strategies in clinical practice.
- A flexible three-part, integrated model for understanding clinical problems that includes:
  - Why clients' ways of relating to their internal responses can become problematic.
  - How rigid efforts to feel or think differently can make clients' challenges worse.
  - Different ways clients can lose their connection to what matters to them.

Kamila is a second-generation Pakistani American, Muslim, heterosexual, cisgender woman who was referred to therapy by her primary care clinician to whom she had reported difficulty sleeping, stomach problems, distractibility, irritability, and muscle pain, particularly in her neck and shoulders. Although Kamila believed her difficulties were physical, her doctor had been unable to determine a physical cause. Because Kamila endorsed symptoms of both generalized anxiety and depressive disorders on a screening form, the primary care clinician suggested therapy. Kamila came to her initial intake saying she was willing to try anything given how much symptoms were interfering in her life. Although she did not describe herself as "anxious," she acknowledged that she had always been "high strung." Kamila explained that her mind was constantly reviewing past events to try to sort them out or running through things she feared could happen in the future to her or members of her family, so that she could avoid problems or be better "prepared" to respond effectively. She emphasized that being a "planner" and a "problem solver" had served her well during school and made her an effective teacher, parent, and household manager. However, in recent years, she had found it harder to "turn off" her mind when she got into bed. Kamila had also started to notice she was often thinking through past or upcoming situations when she meant to be focused on something else, such as work or the person she was with. Kamila described several strategies she had tried to "clear" her mind but admitted they were never successful; in fact she felt her efforts left her more and more distracted, leading her to make mistakes or forget things. She also described snapping at people in her life more and more frequently, which led her to devote even more mental energy to trying to figure out why she was so irritable. Kamila identified a shift in her ability to "manage" her life, which had been precipitated by her husband getting injured at work and going out on disability for 6 months. The increased financial strain for their family was stressful, and she felt even more pressure about her own work (as a high school teacher), since it seemed essential to her family's well-being that she succeed. Kamila shared that she worried about the potentially negative impact that this change in their financial situation could have on their children and that worries and concerns about how to maximize their success and well-being often kept her up nights. She described trying to be cheerful and upbeat with her husband during this time, so that he wouldn't get discouraged. Unfortunately, Kamila's pattern of carrying the responsibility for her family's security and happiness continued even after her husband returned to work. When asked about what she enjoyed in life, Kamila hesitated and then began to cry. But after just a few minutes, she apologized for her "outburst," stopped crying, and shared that she enjoys keeping her family and life in order and on track because it makes her feel she is being a good mother, wife, daughter, and teacher. Kamila disagreed with her primary care physician's assessment of her as depressed, declaring she was much too busy to be depressed. Kamila pointed out that she had everything she needed to be happy, although she acknowledged that she didn't feel that she had the energy or mental capacity to really enjoy any aspect of her life currently, which is why she was seeking help. She admitted feeling hopeless and worn out at times and angry at herself for yelling at her children and not being more cheerful with her family. She worried that her current difficulties were "stressing out" her parents, who shared their concerns after Kamila missed several family gatherings due to her digestive difficulties. She also worried that she wasn't being a good Muslim because she frequently avoided going to activities at her mosque. Kamila hoped that therapy would help her to "get over it," as she saw her preoccupation and worry as signs of weakness. She had been trying everything she could think of to be more patient with her family and her students, to feel better physically, and "be happy," and she was confused as to why nothing seemed to help.

Our first step in therapy with Kamila would be to work with her to develop a shared understanding of how her experiences, reactions, and behaviors are linked together and understandable, even though they may seem confusing or disconnected to her. This individualized conceptualization would be grounded in an overarching acceptance-based behavioral conceptual model, which we describe in this chapter as a foundation for the work that follows. We describe the overall model here that informs ABBT, drawing some links to Kamila to illustrate concepts, and then, in Chapter 3, we explore how to develop an individualized case conceptualization.

OVERVIEW OF THE ACCEPTANCE-BASED BEHAVIORAL MODEL

In our clinical work, we use a three-part general model as a starting point for individualized case conceptualizations (see Figure 1.1). This model of proposed psychological mechanisms is grounded in behavioral theory and draws from the acceptance and commitment therapy (ACT) hexaflex (Hayes, Strosahl, & Wilson, 2012). Each part of the model relates to the others, leading to an escalating cycle of difficulty that can be hard to recognize and break out of on one's own. Biology and history also play a significant role in the development of these challenges, while ongoing environmental events and context influence and are in turn influenced by each element.

First, clinical difficulties stem from the problematic ways that clients (and humans in general) often learn to **relate to their internal experiences.** This relationship can be characterized as reactive and critical, in addition to "fused" (Hayes, Strosahl, & Wilson, 2012), entangled (Germer, 2005), or "hooked" (Chodron, 2007). This involves seeing our thoughts, feelings, sensations, or urges as negative and as self-defining rather than as phenomena that rise and fall. Although Kamila doesn't use the term *anxious* to describe herself, she does see her thoughts and feelings as signs of personal weakness. She also reacts to her thoughts and feelings as though they are accurate, and she assumes she must attend to and respond to each of them. This perspective leads her to become entangled with each worrisome thought and painful emotion that arises.

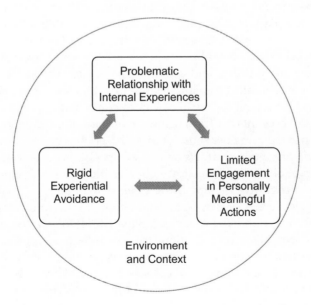

FIGURE 1.1. Acceptance-based behavioral conceptualization of the psychological processes that maintain clinical problems.

The second element of the model is **experiential avoidance,** or rigid emotional, cognitive, and behavioral efforts aimed at helping one to avoid or escape distressing thoughts, feelings, urges, memories, and sensations (Hayes, Wilson, Gifford, Follette, & Strosahl, 1996). Experiential avoidance is a natural consequence of fusion with and entanglement in internal experiences—if some thoughts and feelings are experienced as negative, self-defining, all-encompassing, and persistent, trying to push them away or change them makes a lot of sense. Unfortunately, as described later in this chapter, rigid efforts to get rid of internal experiences often exacerbate these difficulties. In Kamila's case, she tries to "clear her mind" as a way of removing her constant worries. In addition, the worry process itself likely serves an experientially avoidant function (as does her rumination): Kamila often brings her full attention to her worries about the future with the hope of trying to find ways to avoid potential problems and to reduce her fear over the uncertainty of future events. She also hopes that focusing on and working through memories of painful past experiences will reduce her regret over how things went. This habit of worry and rumination may sometimes reduce her arousal or distress in the moment; unfortunately, it also maintains her ongoing sense that she has to remain vigilant for potential threats. Kamila has devoted considerable time and effort toward trying to "fix" or control her thoughts and feelings. Although she notices the costs of this strategy, such as feeling distracted and irritable, she doesn't see any other options. Our assessment of Kamila (see Chapter 2) may help us identify other behaviors and habits that also serve an experientially avoidant function.

The final element of the model is **limited engagement in personally meaningful actions,** which refers to the ways that people who are struggling with their thoughts, feelings, and sensations often become disconnected from the things that matter most to them (i.e., valued action; Wilson & Murrell, 2004), which adds to their distress and dissatisfaction. The time one spends entangled with internal experiences and occupied with change and avoidance efforts is time that is not spent engaged in personally meaningful activities. Kamila feels like she is constantly consumed with activity aimed at keeping her family happy, safe, and secure. Yet, the strategy of trying to think through how to best manage her life actually leaves her less present with her family and less available to participate in events and activities she values. The sadness she expressed briefly in session may actually be an important signal that she is not living in a way that is meaningful and satisfying for her (i.e., values consistent), yet her desire to remain upbeat and cheerful prevents her from using the important information communicated by this emotion, perpetuating her sense of dissatisfaction with her life.

The model we present here draws on several specific acceptance-based behavioral (e.g., ACT [Hayes et al., 2011], dialectical behavior therapy [DBT; Linehan, 2015], and mindfulness-based cognitive therapy [MBCT; Segal, Williams, & Teasdale, 2012]), and general mindfulness (e.g., Germer, Segal, & Fulton, 2013) approaches and cognitive-behavioral models (e.g., Borkovec, Alcaine, & Behar, 2004) to focus on what we consider central, clinically useful elements. We hope this provides a useful framework that you can synthesize with other approaches you use in your clinical practice. We don't provide an in-depth review of the empirical basis for the model here (see Orsillo, Danitz, & Roemer, 2016, and Roemer & Orsillo, 2014, for more detailed reviews), but in Chapter 5 we do present some examples of research that we often share with clients as we introduce and explain the model and apply it to their specific experiences. In this chapter, we present the core elements of the model, with brief mentions of some complexities that we examine more fully later in the book.

A BEHAVIORAL UNDERSTANDING OF CLINICAL CHALLENGES[1]

We conceptualize clinical challenges using a behavioral lens (for more in-depth descriptions of behavioral theory and therapy, see Antony & Roemer, 2011; Tolin, 2016). That is, we see clinical problems as occurring because individuals naturally learn to respond in certain ways, and their responses are maintained by the consequences of these responses. For instance, if someone has had multiple experiences of being ignored when showing genuine sadness and asking for assistance, and being readily responded to when showing anger and demanding help, that person has likely learned that expressing anger is the effective way to get a need met and may continue to respond with anger habitually across situations. It may be that in the current context anger still garners attention, which brings some emotional relief, but it also causes distance and conflict in relationships. Unless the person has an acute awareness of the range of context-specific consequences that follow angry outbursts, they will likely continue to respond in a habitual way. Even if the person is aware of the costs associated with using anger to ask for help, if they have had limited opportunities to learn alternative, more relationally effective methods of effective communication, they may feel like they are stuck. When we can identify the conditions that maintain problematic ways of responding, we can more effectively and efficiently intervene to make changes. Sharing the idea that past learning influences current patterns also provides an opportunity for therapists to validate clients who believe (or who have been told) that their responses are "irrational," "self-defeating," or "pathological" and may help clients to cultivate self-compassion for their own responses. When we are able to see that even our most frustrating and life-interfering habits make "sense" or serve some function, it's much easier to be kind and compassionate to ourselves when we have them and to be open to trying to change them.

From a behavioral perspective, human difficulties arise from a combination of biological predispositions, environmental factors, and learned habits that result in a host of reactions and behaviors that occur automatically, without awareness or apparent choice. Human learning is complex and nuanced, and it occurs in several ways:

- **Direct experience.** For instance, someone who was sexually assaulted might learn to connect (i.e., associative learning) the smell of cologne with danger, which motivates them to avoid people wearing that same scent. We also learn through consequences (i.e., operant learning) that consistently follow particular behaviors and either reinforce (i.e., increase the frequency) or punish (i.e., reduce the frequency) of the behavior. So someone might continue to drink excessively

---

[1] Because we view the factors that create and maintain clinical problems as factors that influence all of us, and to recognize that clinicians also experience clinical problems, we switch between referring to clients and using the term *we* in this discussion. As we describe throughout, we often use *we* or *humans* in our psychoeducation with clients.

because of the immediate reduction in stress they feel when they binge drink (i.e., drinking is negatively reinforced).

- **Modeling and observation.** For example, hearing a parent continually talk about all of the potential catastrophes that could result from one action might lead us to engage in the same process.
- **Instruction.** For instance, being warned about the consequences of showing certain emotions or being advised against "making waves" even when one is treated unfairly may lead one to habitually conceal emotional responses.

Learning how to respond and act from associations, consequences, modeling, and instruction is extremely beneficial and often serves us well—for instance, instruction allows us to learn about real dangers without ever encountering harm. However, learning is context specific; behavioral patterns that are adaptive in one context may be problematic in another. Learning to "put on a happy face" when distressed might keep a child from being physically abused for showing sadness or anger, but masking distress in a romantic relationship could reduce genuine intimacy and make it challenging to get one's needs met. Also, the consequences of behavior are often complex in that many responses have both benefits and costs. For example, although dismissing and pushing away the feelings of sadness that Kamila feels when she notices how little time she spends visiting her parents or being intimate with her husband temporarily relieves her pain, it also prevents her from recognizing that she could make different choices. Finally, we don't always have the sustained awareness of our experience to truly observe and notice our behaviors and their consequences. Often, the habitual responses we develop, like reacting to pain with efforts to suppress, are elicited so quickly, consistently, and automatically that we lose awareness of our full experience.

Clinical problems are often characterized by these kinds of habitual, insensitive (to context), and automatic responses. The three elements of the ABBT model described earlier can be conceptualized as three classes of learned responses that are clinically important targets for intervention:

1. Learned qualities of relating to internal experiences.
   - We can learn to associate our own emotions, thoughts, sensations, and memories with threat, danger, and negative outcomes, leading us to react with criticism and judgment to these natural, human experiences.
   - We can also learn to view our momentary internal experiences as indicators of reality, defining the qualities of who we are at our core and our enduring traits, which amplifies our reactive and critical response to them.
   - Our understanding of, and relationship with, our internal experiences, particularly our emotions, are influenced by our caregivers, the societal messages we receive, and the cultures with which we identify.
2. Learned responses that function to suppress, change, or avoid internal experiences (i.e., experiential avoidance).
   - Clinically relevant behaviors such as avoiding situations or activities that could elicit painful thoughts and emotions, alcohol or drug use, restricted or excessive eating, ruminating, and general inaction may be maintained specifically because they serve the function of temporarily reducing, eliminating, or avoiding distressing thoughts, feelings, or sensations.

3. Learned habits of behavior that limit engagement in personally meaningful actions.
   - Experiential avoidance can lead us to intentionally avoid engaging in valued actions that have the potential to elicit painful internal experiences.
   - Sometimes we may impulsively and automatically take actions that are not particularly valued, due to their experientially avoidant function (e.g., spending hours on the Internet reading about whether a physical symptom we notice is actually a sign of a terminal illness).

We describe each of these in more detail below.

PROBLEMATIC RELATIONSHIP WITH INTERNAL EXPERIENCES

One important element of understanding clients' challenges is examining the way they respond to their internal experiences. Research, theory, and clinical experience highlight a number of ways we all may learn to respond to internal experiences through experiences, modeling, and instruction (from family members and also from broader cultural messages) that can lead to ongoing clinical problems.

Reactivity to and Judgment of Internal Experiences

A common emphasis in many models of clinical difficulties is that internal responses become problematic because of people's reactions to these responses rather than because of the responses themselves (e.g., Barlow, 1991; Borkovec & Sharpless, 2004). A whole range of internal responses may naturally come and go for all of us; however, we sometimes learn inflexible ways of reacting to these responses that may lead them to become more intense, long-lasting, or "sticky," leading to clinical problems. For instance, panic attacks themselves are common occurrences. People who develop panic disorder are those who have come to associate their bodily sensations with danger (interoceptive conditioning). They experience their sensations as a threat, which increases their distress about having sensations and, in turn, their bodily sensations, creating an escalating cycle.

A similar fear and distress can occur in response to a range of internal experiences—for instance, certain thoughts are reacted to as dangerous among individuals with obsessive–compulsive disorder; certain memories are threatening for individuals with posttraumatic stress disorder; and sensations of fullness can be distressing for people with bulimia. Broadly, through classical conditioning, modeling, and instruction, we can learn to experience distress (including fear, but also other emotions and physiological responses) as a reaction to a range of internal experiences. We can also learn these reactions through operant conditioning—for example, being punished for crying may teach us that it is dangerous to feel sad. Learning can lead us to react to naturally occurring distress with added distress and to react to our heightened distress with more distress, creating an escalating cycle that strengthens our reactivity.

Another element of these learned reactions is the critical thoughts and judgments that accompany a range of internal experiences. Clients often present to therapy with habitual judgments that certain emotions, thoughts, sensations, or images are "irrational," "stupid," and the like. In addition to the range of critical judgments that may arise, clients may also notice strong preferences about the types of internal experiences they have (i.e., wanting to feel calm or to have uplifting thought), which is connected to the perception that human/natural responses like anxiety and sadness are problematic, wrong, or bad. These critical judgments may stem from the learned associations, modeling, instruction, reinforcement, or punishment, as described above. For example, we may have been taught that certain responses are "bad" or signs of weakness (from significant caregivers and role models, as well as societal influences). Our inability to observe other people's internal experiences can also lead us to judge our own natural responses as unusual and therefore problematic. Kamila may not realize that her friends and family also worry about things that may go wrong, fret over events from the past, or feel irritated with their loved ones at times. She may view her colleagues as calm and confident because she can't see that they have fears and doubts about

their teaching abilities. This may lead her to judge her own thoughts and feelings and motivate her to hide these internal experiences. Ironically, in doing so, she misses the opportunity to learn that others have similar reactions. Finally, some of us have been taught to believe that it is beneficial to respond to ourselves with self-criticism and that it might motivate us to be our best selves. Those beliefs can contribute to the establishment and maintenance of this habitual way of responding.

> In Chapter 7, we provide psychoeducation on the positive effects of self-compassion, which counters these beliefs.

Fusion and Entanglement with Internal Experiences

Just as we often learn to criticize and judge our internal experiences, we can also learn to respond to them as if they are indicators of truth. If we experience fear, we may view our thoughts, feelings, and physical sensations as evidence that a threat must be present. If we feel anger, we may believe that our emotional response is proof that we have been wronged. Sometimes this way of responding to internal experiences leads us to view them as signs of who we truly are at our core. In other words, if we have the thought "I am worthless," we may assume the thought accurately reflects that fact we have a characterological flaw. Or if we notice fear arising, we make take it is a sign that we have an anxious personality. Relatedly, we often learn to react to these responses as though they are constant and unchanging, rather than transient, situationally specific responses.

This *fusion* between our experience and our perception of reality (and our sense of ourselves) makes internal experiences particularly powerful and feeds the escalating cycle by increasing our reactivity to and judgment of these experiences. If the thought that our partner does not really care about us were just a thought that would arise and fall naturally and did not necessarily reflect reality, it would not be so aversive and distressing.[2] Similarly, if we take our own transient experience of anger toward

---

[2]Thoughts do not have to be clearly false for this defusion or *decentering* to be beneficial. A fused relationship to a thought that accurately reflects a momentary reality would still be problematic in that it would diminish the chances of responding flexibly—choosing rather than reacting automatically.

and absence of affection for our partner as a sign that we are no longer in love, that could lead to overpowering feelings that the relationship is over. If we are fused with our physiological arousal and thoughts about how others will judge us before a social engagement, it can seem like good evidence that we will be rejected if we go and we might end up avoiding the engagement.

Kamila's fusion with her thoughts motivates her to fully engage with every worry or ruminative thought that arises because she views each one of them as significant problems that must be solved. This leaves her feeling constantly on edge and exhausted as she tries to prepare for and respond to every thought that crosses her mind. Further assessment may also reveal that this fusion is affecting the way she views herself, leading to even more heightened distress. When the learned habit of judging internal experiences is paired with the learned sense that internal responses are accurate, self-defining, and enduring, it can lead to chronic self-criticism.

Mindfulness- and acceptance-based models, both within psychology and beyond, highlight the ways that suffering is associated with being "hooked" into our internal experiences, as a result of critical and judgmental reactions to these experiences and seeing responses as more indicative of reality, self-defining, and enduring than they are. Learned reactivity and judgment naturally leads to internal responses and associated reactions looming large in experience so that these internal experiences can become the lens through which we experience our lives, rather than reactions that rise and fall in the midst of other experiences. Phenomenologically, thoughts, emotions, sensations, judgments, and reactions can all weave together to become a net of experiences that become more intense and enveloping the more we react to them, feel defined by them, and wish they would go away. This leads many clients to experience constant distress and to have trouble distinguishing and recognizing specific aspects of their experience. In this way, rather than just experiencing anger, we may have anger, a dislike of anger, and a strong wish for anger to go away.[3] Rather than experiencing a fearful response, we may define ourselves as a fearful person with a fearful personality that we will never escape. Paradoxically, these secondary responses tie us more closely to the very emotions experienced as problematic.

The Role of Experiential Awareness

These natural, learned, problematic, entangled ways of relating to internal experiences affect our awareness of our internal experiences (and are likely also affected by deficits in internal awareness). Here we provide a brief overview of some of the qualities of experiential awareness that are relevant to understanding our clients; we explore these more fully in Chapters 5 and 6 as we describe how we help clients to expand their awareness of their experience as it unfolds.

---

[3]Many theorists have highlighted this type of reaction to responses that intensifies them and is an important target for intervention. Greenberg and Safran (1987) refer to secondary emotions, or emotions that occur in response to adaptive primary emotions. Hayes and colleagues (2012) describe "dirty" pain as the responses that emerge as part of efforts to control "clean" pain, the natural responses to events. We use the term *muddy* emotions to describe these secondary reactions to "clear" emotions, as we describe later.

Narrowed, Selective Attention

Learning that internal responses are dangerous will naturally lead to a narrowed focus on those responses seen as threatening. As a result, clients will often present with an acute awareness of a variety of responses they view negatively (e.g., physical sensations, critical thoughts, feelings of fear), but little awareness of a broader set of responses, such as what leads to the thoughts, feelings, and sensations they are reacting to, or feelings of joy or satisfaction. This narrowed focus also perpetuates the sense that these responses are dangerous or problematic (as well as unchanging and defining), further feeding the cycle.[4] Fusion with these responses also contributes to this narrowed perception of emotional responses as indicators of truth.

Lack of Awareness

Clients may present with alexithymia and may report not really noticing the thoughts and feelings that arise. This lack of awareness or attention to internal experiences may be a consequence of rigidly learned experiential avoidance (described more fully below) that has become so automatic that it is no longer even perceptible. Lack of awareness may, in turn, interfere with an ability to respond to emotions in the moment, contributing to chronic dissatisfaction or unease.

Confusion or Misunderstanding

Learned reactivity and judgment of, fusion with, and entanglement with internal responses often leads clients to habitually have difficulty recognizing or understanding how they're feeling. Clients may mistake one personally threatening emotion (such as anxiety) for another, more personally acceptable one (like anger), or simply not be able to distinguish specific emotional responses among the cascade of distress they experience. If clients habitually try to ignore the subtle signs of emotions they view as dangerous or unacceptable, over time their automatic reactions of labeling and trying to suppress their emotions can create a more intense response that might seem surprising and out of context when it finally enters into awareness (described in more detail below). Two kinds of learned experiences can lead clients to distrust their emotional responses and to consequently miss the important information that these emotions convey. Clients may be repeatedly told by others that the emotions they express are wrong or unacceptable. Since critical judgments, fusion, entanglement, and experiential avoidance intensify natural distress, clients who habitually react to their internal experiences may in fact have strong responses that don't actually provide meaningful information.

> See Chapter 5 for an explanation of the differences between emotional responses that do and do not provide useful information.

Kamila doesn't seem to recognize her feelings of sadness until they are strong, so she is surprised when she is moved to tears in session. Confusion or misunderstanding of internal responses can lead clients to be unaware of the impact events are having on them, and therefore interfere with their

---

[4] A similar selective attention happens in attention to external cues, with hypervigilance to threat cues perpetuating a sense of ongoing danger and reducing attention to nonthreatening cues in the environment.

BOX 1.1. A CLOSER LOOK:
The Importance of Considering Context

Psychological theories, such as the one informing ABBT, often focus on the contribution that internal, underlying psychological mechanisms play in the cause and maintenance of psychosocial problems and distress. However, it is also critically important to consider the impact of the historical and current external experiences and events clients encounter such as loss, illness, injury, discrimination, economic stress, and emotional and physical harm as they naturally lead to intense, understandable emotional responses. As we will discuss throughout the book, in both case conceptualization and treatment, although we emphasize the importance of focusing on the internal factors that can exacerbate these responses (such as judgment, fusion, and entanglement), we also recognize and communicate to our clients how understandable the responses are. As we discuss further, especially in Chapter 4 and throughout the book, validation of the reasonableness of initial responses to stressful, unjust circumstances will help to address some of the learned problematic reactions that we've been describing in this section. Keeping these external realities in mind, while also considering the learning processes and habitual responses that are contributing to our clients' current challenges, is an important aspect of being an effective ABBT therapist.

ability to make meaningful changes. For instance, Kamila can't make changes to increase her sense of satisfaction when she doesn't notice the moments that she feels sad or disappointed. This misunderstanding may stem from critical beliefs she holds about feeling sad, or from habits of attending more to thoughts and sensations than emotions, or from a host of other learning experiences.

In Chapter 5 we expand on the ways that reactivity and judgment can lead to "muddy" emotions, making it harder to notice and understand the "clear" emotions that arise in response to our lives.

EXPERIENTIAL AVOIDANCE

A habitual, critical, fused, entangled relationship with internal experiences can naturally lead to rigid attempts to alter or avoid internal experiences or *experiential avoidance.* Hayes and colleagues (2012) and others highlight the central role that the function of experiential avoidance plays in a wide range of clinical presentations. A host of clinical challenges can be understood as efforts (that inevitably fail in the long-term) to alter the form or frequency of thoughts, feelings, sensations, images, and/or memories. Studies have shown that rigid efforts to avoid internal experiences often have paradoxical effects in that they increase the frequency of targets of avoidance (e.g., unwanted thoughts, feelings, or sensations) and more general psychological distress (see Chapter 5 for a more in-depth discussion). Concealment of emotional expression has similar paradoxical effects (Gross & Levenson, 1997). Kamila seems to be trying to experientially avoid her fear of uncertainty by keeping her mind busy with rumination and worry. Kamila's attempts to push away and conceal her sadness may also reflect experiential avoidance. She also describes trying, unsuccessfully, to "clear" her mind. Unfortunately, these strategies may paradoxically be increasing her general arousal and distress.

Many of the tactics we use to avoid our internal experiences (e.g., drinking alcohol or taking a sedative, shopping for things we don't need, mindlessly watching videos online) can themselves become clinically problematic behaviors that interfere with our quality of life. Sometimes the avoidant function of a behavior is intentional and conscious (e.g., using rituals to reduce obsessions in the moment; trying to avoid thoughts, feelings, and memories associated with traumatic experiences; repeatedly and intentional trying to ignore anger or disappointment that arises when one's partner acts inconsiderately). Other times avoidance strategies can be quite subtle and difficult to notice. For example, we may start an argument with a loved one about the distribution of chores to distract from painful emotions that arise due to the absence of intimacy in the relationship.

Behaviors initially enacted intentionally to reduce distress can sometimes become habitual and automatic; thus, experiential avoidance may evolve to happen outside of awareness and without intention. For example, when 34-year-old Lee first started therapy, he described his solitary lifestyle as a preference, noting that he enjoyed spending quiet nights at home on the weekend with a book and a glass of wine. Over time, it became clear that when Lee was in his 20s, he often turned down social invitations as a way to avoid possible rejection. Lee's habit of declining invitations to avoid potential evaluation by others had become so automatic he no longer considered his options or what mattered to him personally when planning his leisure time.

Behaviors enacted to reduce or avoid distress, like drinking too much, maxing out a credit card, spending all weekend watching videos, or turning down a social invitation, can obviously create life problems and general additional emotional distress. However, because immediate consequences are more powerful shapers of behavior than longer-term consequences, the long-term negative effects of these behaviors don't typically act as deterrents. Instead, they are actually more likely to trigger additional attempts at experiential avoidance, escalating this cycle.

Some common internal processes may also reflect efforts at experiential avoidance. Chronic excessive worry (repeatedly considering potential negative outcomes in the future) may function in part to reduce various types of distress (e.g., more upsetting topics, physiological arousal, uncertainty, or unpredictable, distressing contrasts in emotional experiences; see Borkovec et al., 2004; Mennin & Fresco, 2014; Newman & Llera, 2011, for reviews). Tom Borkovec proposed that worry may lead people to a sense of being braced, or feeling suspense, which is less unsettling than being surprised or caught off guard. Although the worries themselves also become an internal experience that people often find undesirable and want to get rid of (leading to a second layer of efforts at experiential avoidance), the habit of engaging in thinking to try to "prepare" (as Kamila describes) for the unknown and gain some sense of control can be very hard to change. Rather than exerting more effort to try to control these thoughts, meaningful change often involves recognizing these patterns and then letting go of these efforts to be prepared and "in control." Other types of rigid thinking, like rumination, may serve a similar avoidant function, with the constant rehearsal of past events reducing strong feelings of sadness, shame, or regret associated with them, while paradoxically maintaining focus on these events. Again, these strategies can be intentional, but they also can occur out of habit and outside of awareness; they often fall someplace in between,

BOX 1.2. TO SUMMARIZE:
Consequences of Rigid Experiential Avoidance

- **Paradoxically increases distress/arousal/frequency of targeted thoughts.**
  - Trying to change or avoid the way we think or feel, our memories or imagined futures, as well as our bodily sensations, can lead these internal experiences to become more frequent and distressing.
- **Increases critical judgments of our internal experiences and triggers additional attempts at avoidance.**
  - When experiential avoidance efforts fail and paradoxically produce more frequent and intense distress, we can become even more critical and reactive toward our internal experiences because our heightened responses seem even more overwhelming, confusing, and aversive.
  - This increased distress and intensified reactivity triggers even more attempts at experiential avoidance, creating a cycle in which the more distressing or unwanted an experience is, the harder it is to suppress, and the more those efforts to suppress increase the distress associated with the experience.
- **Reduces awareness and clarity of internal experiences.**
  - When our emotions are intensified by critical reactions and attempts at experiential avoidance, and when we habitually try to avoid or suppress how we feel, we naturally become more unaware of and confused by our emotions.[*]
- **Interferes with functional value of emotional responses.**
  - Habitually avoiding emotional experiences, or frequently experiencing our emotions as intense and confusing, prevents us from hearing the "message" emotions convey and could cause us to miss an opportunity to take an action that could improve our lives.
  - Suppressing the expression of our emotions to others.
    - Inhibits our ability to receive validation and support from others.
    - Prevents us from learning that others struggle in similar ways (which intensifies our critical judgments about our experience).
    - Makes it harder for others to understand our wants and needs, which can reduce relationship satisfaction.
- **Interferes with new learning about internal responses.**
  - When we successfully avoid or suppress our emotions, memories, thoughts, or sensations, we miss an opportunity to learn that they may not be as dangerous, damaging, or long-lasting as we fear. Ironically, the more frequently and successfully we avoid internal experiences, the more we come to see them as things that must be avoided.
- **Interferes with broader functioning by influencing engagement in values-based actions.**
  - When we are entangled with our internal experiences and consumed with attempts to change or avoid them, it takes time and attention away from things that matter to us personally.
  - When our attempts to change, escape, or avoid internal distress aren't sufficient, we may start avoiding situations or activities that we value because they could trigger unwanted thoughts, emotions, and sensations. (This consequence is described in more detail below.)

[*]See Chapter 5 for an in-depth discussion of clear versus muddy emotions.

with clients reporting beliefs that the strategies can be useful, but also finding them distressing and unwanted.[5]

We have described numerous negative consequences of rigid experiential avoidance throughout this chapter; we summarize these consequences in Box 1.2.

LIMITED ENGAGEMENT IN PERSONALLY MEANINGFUL ACTIONS

Although clients often come to treatment with complaints about their internal experiences—feeling anxious, depressed or irritable, consumed with thoughts, physically tense or aroused—their broader goals for therapy are usually to feel more satisfied in their lives. The common misconception that we need to feel differently to act differently leads to the desire to get rid of the internal experiences we perceive as affecting the way we live our lives. For example, a client may want to meet new people and believe that they need to feel more "self-confident" in order to do so. This leads to "increased self-confidence" as a common goal for treatment, when, in fact, a more attainable goal would be "meeting new people, and making new connections." This makes this final element of an acceptance-based behavioral model—limited engagement in what matters to the client—a particularly important part to explore with clients.

Obvious and Subtle Avoidance

The impact of having a problematic relationship with internal experiences and repeatedly engaging in experiential avoidance on behavioral engagement is often clear and obvious. For example, Jack, a veteran with posttraumatic stress disorder (PTSD), isolates himself in his home to avoid the anxiety he experiences in crowds or with other people, leading to disconnection from his family and other sources of support, and significantly limiting his ability to engage in work or other activities that used to be meaningful to him. Similarly, Kamila frequently misses family gatherings despite valuing these relationships because she doesn't want to leave her house when she is experiencing gastrointestinal distress (intensified by her worry and stress).

Like experiential avoidance, behavioral avoidance commonly protects against short-term risks but increases the risk of longer-term losses and disappointments. Clients may avoid situations, distract themselves, or hold back emotionally in certain contexts as a way of avoiding distress from potential rejection or hurt. Paradoxically, these protective actions often trigger more distress. For example, Edgar wants to be in an intimate relationship, but he feels that any sign of disinterest by others is an indication of his fundamental unworthiness and inability to be loved, so he refrains from taking

---

[5] A common misconception about mindfulness- and acceptance-based behavioral approaches is that they suggest that individuals should never make a choice or take an action to try to improve their mood. We all regularly engage in efforts to alter our thoughts or feelings. Both research and personal experience show that efforts to regulate emotions can be beneficial rather than harmful. In Chapter 5, we explore the complexity of the distinction between beneficial emotion regulation and problematic experiential avoidance, identifying ways we help clients develop their ability to intentionally, flexibly, with self-compassion, modulate attention and internal experiences without attaching to any intended internal outcome, and instead focusing on choosing personally meaningful actions.

any actions that would put him in situations where he could be rejected by a potential partner. Although this choice immediately reduces his risk of rejection, it also increases the chance that he will never find an intimate partner.

The impact of experiential avoidance on engagement can also be much subtler. When restrictions in behavior are automatic and habitual, clients may not be aware of the role their own choices are playing in the long-term dissatisfaction they are experiencing. We may find, for instance, that Kamila has been unintentionally avoiding seeing her parents and attending her mosque because she doesn't want others to be worried about her. Yet that separation is removing meaningful familial, spiritual, and community sources of support from her life.

Behavioral excesses that function to reduce distress (i.e., attempts at experiential avoidance), like hair pulling or substance use, can also directly reduce engagement in valued action in ways that are not always obvious. Simply put, time spent engaging in these behaviors is time away from other meaningful activities. For example, a client might see no harm in spending the weekend binge watching a favorite series. What can be challenging to notice is that the time the client spends watching television over the weekend is time away from taking a walk in the park or socializing with others.

Another way avoidance of valued actions can be subtle is when we repeatedly engage in important, valued tasks at the expense of other equally valued tasks that are more anxiety-provoking or painful. For example, Wesley diligently worked on writing his column and responding to his emails every day, telling himself that it was important to him that he be a responsible correspondent. When he thought about spending time working on the book he was writing, he felt a rush of anxiety and a cascade of thoughts that he was an imposter and didn't have anything worthwhile to say. To escape those uncomfortable sensations, Wesley would immediately turn his attention back to writing his column or responding to emails and would feel a sense of relief. However, he grew increasingly sadder and more disappointed in himself as the book he cared about remained unwritten.

The Quality of Engagement in Valued Activities

Our struggle with emotions, thoughts, and sensations can also subtly impact the *quality* of our engagement in activities we care about and degrade our life satisfaction. This consequence is particularly frustrating because clients intentionally engage in valued actions, yet they don't feel fulfilled. One common form this takes is when we are distracted and disconnected while participating in valued activities. Leia devotes time and energy to her work, volunteers for numerous organizations, and has a broad social network, but she is rarely present in these activities, which leaves her with a general sense of dissatisfaction. Similarly, Kamila describes feeling like her limited mental capacity, likely a result of her entanglement with worries and rumination, keeps her from fully engaging in important aspects of her life.

The scope of our attention also affects the quality of our engagement. Cognitive theories of emotional disorders highlight the ways that people often attend to, interpret, and remember events in biased ways that feed a heightened sense of threat or harm. This narrowed attention can affect the experience of our involvement in valued activities. If Kamila notices any negative cues that arise while she's with her children, and fails to notice cues that they are safe, happy, or satisfied, she will be more worried and will enjoy her time with her children less.

Another quality we sometimes bring to valued activities that prevents us from truly experiencing them is a desire for experiences to unfold in a particular way. For example, Ellie spent much of her time during "date night" with Jade focused on how things were not going as planned. Ellie had a slight headache, Jade was a bit distracted with thoughts about work, and the bottle of wine they ordered was too expensive and not very tasty. Rather than acknowledge her judgments and disappointment while also bringing her attention to Jade and fully experiencing their time together, Ellie became hooked by her experience and grew more and more frustrated. This kind of rigid attachment to the way things or people should be can interfere with our ability to be fulfilled by engagement in valued activities.

A closely related phenomenon is when we hold values that require us to be able to control things out of our control. Clients may have a clear sense that their lives would be enriched if their boss took a different approach to management, or their partner was more demonstrative, or their aging parents more self-sufficient. Yet, actions they take aimed at changing others may not be effective. Cassandra struggled with the way her coworkers interacted on team projects. She wanted them to communicate clearly and promptly, and to express appreciation for the work of other team members. Her many attempts to encourage them to change their behavior were unsuccessful, and she gradually began to invest more time in getting them to change than she did carrying out her team activities in a way that was consistent with her own values. Her very understandable focus on other people's actions became such a central focus that her own actions became less satisfying to her, further perpetuating her distress and interfering with shared goals.

Sometimes it is the specific actions we take in valued domains that minimizes our ability to gain satisfaction and meaning from our behavior. Although Kamila devotes significant time and energy to parenting and teaching, her actions often take the form of worrying about her children and ruminating over her performance at work. Not surprisingly, she does not find these actions fulfilling. Other times conflicting actions undermine our satisfaction. For instance, Jorge, who both values relationships and fears abandonment, went through the motions of initiating a new relationship, but he keeps himself distant emotionally when he is with his partner as a way of avoiding this feared outcome. Paradoxically, this distancing (an attempt to avoid abandonment) leads Jorge's partner to distance in return, which Jorge experiences as abandonment, confirming his fear and reinforcing his distancing behavior.

Disconnection with Values

Finally, our struggle with internal experiences can sometimes make it challenging for us to even identify what matter most to us personally. The option of reflecting on what we value and making choices accordingly can easily become overshadowed by our attempts to identify potential threats and avoid dreaded outcomes. Because Kamila's energy and focus are aimed at preventing her family from pain and harm, she no longer pursues activities simply because they matter to her.

External Barriers to Valued Actions

In the ABBT model, we focus on the ways in which a problematic relationship with internal experience and experiential avoidance limit us from fully engaging in valued activities. However, an important part of treatment involves identifying external barriers, validating their considerable impact, and helping clients to find ways to live consistently with values even when they face barriers that are real, unfair, unjust, and problematic. Clients may reasonably be frustrated by external constraints on their life—a type of discrimination they face in their workplace, economic constraints that make it harder for them to meet the needs of their children, physical limitations that make it more difficult for them to contribute to community efforts that matter to them; our conceptualization needs to incorporate, recognize, and validate these barriers. Then we can work together to find ways to engage in meaningful actions despite these unjust constraints.

 We explore these important considerations in depth in Chapter 10.

We summarize the ways in which clients may limit their engagement in valued actions in Box 1.3.

BOX 1.3. TO SUMMARIZE:
The Ways Clients May Limit Their Engagement in Valued Actions

- Clients may actively and intentionally avoid activities and situations they find personally meaningful.
  - Like experiential avoidance, behavioral avoidance commonly protects against short-term risks but increases the risk of longer-term losses and disappointments.
  - Over time, these patterns can become more automatic and happen out of awareness.
- Behaviors like substance abuse and mindless Internet surfing that serve an experiential avoidance function can take time away from engagement in valued activities.
  - They can cause problems in valued domains of living.
- Clients sometimes avoid valued actions or domains by focusing excessively on values in one specific area.
- The quality of engagement in valued actions can interfere with clients' sense of fulfillment.
  - Clients may be distracted and disconnected during valued activities.
  - Clients may focus narrowly on threat.
  - Clients may be preoccupied with a desire for things to be different than they are.
  - Clients may be focused on changing things that are out of their control.
  - Clients may equate worrying about something they care about with taking action in that domain.
- We may lose touch with what matters most to us.

CULTURALLY INFORMED CONCEPTUALIZATION

So far, we have focused on the general ABBT model. In Chapters 2 and 3, we describe how to design and conduct an assessment that will allow for the development of a tailored case conceptualization to guide individualized treatment. As with all approaches to case conceptualization, consideration of aspects of identity, culture, and context should be integrated throughout our application of an acceptance-based behavioral model to an individual client (see Hays, 2016; Okun & Suyemoto, 2013; Sue & Sue, 2016) for more in-depth discussions of this important component of case conceptualization). As Okun and Suyemoto (2013) describe, drawing in part from Bronfenbrenner (1979), this includes understanding clients within their family/intimate relationships, extrafamilial relationships, neighborhood and community contexts, and sociocultural and sociostructural systems, as well as universal contexts. It also includes attending to a range of influences, including relationships, environmental factors, ideology and practices, and identities. Kamila's identity as a second-generation Pakistani American, Muslim, heterosexual, cisgender woman who has current educational and economic privilege, but a family history of economic struggle and educational marginalization, who lives in a predominantly white suburb of a Midwestern city, likely shapes all aspects of her experience and may influence her judgments of her own responses, her strategies for managing her distress, and her behavioral choices in response to this distress. For example, in our interview, we may discover that her anxiety in response to her husband's job loss and their altered economic status was tied to her own experiences growing up under constant economic strain. Understanding and exploring this background will help us to develop a strong therapeutic alliance with Kamila and help her to cultivate compassion for her very reasonable reactions, while also potentially decentering from those reactions as she is able to see their source more clearly and recognize some of the contextual differences between her upbringing and her children's context, which may reduce the sense of threat that stems from these learned associations. Similarly, we may learn that her sense of needing to be in control and "on top of" everything is tied to her experience as a woman of color, receiving both explicit and implicit messages throughout her life that she is seen as less competent and so has to strive even harder. Explicitly identifying this context and lived experience again provides validation, understanding, and compassion for the specifically charged context of these natural reactions that can help with cultivating self-compassion, and disentangling from the automatic, habitual responding. We may also learn that her exposure to anti-Muslim rhetoric and actions has contributed to her heightened general sense of threat and danger for herself and her family, providing a learning-based explanation of her sense of apprehension and concern that can also enhance her self-compassion and the working alliance.[6]

---

[6] Although this specific case example highlights how marginalized identities may shape a case conceptualization, in part because these influences are often underemphasized, so that their recognition in therapy is particularly important, contextual and developmental factors can help to make sense of all clients' clinical presentations. These factors should always be incorporated in the conceptualization of a clinical case.

GOALS AND METHODS OF INTERVENTION

Drawing from the integrated model presented above, the overarching aims of ABBT are to (1) alter individuals' relationships with their internal experiences by cultivating an expanded awareness and a compassionate, decentered stance toward internal experiences; (2) reduce rigid experiential avoidance by increasing acceptance of/willingness to have internal experiences; and (3) increase mindful engagement in personally meaningful behaviors (see Figure 1.2). The methods used to achieve each of these goals are described in detail throughout the book. Below, we provide a brief overview.

ALTERING INDIVIDUALS' RELATIONSHIPS WITH THEIR INTERNAL EXPERIENCES

We work to alter clients' relationships with their internal experiences by helping clients to **expand** and **clarify** their awareness of their thoughts, feelings, and sensations so that they have a broader, more attuned awareness of responses as they arise. A central focus is on cultivating a **compassionate** (nonjudgmental) response to these experiences as they arise, in order to reduce reactivity, fear, and judgment that have been found to increase distress, motivate experiential avoidance, and interfere with functioning. Relatedly, we help clients to cultivate a **decentered** relationship to thoughts, feelings, and sensations, so that these are seen as naturally occurring and transient experiences rather than as indicators of a permanent, unchanging truth.

For instance, Kamila, who habitually experiences worrisome and ruminative thoughts, as well as physical symptoms of anxiety, and experiences these as evidence of her inability to cope, would engage in a range of practices designed to help her notice the thoughts and sensations as they arise, bring compassion to herself for experiencing them, see them as overlearned reactions that elicit a range of reactions and judgments

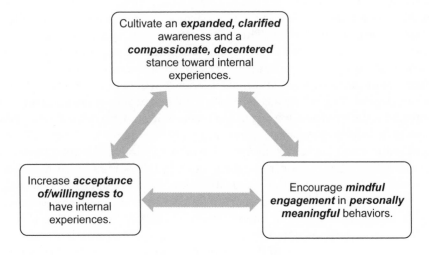

FIGURE 1.2. Goals for ABBTs.

but that do not in and of themselves define her, and expand her awareness such that she could notice other experiences and sensations, such as feelings of sadness, as well as moments of joy or satisfaction, as well as the way these reactions rise and fall.

Several types of interventions can be used to assist in meeting this goal. The **therapeutic relationship** will provide a vital context for enhancing understanding, providing validation, and modeling compassion and decentering to promote this new way of responding (Chapter 4). **Psychoeducation** helps clients understand the nature of internal experiences (and specifically the function of emotions) and the role that these types of relationships to internal events can play in sustained distress and restrictions in our lives (Chapter 5). **Self-monitoring** can also help to enhance clients' awareness of the range and unfolding of their internal experiences, the way these experiences rise and fall, and how they are connected to contexts and behaviors (Chapters 5 and 6**). Experiential practices** help cultivate these ways of relating to internal experiences. A range of mindfulness (commonly defined as "paying attention in [a] particular way, on purpose, in the present moment, and nonjudgmentally" [Kabat-Zinn, 1994, p. 4]) practices can be used. We combine formal (i.e., specific, planned practice of a particular technique to develop the skill) and informal (applying skills to daily living) mindfulness practices, both within and between sessions (Chapters 6 and 7). We also use defusion strategies from ACT, such as labeling thoughts and feelings, to bring awareness to them as separate rather than fused experiences (Chapter 4).

Reducing Rigid Experiential Avoidance by Increasing Acceptance of/Willingness to Have Internal Experiences

The second goal of treatment is to **increase acceptance of/willingness to have internal experiences.** We help clients bring awareness to the range of obvious and subtle behaviors and symptoms that may function as efforts to escape or avoid internal distress. We distinguish between acceptance and resignation, with acceptance referring to not fighting against a reaction that is already present and resignation suggesting that that one should give in to the idea that nothing will ever change. We encourage clients to expand their repertoires by practicing and learning how to choose, rather than react, in a potentially evocative situation. This goal relates closely to the previous goal in that developing a new, disentangled, relationship with internal experiences will naturally decrease the habitual pull to rigidly avoid or escape distressing experiences. Cultivating a curious, inviting stance toward internal experience will help to reduce experientially avoidant tendencies and enhance acceptance. Conversely, reducing experiential avoidance will also reduce judgment and entanglement with internal experiences. Many of the methods described above also target this goal of treatment.

Psychoeducation presents examples of ways that trying to control internal experiences can increase rather than decrease difficulties. We encourage clients to look to their own experience to see whether this is true for them. We help clients to increase flexibility by noticing how internal experiences pull for particular actions, yet we can separate from these action tendencies and choose responses rather than reacting (Chapters 5 and 8). Monitoring helps clients to observe how experiential avoidance affects their lives and to identify early cues to opportunities to practice an accepting, rather than avoidant, response (Chapters 5 and 6). Mindfulness- and acceptance-based experiential practices help to develop the skill of acceptance, increasing clients' flexibility in the ways they respond to contexts that elicit intense reactions (Chapters 6 and 7).

Increase Mindful Engagement in Personally Meaningful Behaviors

Finally, we **encourage mindful engagement in personally meaningful behaviors.** This goal involves helping the client identify and clarify what matters to them, bringing their awareness to moments when choices could be made based on these values and encouraging action in desired directions. All the methods that promote the first two goals also serve this goal in that engaging in chosen action is facilitated by a disentangled, defused relationship to one's experience and an ability to choose a nonexperientially avoidant response. Nonreactive, decentered awareness can allow one to *reflectively* see what matters, rather than *reflexively* endorsing values based on societal pressure or fears (Shapiro, Carlson, Astin, & Freedman, 2006).

In addition, **psychoeducation and monitoring** (described in Chapter 8) help bring a client's attention to what is important to them, setting the stage for chosen action. **Writing exercises** (also described in Chapter 8) serve to clarify values. **Between-session behavioral exercises** (described in Chapter 9), in which actions are chosen and planned for, engaged in, and reviewed, allow clients to expand their behavioral repertoire and engage more fully in their lives. These behavioral changes often elicit new types of problematic relationships with internal experiences and impulses to experientially avoid, feeding back into the previous two goals. Chapter 10 explores how to address barriers to making meaningful changes that often arise.

CHAPTER 2 ❦❧❦❧❦❧❦❧❦❧❦❧❦❧❦❧

Gathering Clinical Information to Prepare a Case Formulation

Clinicians recognize the value of gaining a good understanding of a client's presenting concerns, current context, personal and family history, cultural identity, strengths, and challenges before beginning therapy. Careful and systematic assessment not only guides the development of a useful case conceptualization and an informed treatment plan, it also helps validate the client's experience and develop a strong therapeutic alliance. Occasionally, when therapists start to integrate ABBT into their clinical work, they assess clients as they always have, waiting until the first "therapy" session to work from an ABBT perspective. We discourage this strategy because an ABBT-informed assessment provides rich information about how the ABBT model applies to a client's specific presenting concerns and yields examples that can be used throughout therapy to help clients when they are struggling to see the relevance of certain concepts.

What you will learn

- ❧ How to design a comprehensive assessment plan that can inform case conceptualization and treatment from an ABBT perspective.
- ❧ Specific examples of questions that can be used to assess processes related to the three parts of the ABBT model.
- ❧ ABBT relevant measures that can be used to supplement the clinical interview.

The first question most therapists ask when meeting with a new client is some variation of "What brings you into therapy?" Assessment from an ABBT perspective is no exception. In contrast, the follow-up questions therapists ask after listening to their clients' responses to that universal question are highly influenced by theoretical orientation. Therapists working from an ABBT perspective intentionally design their assessment to explore whether or not some or all the model elements seem to account for the clients' presenting concerns. Gathering this information helps therapists determine if ABBT is the best fit for the clients' needs.

A theoretically informed interview, supplemented with self-report measures chosen to directly tap into core ABBT constructs and careful listening and behavioral observation, can help the therapist gather the information needed to develop an informative and cohesive formulation. A well-planned and skillfully executed assessment can also be therapeutic in and of itself. The way therapists closely listen and attend to their client's experience, which questions are asked and how they are worded, and therapists' in the moment reactions can all have a meaningful impact on the client and the therapeutic relationship.

> Chapter 4 describes an ABBT perspective on the therapeutic dialogue and provides suggestions as to how to model the treatment and cultivate a strong therapeutic relationship. We encourage therapists to adopt this style during the assessment.

Box 2.1 includes a summary of the types of information the ABBT therapist tries to gather during the clinical interview. Throughout the chapter, we provide a number of potential interview questions and refer to several measures (see Appendix A for a table of these measures) that can be used in an ABBT assessment. Therapists should select items from this pool to craft an individualized assessment plan that best meets the needs of a particular client, based on their personal characteristics and presenting concerns, and that is consistent with priorities and constraints in the treatment setting.

BOX 2.1. TO SUMMARIZE:
Domains to Assess during an ABBT Assessment

- ABBT model-specific processes
  - Internal experiences or responses (thoughts, emotions, physiological sensations, memories/images) that the client finds particularly painful or challenging.
  - The client's relationship with their internal experiences.
  - Behavioral and internal, obvious, and subtle strategies that are used to change, escape, or avoid internal experiences.
  - The extent to which the client is aware of and engaged in personally meaningful activities.
  - The costs associated with a problematic relationship with internal experiences, experiential avoidance, and values inaction.
- The client's goals for treatment.
- Information about the client's current context, as well as factors and experiences that may be triggering challenging internal experiences.
- Cultural identity and its impact on current context and history.
- Relevant psychosocial, family, and treatment history (including previous experience with mindfulness).
- The strengths the client brings to therapy.

Although this chapter focuses on assessing the constructs and domains most relevant to an ABBT formulation, we often supplement the assessment with screeners or a semistructured interview to assess for the presence of other psychosocial difficulties that could otherwise go undetected. Clients with significant trauma histories, substance misuse, or self-injurious behavior may be reluctant to share that information unless they are asked directly in a compassionate and professional manner. Symptom-specific questionnaires can also be used to provide more information about the nature and severity of psychological symptoms, which can be useful for tracking progress.

Of course, model-consistent information does not need to be gathered through direct questioning. Frequently, clients provide ABBT-relevant information in the course of telling a story or describing a recent stressor. Therapists should carefully listen for details about the client's experience and style that may be relevant to the conceptualization. Behavioral observation can also provide invaluable information.

ASSESSING PROCESSES UNDERLYING THE ABBT MODEL

Internal Experiences or Responses That the Client Finds Particularly Painful or Challenging

Interview and Observational Strategies

Clients differ in their ability and willingness to reflect on and share their internal experiences. Although some clients are clear and open in describing their struggle with sadness, worries about the future, bothersome physical sensations, or intrusive memories, others struggle to name and describe their experience. Clients might use more general terms that require careful follow-up, for example, saying that they are stressed, overwhelmed, or just not satisfied with their life. Occasionally clients use the name of a psychological disorder to explain their current state such as saying, "My depression came back," or "I've been really obsessive-compulsive over the past month."

An ABBT therapist asks questions that help the client, as best as they can, break their internal response into different components, including emotions, thoughts, physical sensations, memories/images, and behaviors. If a client describes a particular response that is challenging—for example, the emotion of anger or the sensation of blushing—the therapist will probe to ask about associated responses across the different channels of responding. Questions might include:

- "When you notice you are having feelings of _____ (*emotion*), do you also notice certain thoughts that come to mind?"
- "Where do you notice _____ (*emotion*) in your body?"
- "Are there certain behaviors you are more likely to engage in when you experience _____ (*emotion*)?"
- "When you start to notice _____ (*physiological sensations*) in your body in a social situation, do you notice any emotions that arise?"
- "What thoughts come to mind when you feel _____ (*physiological sensations*)?"
- "Are there actions you take or actions/situations you avoid when you feel _____ (*physiological sensations*)?"

Measures

Clinicians can use any of a number of different questionnaires to gather more information about the nature and severity of a client's challenging internal experiences. One option is to use broad measures of psychological functioning as screeners. For example, the DSM-5 Level 1 Cross-Cutting Symptom Measure (self-rated version; Narrow et al., 2013) is a brief measure that assesses a variety of different symptoms, including depression, anger, mania, anxiety, somatic symptoms, and repetitive thoughts and behaviors. The 18-item version of the Brief Symptom Inventory (BSI-18; Derogatis, 2000) measures three of the most common symptom presentations: somatization, depression, and anxiety. Similarly, the Depression Anxiety Stress Scales—21-Item Version (DASS-21; Lovibond & Lovibond, 1995) is a 21-item measure that yields separate scores of depression, anxiety (i.e., anxious arousal), and stress (e.g., general anxiety and tension).

Another option, particularly if the therapist has a clear idea of the client's area of struggle or wants to follow up on information from a screener, is to use symptom-specific measures. For example, the Social Interaction Anxiety Scale (SIAS) and the Social Phobia Scale (SPS) provide a more in-depth assessment of generalized social interaction anxiety and specific fears of scrutiny associated with social anxiety, respectively (Mattick & Clarke, 1998). Resources that can be used to identify specific measures include websites such as the Registry of Scales and Measures (Santor, 2017) at *www.scalesandmeasures.net* and HealthMeasures, at *www.healthmeasures.net/index.php*, and books such as the *Handbook of Psychiatric Measures* (Rush, First, & Blacker, 2008) or the *Practitioner's Guide to Empirically Based Measures* series that include texts on topics such as anxiety (Antony, Orsillo, & Roemer, 2001) and depression (Nezu, Ronan, Meadows, & McClure, 2000).

Relationship with Internal Experiences

In ABBT, the relationship a client has with their internal experiences is presumed to play a major contributing role in their distress and reduced quality of life. Yet, clients rarely talk about their problems this way. The best way to assess a potentially problematic relationship with internal experiences is listening for statements like those in Table 2.1 that may suggest the presence of these underlying problematic patterns and exploring them with reflective listening statements.

If a client doesn't naturally describe their relationship with internal experiences, general questions that can sometimes open up a discussion about this topic include:

- "How do you respond when you notice _____ (*challenging internal experience*) arise?"
- "What is it like for you when you feel that way or notice that thought?"
- "Do you ever get angry or frustrated with yourself for experiencing _____ (*challenging internal experience*)?"
- "Does it worry or frighten you when you experience _____ (*challenging internal experience*)?"
- "When you experience _____ (*challenging internal experience*), do you ever wish you didn't think or feel that way?"

- "When you notice _____ (*challenging internal experience*) arising, does it seem like a response to a particular challenge or stressor that will recede over time, or does it seem more like a part of your personality?"
- "Do you feel defined by _____ (*challenging internal experience*)?"
- "Do you ever get consumed by worries or other challenging thoughts?"
- "Do you ever get immersed in thinking about why you struggle with _____ (*challenging internal experience*) or worry about how your struggle is going to impact your life?"
- "Do you ever feel confused about what emotions you are feeling in a situation?"

TABLE 2.1. Assessing Problematic Relationship with Internal Experiences

Statements to listen for	Problematic patterns they may reflect	Reflective listening responses
"I am angry at myself for caring about him when he obviously isn't interested in me." "I am a bad person for feeling disappointed that my friend got the promotion instead of me." "I am afraid that if I let myself get angry at my partner, I'll forget what I love about her."	Responding to an internal experience with fear or distress	"It sounds like you're uncomfortable with your emotional response in that situation."
"It is stupid of me to feel this way." "I am an evil person for getting so angry about this." "I am a loser for loving someone who does not love me" "I am such a baby for feeling scared in this situation."	Criticizing self for having an internal experience	"You find yourself criticizing yourself for feeling the way you do."
"I am just a negative person." "I can't advance in my career until I get my anxiety under control." "I will never make new friends unless I feel more self-confident." "Feeling sad reminds me I am trapped by my depression."	Feeling defined by, or fused with, an internal experience	"You feel defined or held back by your thoughts and feelings."
"I lay in bed for hours worrying about all of the terrible things that could happen to my daughter while she is at college."	Being entangled in thoughts	"Your attention gets pulled into a cycle of worry."
"I constantly find myself checking my heart rate to see if I'm okay." "My partner always asks how I feel–I would tell her if I knew!" "I have no idea why I got so angry at work."	Altered awareness	"Your attention gets pulled toward those sensations." "It's difficult to tune into what you are thinking or feeling."

Assessing Experiential Avoidance

Interview and Observational Strategies

As described in Chapter 1, clients use a broad array of strategies in an attempt to change, ignore, or avoid painful internal experiences. Sometimes clients are acutely aware of the fact that they engage in experiential avoidance. In fact, the inability to be "successful" in one's attempts to control emotions, thoughts, physical sensations, and images is often what motivates clients to seek therapy. Many clients explicitly present to therapy with the goal of reducing feelings of anxiety or sadness, pushing away memories of a traumatic experience, or preventing anger from arising in challenging interactions. Clients might also describe internal strategies for experiential avoidance, like distraction, self-instruction, and self-criticism, so it can be helpful to listen for statements such as "I just try to put it out of my mind" or "I try to focus on the positive!" Finally, clinicians should attend to behavioral patterns that could function as avoidance such as a client describing drinking a few glasses of wine each night to unwind or exercising to "burn off" anger.

If clients don't explicitly talk about their desire to avoid internal experiences, it can still be helpful to assess this domain with questions like:

- "What sort of coping strategies have you tried when you notice _____ (*challenging internal experiences*)?"
- "Have any been particularly helpful?"
- "Are there any downsides to those strategies?"
- "Sometimes people develop habits that seem like they help them escape _____ (*challenging internal experience*) at least in the short term, like having a few drinks, eating comfort foods, watching TV, surfing the web, browsing social media, and gaming. Do you have any habits like those?"
- "Do you ever try to distract yourself when you notice _____ (*challenging internal experiences*)?"
- "Do you ever try to talk to yourself to change what you are thinking about or feeling?"

Keep in mind that experiential avoidance strategies may be subtle and difficult to assess in early sessions. One place to look for behavior that may serve an experiential avoidance function is in any sort of problematic or "self-destructive" behaviors a client might report. Table 2.2 lists some examples of presenting concerns or behavioral patterns that could be serving an experientially avoidant function.

Clinical sensitivity is required when assessing whether behaviors a client describes as bothersome and out of their control also serves to reduce their distress. Clients may feel invalidated if a therapist suggests that the very problem for which they are seeking therapy (e.g., alcohol misuse, relationship problems) is helpful or adaptive in some way. Before exploring whether a challenging behavior also serves an experiential avoidance function, the therapist should validate the client's experience. For example, a therapist might say:

"It sounds like these periods of dissociation that happen while you are in class are distressing and frightening and that they make it really hard for you to follow along and learn the material. I know you also mentioned that being around so many people in such a large lecture hall brings up memories of the fire and how scared you were trying to move through the crowd to exit the club to safety. What happens to the memories and feelings of fear when you dissociate? Have you ever noticed that the dissociation reduces some of distress you feel in that moment, even though it is also distressing to experience?"

A final point to keep in mind about experiential avoidance is that even behaviors that seem useful and adaptive on the surface can be examples of experiential avoidance for a particular client. For example, Hirsch finds the physical symptoms of anxiety—increased heart rate, shortness of breath, sweating—very uncomfortable and frightening. He works out vigorously at the gym each morning because the daily ritual both "settles him down for the day" and improves his fitness. On the surface, it seems like the "settling" part of exercise is just an added benefit. But some information Hirsch's therapist gathered during the assessment made her consider that, for him, exercise might be a form of experiential avoidance. Hirsch reported that his anxiety became considerably more impairing about a month before he contacted the therapist. At that time, Hirsch sustained a knee injury that interfered with his normal workout routine. Hirsch told his therapist that because he could no longer "work off his anxiety," he became extremely nervous about upcoming social and work situations and often canceled them.

Exercise in and of itself is not a form of experiential avoidance. But rigid adherence to any healthy habit with the goal of managing challenging internal experiences may cause an otherwise helpful activity to become problematic. When conducting an ABBT assessment, therapists should pay attention to the *function* of different behaviors, not just their *form*.

TABLE 2.2. Presenting Concerns or Behavioral Patterns That Could Be Serving an Experientially Avoidant Function

Presenting concern/problematic behavioral pattern	Possible avoidant function
Sebastian knows he spends too much time playing games on his phone.	It helps relieve his loneliness when he is home alone.
Molly is concerned about her drinking.	It helps her feel less angry about her partner's unwillingness to help with household chores.
Carl is really struggling with his weight.	Bingeing on comfort food is one of the few things that calms him down after a difficult day.
Luis constantly seeks reassurance from Isabella, even though it causes conflict in their relationship.	He is afraid to feel uncertain.
Opal wears baggy clothing.	Form-fitting clothes increase her awareness of her body shape and size, which cues unwanted feelings of shame and disappointment.

Measures

Appendix A provides examples of self-report measures that can be used to assess a client's relationship with their internal experience and their tendency to engage in experiential avoidance. For instance, the Twenty-Item Toronto Alexithymia Scale (Bagby, Parker, & Taylor, 1994) is a questionnaire that measures difficulties identifying and describing emotions, a tendency to minimize emotional experience, and a pattern of focusing attention externally. There are questionnaires that assess fear of emotions (Anxiety Sensitivity Index-3: Taylor et al., 2007; Affective Control Scale: Williams, Chambless, & Ahrens, 1997), difficulties tolerating uncertainty (Intolerance of Uncertainty Scale: Freeston, Rhéaume, Letarte, Dugas, & Ladouceur, 1994), fusion with internal experiences (Experiences Questionnaire: Fresco et al., 2007; Cognitive Fusion Questionnaire: Gillanders et al., 2014; Thought–Action Fusion Scale: Shafran, Thordarson, & Rachman, 1996), and self-compassion (Self-Compassion Scale: Neff, 2003).

Many measures of mindfulness (e.g., the Five Facet Mindfulness Questionnaire: Baer, Smith, Hopkins, Krietemeyer, & Toney, 2006; Philadelphia Mindfulness Scale: Cardaciotto, Herbert, Forman, Moitra, & Farrow, 2008), and emotion regulation (e.g., Difficulties in Emotion Regulation Scale: Gratz & Roemer, 2004) have subscales that tap into both the client's relationship with internal experiences and their attempts to engage in experiential avoidance (or the opposite, acceptance). However, there are also measures that focus specifically on efforts to control thoughts (Thought Control Questionnaire: Wells & Davies, 1994; White Bear Suppression Inventory: Wegner & Zanakos, 1994) and broad measures of experiential avoidance (Acceptance and Action Questionnaire–II: Bond et al., 2011; the Brief Experiential Avoidance Questionnaire: Gámez et al., 2014).

Awareness of and Engagement in Personally Meaningful Activities

Interview and Observational Strategies

A final component of an ABBT model to assess is the extent to which clients are aware of, and connected with, activities that matter personally to them. The process of assessing values and barriers continues throughout therapy, and we delve deeper into defining values, differentiating them from goals, and exploring challenges that often arise in the values articulation process in Chapter 8. During our initial assessment of a client, we typically focus on simply understanding what matters to our clients and how they are functioning in different life domains (e.g., relationship, work/school/household management, self-nourishment and community activities). If the client does not naturally provide this information, consider asking one or more of the following questions:

- "What are some ways of being in your life that are important to you?"
- "What matters most to you personally?"
- "Tell me about some of the important relationships in your life."
- "Does your struggle with _____ (*challenging internal experiences*) impact your relationships?"

- "Tell me about your current experiences at _____ (*depending on client's context, work, school, or household management*)."
- "Does your struggle with _____ (*challenging internal experiences*) impact that domain of your life?"
- "What are other activities in your life that are important to you?"
- "How do you spend your free time?"
- "What are some of the ways you take care of yourself?"
- "Does your struggle with _____ (*challenging internal experiences*) affect those domains of your life? In what ways?"
- "How much time do you spend in activities that you feel '*must*' or '*should*' be done?"
- "How present or 'in the moment' do you feel when you are interacting with others or engaged in activities?"
- "Do you ever feel like you can't take in your entire experience because your attention is pulled toward what might be difficult or challenging about a situation or activity?"

In Chapter 1, we discussed two qualities that clients sometimes bring to valued activities that prevent them from truly experiencing these moments: a desire for experiences to unfold in a particular way and a desire to control things that are not entirely under one's control. ABBT therapists listen carefully during the assessment for statements that might reflect these qualities. Some examples can be found in Table 2.3.

TABLE 2.3. Assessing Qualities of Engagement in Valued Action

Statements to listen for	Problematic patterns they may reflect	Reflective listening responses
"I don't want to feel irritated when I am volunteering."	Wanting to have a different experience	"It sounds like you're uncomfortable with your emotional response in that situation."
"I want to feel more patient when I am playing with my kids."		
"I would like to feel happy and fulfilled at work."		"You wish you felt different."
"I don't want to have doubts when I am in church."		"You don't want to have the emotional responses you have."
"I don't want to feel jealous or resentful when my friend gets more attention that I do."		
"I can't be the kind of student I want to be when my professor is so unfair."	Wanting to control things out of one's control	"You think you know what needs to change for your life to improve, but you don't know how to make the changes."
"I would be completely satisfied in my relationship if my partner was a little less self-focused."		
"It's impossible for me to be happy knowing my son is suffering with his illness."		

Measures

Questionnaires like the Valued Living Questionnaire (Wilson, Sandoz, Kitchens, & Roberts, 2010) and the Bull's-Eye Values Survey (Lundgren, Luoma, Dahl, Strosahl, & Melin, 2012) can also be used to gather information about the content of clients' particular values, the importance of specific values domains, the extent to which the client lives consistently with values, and the ability to persist in values-driven behavior even in the face of obstacles. The Valued Living Questionnaire is by far the most widely used measure to assess values. Wilson and Murrell (2004) describe three clinically notable profiles that can be derived from the Valued Living Questionnaire. The first common profile reflects a high discrepancy between ratings of importance and ratings of consistency in one or more valued domains. For example, a client who is currently out of work on disability due to symptoms of major depressive disorder and who cares about being challenged and contributing in the workplace might rate this domain as highly valued and inconsistently pursued. Clients with this profile are likely to report significant psychological distress and to appear immobilized with regard to moving forward and making changes in valued domains.

Another pattern worth noting is one of extremely low importance scores across most or all valued domains. For instance, a client who is extremely isolated, with a history of social rejection, might uniformly rate family, intimate relations, parenting, and friendship as all unimportant. Sometimes this pattern of "not caring" may actually reflect a desire to avoid the pain associated with acknowledging a wish to be connected with others (Wilson & Murrell, 2004). In these cases, the clinician can gently explore if "not caring" is preventing the client from pursuing these important life domains.

A final notable pattern is that of extremely high total importance and consistency scores. This pattern of endorsement may reflect the client's desire to present themselves in a socially acceptable way (Wilson & Murrell, 2004). In our own practice, we have seen a number of clients who endorse many values as highly important and report that they are consistently acting in accordance with these values but describe significant psychological distress. For example, although Kamila from Chapter 1 was living a life that on the surface seemed consistent with her values, her ability to derive a sense of fulfillment and meaning from her daily life was considerably diminished.

Costs Associated with a Problematic Relationship, Experiential Avoidance, and Values Inaction

As we assess the different elements of the ABBT model, not only is it important to understand the frequency, form, and function of different behaviors (e.g., critical reactivity in response to painful emotions, marijuana use to dull feelings of sadness and loss, avoidance of social activities), it's also essential to assess the consequences. This information informs case conceptualization and helps strengthen the rationale for why a client might want to consider developing new habits of responding.

In Table 2.4, we include examples of client problems that may be partially caused or maintained when clients develop habitual ways of responding in response to their problematic relationship with their internal experience, experiential avoidance, and low engagement in values-driven action. We also include sample questions that can be used to assess for their presence.

TABLE 2.4. Questions to Assess the Costs of ABBT-Relevant Behavioral Patterns

Secondary problems that can arise	Questions to elicit them
Reduced awareness and clarity of internal experiences	"Throughout the day, how tuned into your thoughts and emotions are you?"
	"Are there times when you are confused or surprised by the appearance of a strong emotional response?"
	"Are you ever surprised to learn you are more upset than you thought you were?"
Misconceptions about internal experiences	"What do you think would happen if you didn't _____ (engage in avoidant behavior; e.g., take a Xanax when you felt panicky)?"
	"What do you think would happen If you allowed yourself to _____ (take an action that is typically avoided; e.g., be intimate with someone and memories of the rape were triggered)?"
Attentional disengagement	"How has your concentration been recently?"
	"Do you have trouble staying on task or paying attention?"
Interpersonal problems related to struggles with internal experiences	"How are your relationships with others?"
	Examples of relationship problems to listen for: • Client is seen as self-centered because he is often entangled with social evaluative thoughts when interacting with others • A client's partner sees the client as distant and withholding because the client lacks awareness of her thoughts and feelings and struggles to share them • A client feels that his friends are fed up with his need to seek reassurance from them
Inhibited ability to receive validation and support from others	"Do you feel like there are people in your life who truly understand what you are feeling or struggling with?"
	"Do you feel like there are people you are close with who face similar struggles?"

IDENTIFYING TREATMENT GOALS

Generating preliminary treatment goals with a client is a critical component of assessment, but it can sometimes be tricky. Although some clients describe their goals when they first contact a therapist (e.g., "I am looking for someone to help me be more assertive in my interactions with friends"), others are perplexed by the question, responding with something like "I know I need to be in therapy, but I haven't really thought about particular goals." One somewhat unique challenge for ABBT therapists is that often clients present with goals that are somewhat to very inconsistent with this approach. For example:

- "I am dealing with so much in my life, I need therapy for emotional support."
- "I am looking for a place to vent about all the frustrations I encounter at work."

- "I want to understand why I have had problems with alcohol my whole life, while my sister is completely abstinent."
- "I want to be less anxious and more confident."
- "I want to increase my self-esteem."

ABBT therapists absolutely provide their clients with emotional support, along with empathy and validation. But they also help clients to develop skills and make behavioral changes that hopefully persist beyond therapy termination. A brief exploration of a client's history can both inform case conceptualization and personalize psychoeducation about how learning contributes to the development of challenging habits like experiential avoidance. On the other hand, an in-depth analysis of the factors that "caused" the client's current problems may not be helpful, particularly if session time is limited. It is also most likely impossible to do accurately. Humans don't have the capacity to self-observe and remember all of the instances of associative or operant learning they encounter throughout their lifetime. Clients seeking a definitive understanding of the exact cause of their behavior can get caught in an endless search that prevents them from fully engaging in their lives. Even clients who believe they do understand "why" they are struggling rarely feel satisfied as a result of "knowing." A general understanding of the factors that can lead to certain challenges may help to validate clients' experiences, but directly targeting the factors that currently maintain these challenges and practicing new ways of responding are essential components of ABBT.

Clients frequently present to therapy with the goal of "getting rid of" the thoughts, feelings, and sensations they believe are interfering with their lives. Unfortunately, these types of goals are inconsistent with several assumptions underlying ABBTs such as:

- All humans experience the full range of emotions.
- Once an association is learned (e.g., vulnerability and weakness), it is never unlearned—although new associations (e.g., vulnerability and intimacy) can be learned.
- It is not always possible to directly control internal experiences.
- Attempts to control internal experiences often produce more distress and restrict valued activities.
- One can have a full and meaningful life and still experience painful thoughts and emotions.

If a client's stated goals can't be reasonably met in therapy, probing a bit deeper can usually provide opportunities to adapt the goal to one that is more attainable. Of course, the therapist always begins by validating the reasonableness of the client's initial goals before probing further. Table 2.5 lists examples of these inquiries.

Often these questions help clients to articulate treatment goals that are addressable using ABBT. For example, Lucia came in with the following goals:

- Reduce my anxiety.
- Let things go easier instead of ruminating about them.

- Stop making impulsive decisions.
- Improve my relationships; build more relationships.
- Take better care of myself.

During the assessment meeting, Lucia's therapist worked with her to elaborate and draw them out a bit to:

- Reduce my anxiety.
  - Feel less anxious on a day-to-day basis.
  - Don't get so caught in my worries.
  - Don't let anxiety stop me from doing things.
  - Improve my self-confidence.
- Let things go easier instead of ruminating about them.
  - Stop being so hard on myself.
  - Reduce procrastination.
- Stop making impulsive decisions.
  - Consider what matters most to me personally.
  - Find a way to make choices based on what matters rather than impulsively.
- Improve my relationships; build more relationships.
- Take better care of myself.
  - Cut back on my drinking.

In Chapter 3, we describe the ways in which Lucia's therapist integrated these goals into the ABBT model and discussed them with Lucia. We also provide guidance for how to talk with clients about goals that may not be achievable through ABBT.

TABLE 2.5. Potentially Helpful Questions Aimed at Shaping ABBT-Consistent Goals

Initial Therapy Goals	Potentially Helpful Questions
"I am dealing with so much in my life, I need therapy for emotional support."	"Who are your current sources of emotional support?"
	"What prevents you from getting the emotional support you need from people in your life?"
"I am looking for a place to vent about all the frustrations I encounter at work."	"What are some of the other coping strategies you have for dealing with frustration?"
	"What sort of work environment would you like to be in? "
"I want to understand why I have had problems with alcohol my whole life, while my sister is completely abstinent."	"How do you think your life would be different if you gained that understanding?"
"I want to be less anxious and more confident."	"How would your life be different if you were less anxious and more confident?"
"I want to increase my self-esteem."	"What would you do differently if you had high self-esteem?"

ASSESSING THE CLIENT'S CURRENT CONTEXT

Usually, after assessing the areas that we've described so far, therapists have a good initial understanding of the client's current roles and functioning across important life domains. However, we are careful to fill in any missing pieces to ensure we have a sense of the client's day-to-day experience and routinely ask several facets of current experience: the client's current living arrangement; the key people in the client's life and the quality of each relationship; the different activities that fill our client's day, including work, school, household responsibilities, community activities, recreational pursuits, and self-care and nourishment; the client's current health status; any psychological treatment they may be currently receiving; and current use of psychotropic medication.

Sometimes it is challenging to transition from presenting concerns to an assessment of the client's context and history. One example of how to move into this part of the assessment is to say something like:

> "Now that I have some sense of the kinds of things you have been struggling with and your reasons for seeking therapy right now, and some of the hopes and goals you have for treatment, I would like to learn more about who you are as a person . . . the values you currently hold, your background, and anything else about you and your life experiences that you think is important for me to know about. If I ask you any questions that you are not comfortable answering, please feel free to let me know."

Therapists also need to have a good understanding of the current stressors and challenges in their clients' lives. This helps to establish an understanding therapeutic relationship, guide expectations, and make choices as to how to best pace therapy (as some clients may have less time and fewer resources to engage in regular practice outside of therapy). A number of external stressors can trigger painful thoughts and emotions and serve as barriers to values consistent actions: dealing with racism and other forms of discrimination and marginalization, financial concerns, legal concerns, health concerns, transportation difficulties, parenting or eldercare responsibilities, relationship conflicts, problems at work or school, or significant life transitions (e.g., new baby; death of a partner, family member, or close friend; family member moving in; need to find a new place to live; recent breakup or divorce; being laid off from work or unemployment).

CULTURAL IDENTITY AND ITS INTERACTION WITH CURRENT CONTEXT AND HISTORY

In order to build strong therapeutic alliances, generate accurate case conceptualizations, and develop acceptable and effective treatment plans, ABBT therapists must explore their clients' cultural identities and consider the impact of current and historical environmental factors on their clients' psychosocial functioning and perspectives on therapy. Bringing cultural responsivity to assessment is an important area of growth for many therapists and something we repeatedly return to in order to strengthen our practices.

Cultural identity encompasses a broad array of factors that influence our world-view through learned and transmitted beliefs, values, social norms, and behaviors. Pamela Hays (1995, 2016) developed the ADDRESSING model to capture the multi-dimensional nature of cultural identity. Several cultural influences are important to consider in case formulation and treatment (adapted from Hays, 2016, with a few addi-tional items): age and generational influences, developmental disabilities, acquired disabilities, religion and spiritual orientation, ethnic identity, racial identity, socio-economic status, educational background, sexual orientation, indigenous heritage, national origin (including citizenship status and immigrant generational status), and gender identity.

The meaning and relevance of aspects of cultural identity vary considerably across individuals. For example, although both Leticia and Maria identify as women of color, they differ in how salient that identity is for them and what it means to them. Cultural identity is also fluid and dynamic over time and across situations, such that particular aspects of one's identity may be more or less salient depending on the circumstances. For example, although Imani is acutely aware of her race at school, given that she is one of the few students of color in her classes, among her friend group, her identity as a gay woman is most salient.

In seeking to understand the unique experiences a client might have due to their cultural identity, we also need to consider intersectionality (Crenshaw, 1991). This con-cept refers to the ways in which multiple overlapping aspects of one's cultural identity intersect to influence the extent to which one experiences discrimination and oppres-sion. Although members of a particular group defined by one factor (e.g., race, socio-economic status) may have some shared experiences, every client's lived experience is unique in that it is influenced by all of the interconnected and interacting aspects of their identity. For example, although women living in the United States have some shared experiences in that they do not hold the same power and privilege as men, the experience of women of color differs considerably from that of white women due to race-related social inequities, systemic oppression, and discrimination.

Cultural identity is particularly relevant to ABBT in that cultural factors can play a significant role in how one views one's emotions and emotional expression, comfort level with engaging in mindfulness practice, and types of values (e.g., individualistic or interdependent) that are personally held. Yet, the assessment of cultural identity can be challenging. On the one hand, asking a client about their cultural identity can demon-strate an understanding and appreciation for the influence of culture on psychosocial functioning as well as a willingness to openly discuss cultural issues. On the other, when there are differences in identity and associated power and privilege between the therapist and client, the conversation can be uncomfortable. An awareness and under-standing of one's own cultural identity, privilege, biases, and blind spots, along with a willingness to engage in ongoing efforts to research and learn about other cultures, can facilitate this process. Some of the common stuck points to watch for when preparing to engage in an assessment of cultural identity can be found in Box 2.2.

When assessing cultural identity, therapists need to be sensitive to concerns that clients may have about the conversation. For example, members of some cultural groups may feel like this line of questioning is an invasion of their privacy, and they may be uncomfortable disclosing information about their family. Clients who identify with cultural groups marginalized by some members of the cultural group to which the

BOX 2.2. TO SUMMARIZE: Common Stuck Points to Watch for When Assessing Cultural Identity

- Minimizing the relevance of cultural factors.
- Avoiding a discussion of cultural identity out of fear or guilt.
- Assuming a client's cultural identity without asking.
- Assuming cultural identity is only relevant to people from certain racial or ethnic groups.
- Assuming that whatever feature or features of the client's culture identity is most salient to you is also most salient to the client.
- Relying on a client to educate you about a particular cultural group.
- Assuming that modal characteristics of a group to which a client belongs necessarily apply to them without exploring client's individual experiences.
- Ignoring or minimizing the impact of culture-related stressors (e.g., discrimination, inequities in pay, access to education and health care, sentencing and incarceration rates, deportation fears).
- Overlooking intersectionality or the ways in which different forms of inequality and discrimination overlap and compound one another.
- Failing to acknowledge external barriers (e.g., poverty) to living in values-consistent ways that may be associated with cultural identity.

therapist belongs may worry that their therapist holds certain biases or that discussing an issue could perpetuate stereotyping.

For example, Jia, a Chinese American woman who was seeking treatment for depression, was hesitant to discuss her family history with her White male therapist. Jia's mother Mei was an extremely strict parent who exerted considerable control over the behavior and activities of her children. Jia believes that her mother developed this parenting style during Mei's own childhood; Mei's parents were extremely permissive, and Mei believes her parents' leniency is what allowed Mei's brother to develop a problem with drug use. Although Jia believes that her relationship with Mei is a factor in her depression, she is worried that by describing Mei's approach to parenting she will be perpetuating the stereotype of the Chinese American "tiger" mom.

Jayla's preference was to see a Black, female therapist, but the clinic closest to her work, and thus most convenient for her, did not employ any women of color. Jayla sat nervously in the waiting area, wondering whether or not her new therapist would be able to understand the impact of racism on Jayla's social fears. As she waited, Jayla overheard a conversation between two employees of the clinic. They were talking about a recent case in the news in which a student was suing a university over their admissions policy. Jayla heard one of them say "Everyone can succeed in this society if they work hard enough. The most qualified student is the one who should get accepted." As she grew increasingly uncomfortable with the clinic setting, Jayla left the common area to head toward the bathrooms to give herself a moment alone; however, she ended up leaving the building.

Both Jia and Jayla understandably have concerns about their therapists' cultural responsivity and competence that may inhibit them from fully describing their experiences (or in Jayla's case actually keeping a therapy appointment). Being sensitive to the factors that might cause a client to hold back parts of their experience due to a lack of comfort and trust, acknowledging the reality of systemic inequities, injustice, and stereotypes, and demonstrating respect and interest in a client's cultural identity make it more likely that a strong therapeutic alliance can ultimately be formed.

Assessment of cultural identity is a process that will likely unfold over the course of ABBT therapy. However, it is helpful for the therapist to begin to gain an understanding of the client's cultural identity in their first encounter. We typically do this in two ways: we use self-report to assess aspects of the ADDRESSING framework as part of the intake process, using culturally responsive language (e.g., Wadsworth, Morgan, Hayes-Skelton, Roemer, & Suyemoto, 2016), and then we follow up with questions in session (Box 2.3). The extent to which the assessment focuses on upbringing compared to current context should be determined by the client and their current context.

BOX 2.3. Questions That Can Be Used to Initiate a Discussion about a Client's Cultural Identity

- "Would you be willing to tell me a bit about your upbringing?"
  - "Where did you grow up?"
  - "Who were the important people in your life? Are they still a big part of your life today? How do you think they influenced the person you are today?"
  - "What were the most important values you learned growing up? How similar are the values and beliefs you hold today to those of your family?"
  - "How were difficult emotions handled in your family?"
  - "What roles did different members of your household assume?"
  - "Did your family have the resources needed to meet basic needs?"
  - "What about recreation or vacations?

If we have given out a self-report measure, we will review responses regarding specific aspects of identity (e.g., race, gender identity, sexual orientation) and ask clients how important each aspect is to them. Alternatively, we might ask something like:

- "Often, aspects of identity like age, race, ethnicity, gender identity, or sexual orientation are an important part of our lived experience. What are some aspects of your identity that are particularly important or central to you?"
- "Are you a part of any larger communities? What are some of the benefits of belonging to those communities?"
- "Have you ever been treated poorly or unfairly because of your beliefs or characteristics of your identity like race, ethnicity, gender identity, or sexual orientation?"
- "How do the important people in your life view psychological concerns? Therapy? What other ways do they support their own and others' well-being?"
- "Is there anything else about your upbringing, culture, or identity that you think is important for me to know?"

CLIENT HISTORY

A number of resources exist to guide clinicians through the process of obtaining a client's history and the domains typically covered (e.g., Jones, 2010; Sommers-Flanagan & Sommers-Flanagan, 2016; Zuckerman, 2012). Here we focus on specific aspects of a client's history that facilitate the ABBT formulation and treatment planning process. Assessing a client's cultural identity often yields a good amount of useful information about the client's history. Below we touch on the types of questions we may ask if we need additional information to fill in some gaps.

Assessing Experiences That May Influence Relationship to Internal Experiences

ABBT therapists seek to understand experiences in the client's learning history (or current context) that may have contributed (or may still be contributing) to the development or maintenance of their reactions to responses and habits of experiential avoidance. For example, therapists might ask clients:

- "How were difficult emotions handled in your family?"
- "How did your parents or caretakers typically express their distress?"
- "As a child, were you invited to share your emotional responses with your parents or caretakers?"
- "How did the important people in your life respond when you expressed difficult emotions? What advice did they give for responding to, or coping with, those challenging emotions?"

Learning about the most important and influential people in a client's life can be extremely valuable; it can be particularly helpful to explore the ways in which parents or other caretakers approached difficult emotions and the strategies for coping with emotions that they shared with the client. In this process, it's important not to judge different parenting styles and to keep in mind that all parenting styles may have served a reasonable function given the parents' context. Instead, the goal is to consider possible explanations for rigid strategies that may not be currently serving the client well, in order to generate understanding and self-compassion. Table 2.6 provides some examples of experiences a client may have during childhood that could contribute to learned habits of responding.

Of course, a client's learning history is not limited to their childhood. Thus, therapists may want to ask about other people in their clients' lives who may have influenced their views about emotions and other internal experiences. For example, Hae used to "walk on eggshells" when her partner came home from work until she got a sense of how his day at work went. If he had a challenging day, she was careful not to upset him as he often became verbally and sometimes physically abusive, when mad. In the context of this relationship, Hae learned that certain emotions were associated with danger, and she developed a habit of trying to suppress any emotions she perceived to be negative.

TABLE 2.6. Historic Experiences That May Contribute to ABBT Conceptualization.

Experiences to listen for	Examples
Being punished for expressing emotions	Kelce was often spanked by her mother for expressing sadness or frustration.
Witnessing someone close model avoidant coping	Jared's father died suddenly in a car accident. After the funeral, Jared's mother assured Jared that everything was going to be "fine" and that they should just put the experience behind them. Once, when Jared tried to ask his mother some questions about his father, Jared's aunt intervened—pulling him aside and warning him not to upset his mother.
Being instructed by someone close to change one's thoughts or feelings	Terrell was afraid of the dark, and he frequently worried about what would happen to his family when they were sleeping. His grandmother repeatedly warned Terrell to quit his worrying, and act like a "big boy."
Being labeled for experiencing certain emotions	Claire found the adjustment to middle school very painful. She was repeatedly excluded from social events and was the subject of rumors on social media. Whenever Claire tried to talk to her mother about how sad and lonely she felt, Claire's mother would call her "Debbie Downer" and tell Claire that she brought these problems on herself by being such a negative person.
Being taught that ruminating or worrying are effective problem-solving strategies	Wei's mother constantly expressed her worries about his health and well-being. When a schoolmate was diagnosed with leukemia, Wei's mother criticized the child's parents for being too carefree, warning Wei that such an outcome was likely when parents let their guards down.

Previous Treatment

Discussing a client's previous engagement in therapy can provide a wealth of information about their beliefs and feelings about psychotherapy, expectations, and commitment to making changes. This dialogue can also help to identify other providers whom the clinician may want to consult (with the client's permission) to expand their understanding of the client's psychological functioning. We routinely ask our clients to describe their previous therapy, to note which methods and strategies they found most effective, and to describe any components they found less useful.

A few aspects of previous treatment are of particular interest to ABBT clinicians. First, we want to explore what the roles of the client and clinician were in previous psychotherapy experiences. Although both ABBT clinicians and those working from more of a nondirective humanistic approach take a similar accepting and validating stance toward the client, ABBT is a behavioral approach that requires the client to actively participate in skill development, practice, and application outside of weekly sessions. Clients with a history of more nondirective therapy may be surprised by, or disinterested in, this essential component of ABBT. An assessment of the client's previous experience and satisfaction with nondirective therapies sets the stage for a productive discussion during treatment planning and contracting about the unique and sometimes challenging aspects of ABBT.

In our own practice, we work with a number of clients who tell us they previously tried other types of cognitive-behavioral therapy (CBT). Because CBT is such a broad umbrella, it can be helpful to find out a bit more about the nature of the therapy clients received, along with what they did and did not find helpful. Although ABBT shares many similarities with other CBTs, we've encountered some clients whose previous therapy experiences don't easily fit with an ABBT rationale. For example, a client may have worked with a CBT therapist who placed a strong emphasis on the importance of changing the content of thoughts in cognitive restructuring or who prioritized fear reduction over behavioral action during exposure therapy. Getting a clear understanding of how ABBT may and may not overlap with other forms of CBT a client has received in the past allows a therapist to proactively address questions or concerns that may arise during the treatment planning process.

Finally, therapists should assess the client's history of psychotropic medication, including both the type of medication and the dosage. Clients who struggle with their internal experiences are often prescribed medications and directed to use them as needed to manage an array of symptoms, including sleep difficulties, anxiety, and agitation. During treatment planning, we often consider the benefits and costs of adjunctive medication; understanding the client's history can inform this discussion.

Previous Experience with Mindfulness

As mindfulness, meditation, yoga, and other Eastern spiritual practices become more popular in Western culture, more and more clients present to treatment with some exposure to or history with mindfulness practice. Although having some experience with mindfulness can be quite beneficial in preparing clients to start ABBT, some clients have had negative experiences with these approaches that could interfere with psychotherapy. For example, we have worked with clients who were frustrated by their previous attempts to practice mindfulness because they thought they needed to completely clear their minds to truly benefit from the practice. Other clients have told us that the way mindfulness practice is portrayed in the media makes it seem an exclusive activity available only to a specific segment of the population and something that would not help with "real-life" problems. Although we discuss how to specifically address misunderstandings about, and challenges with, mindfulness as it is introduced during therapy in Chapter 6, it's important to assess clients' previous experiences with mindfulness, including what they have heard about it or found helpful or difficult in their own practice, and use that information when developing and providing a rationale for ABBT treatment.

CLIENT STRENGTHS

Understanding some of the strengths a client brings to treatment helps build the therapeutic relationship and informs treatment planning. To do so, therapists must listen for characteristics and ways of relating to people or their lives that please clients, areas in their lives they find satisfying, experiences and achievements they are proud to describe, values they hold, and future opportunities that excite them. Clients often come to treatment with narrowed, critical views of themselves resulting from fusion with their distressing internal experiences. Asking specifically about strengths can help clients to broaden their perspective and encourage them to attend to the ways in which their personal characteristics and their environment may be leveraged in order to facilitate the life changes they hope to make (Box 2.3). This information also helps the therapist plan early behavioral assignments that are most likely to be successful and reinforcing, supporting future change efforts.

BOX 2.4. **WHEN TIME IS LIMITED:**
Assessment

The breadth and depth of assessment conducted in settings that provide short-term therapy, of course, need to be adjusted. Depending on client need and setting constraints, brief encounters can focus on skill development in one area (e.g., mindfulness practice, values work) or introduce the client to the broader model and provide a few tools that can be used to target all three mechanisms. Sometimes assessment guides that choice (e.g., a client already engaged in valued activities may benefit from cultivating more present-centered compassionate responses while in those activities). Other times it is defined in advance (e.g., when screening clients for a group focused on valued identification and action). These choices will, of course, inform assessment. Below are a few general points to keep in mind, particularly when conducting a more client-centered assessment:

- Familiarity with the ABBT model can help the therapist intentionally focus assessment on the most relevant information.
- Consider developing a brief ABBT-informed assessment packet that can be completed and reviewed before the first session.
  - If you are in a specialized setting (e.g., an anxiety clinic), include the most relevant symptom measures; otherwise consider a questionnaire that screens for a variety of psychological problems.
  - In addition, ask the client to list their top three concerns and treatment goals.
  - Choose measures of key ABBT constructs (e.g., Difficulties in Emotion Regulation Scale, Valued Living Questionnaire).
- During the clinical interview, prioritize the identification of ABBT-relevant psychological mechanisms currently maintaining presenting concerns over gathering a comprehensive history.
  - Once the client describes their relationship with their internal experiences, consider asking an open-ended question to see if the client can identify past experiences that may have taught them to respond that way.
- Always include at least one open-ended question that invites the client to describe any aspects of their upbringing, culture, identity, current (including systemic bias), or historical context that are important for you to know about.

CHAPTER 3 ✦✦✦✦✦✦✦✦✦✦✦✦✦✦✦✦✦

Sharing Case Formulation and Treatment Plan
SETTING THE STAGE FOR THERAPY

ABBT isn't a formulaic approach to therapy with a prescribed set of clinical methods that are uniformly applied to each client; rather, it's a model that informs the development of a personalized treatment plan designed to target the mechanisms maintaining a client's psychological problems and improve their quality of life. Case formulation guides this process of exploring how the ABBT model might contribute to an understanding of the psychological *mechanisms* that caused and are maintaining a client's current concerns given the unique contextual features of their past and current experiences. Case formulation also informs how ABBT strategies might be tailored to address a client's unique presenting concerns.

What you will learn

- ✦ How to use assessment data to develop a case conceptualization and treatment plan from an ABBT perspective.
- ✦ How to present the conceptualization to your client and collaboratively reach a shared understanding of their presenting concerns and treatment goals.
- ✦ How to develop a treatment plan and share it with the client.
- ✦ How to develop a formulation in contexts where clinicians have very limited time to conduct assessments.

A STEP-BY-STEP APPROACH TO DEVELOPING A CASE FORMULATION

We recommend that therapists develop a preliminary case formulation following the initial assessment that informs treatment planning and is shared with the client before treatment starts. Offering clients a professional perspective on what might be

45

contributing to their presenting concerns, providing a personalized rationale for why ABBT may be a good fit, and asking for feedback allow us to correct any misunderstandings and fill in any gaps in knowledge we may have about our clients' experiences. It also lets clients know that we have heard their concerns, we care about their unique experiences, and we believe that treatment will be helpful.

We treat our initial case formulation as a working hypothesis to be revisited in collaboration with clients and in our own reflection throughout treatment, as our understanding of our clients and their experiences deepens. If a client is fully engaged in treatment but is not progressing, we consider what might be missing in our formulation. When we encounter treatment challenges or stuck points, we turn to our formulation to try to understand their cause and how to best address them. Box 3.1 provides a summary of the different functions an individualized case formulation may serve.

Developing an ABBT formulation requires a good understanding of the theory and familiarity with the treatment. Although Chapter 1 provides an overview of the general ABBT model, there are a number of caveats and complexities we touch on throughout the book. We recommend reading the book in its entirety before using ABBT in practice. Below we describe how to use Therapist Form 3.1, *Case Formulation Worksheet,* to organize the information gathered during the assessment; and Therapist Form 3.2, *Case Formulation Narrative Template,* to build a basic preliminary case formulation. You should start by noting your client's presenting concerns on the top of Therapist Form 3.1.

BOX 3.1. TO SUMMARIZE:
The Functions an Individualized Case Formulation Can Serve

- Validates clients' experiences.
- Offers a potential explanation for clients' problems that may help reduce their self-criticism and self-blame.
- Provides a rationale for why a particular treatment strategy may be helpful.
- Informs the therapists' choice of specific clinical strategies.
- Offers guidance when treatment obstacles arise.
- May offer clients hope that the changes they want to make are possible.

DEVELOPING THE CASE FORMULATION

Organizing Information from the Assessment Using Case Formulation Forms

Item 1: Challenging or Painful Inner Experiences and Contextual Triggers

Start by identifying some of the emotions, thoughts, images, and physiological responses associated with your client's presenting concerns and enter them into the table under Item 1A. Next, think about what could be triggering these responses and make a note in the table under Item 1B. First, consider events or experiences in the client's **current** life that would naturally lead to the responses in Item 1A. For example, clients who have recently lost someone or something they care about would be expected to feel sad, and clients whose rights have been violated will justifiably feel angry. Next, consider **past experiences** that could trigger the client's responses. For example, someone with a history of childhood sexual assault might feel disgust or anger from that event. Finally, consider any worries or concerns your client may have about the **future** that might be eliciting some of their current emotions, thoughts, or sensations. For example, a client who is worried their partner might contract a terminal disease and die might be struggling with fear.

When completing Item 1B, remember to consider the client's cultural context and events or experiences related to cultural identity that could elicit strong emotional responses. For example, consider the frequency of first-hand and witnessed experiences of microaggressions, racial bias, discrimination, and systemic oppression that people of color continuously encounter that would naturally cue a range of painful emotional responses. Children of immigrants may experience intergenerational conflicts that can trigger emotions like guilt and anger. Clients who identify as gay may have histories of having been taunted and ridiculed as children and/or experiences of being beaten, harassed, or marginalized as children or adults. Clients with different abilities or chronic illness, and those who live in poverty may face unique challenges and stressors in their activities of daily living.

Item 2: Client's Relationship with Internal Experiences

There are several ways a client might relate to their internal experiences, such as with fear and distress, critical reactivity and judgment, or fusion (i.e., responses experienced as truth; responses experienced are enduring parts of self). Use the table in Item 2A to provide client-specific examples of any of these ways of relating to inner experiences that you learned about through your assessment.

Also consider the patterns of awareness commonly associated with learned problematic ways of relating to internal experiences and experiential avoidance efforts. For instance, clients may be narrowly focused on threat cues or signs that others are negatively evaluating them; they may report an inability to notice and describe their internal experiences or a pattern of being confused by them. If the client you are working with demonstrates any of these patterns, note examples in the table for Item 2B.

Item 3: Experiential Avoidance

Clients use a broad array of strategies in an attempt to change, ignore, or avoid painful internal experiences. Both overt behaviors and internal strategies can be used as a means of escaping or avoiding painful thoughts, emotions, and sensations. Avoidance strategies may have clear negative consequences (e.g., self-injurious behaviors) or consequences that are subtler (e.g., spending hours on the Internet at night reading about ways to be a better parent, checking instead of spending time with children). In Item 3, record examples of behaviors and patterns of responding that your client shared that may reflect their attempts to engage in experiential avoidance along with associated consequences.

> Consider the list of consequences of emotional avoidance from Chapter 1, the costs associated with emotional avoidance described in Chapter 2, and the patterns of attention from Item 2B of the case formulation worksheet.

Item 4: Limited Engagement in Personally Meaningful Actions

Drawing from your assessment, consider whether or not your client has a clear sense of what they value in the three life domains listed in the table (e.g., relationships, work/school/household management, self-nourishment, and community activities) and make a note of this in the first column of the table Item 4A on the *Case Formulation Worksheet*. For each domain also consider how satisfied your client is (e.g., not at all, somewhat, extremely) and how consistently they engage in meaningful activities (e.g., rarely, regularly), noting your impressions in columns 2 and 3.

For Item 4B, reflect on some of the challenges that might prevent your client from being satisfied and fully engaged in the things that matter to them. In the first column, make note of any information from your assessment that suggests your client's entanglement with their internal experiences, attempts to avoid or suppress painful responses, or worry and rumination distract them from gaining fulfillment from their valued life experiences. Next, consider whether your client's desire for things to be different than they are interferes with their ability to be present and engaged in valued activities. If so, make some notes in the second column of Item 4B that reflect client-specific examples. Finally, consider the extent to which your client believes that someone else must change how they feel or behave in order for your client to experience fulfillment in a life domain. If relevant, describe this in the final column of Item 4B.

 Chapters 5 and 8 go into these topics in more detail.

Item 5: Influence of History and Current Context on Relationship with Internal Experiences

In Chapter 2, we suggested that you explore the potential influence of your clients' family history, cultural context, and current relationships on how they relate to their emotions, thoughts, and bodily sensations. Review this information, particularly considering the ways clients' cultural identities may impact how they view, talk about, and respond to emotions. Using the table below Item 5, identify any "lessons" your client learned about ways of responding to internal experiences and/or control strategies. Then briefly describe the influences (i.e., grandparent, teacher, society) that contributed to that learning.

Using the Case Formulation Template

The next step in creating a case formulation is to use the worksheet to develop a coherent narrative. On the one hand, case formulations are, by definition, unique and personalized. On the other hand, it can be helpful, especially when one is just learning a new approach to therapy, to follow a general structure. Therapist Form 3.2, the *Case Formulation Narrative Template*, is an extremely "bare-bones" guide that we hope you will find helpful as you consider how to conceptualize your own clients' presenting concerns from an ABBT perspective, given their specific presenting concerns and behavioral patterns and their unique life experiences and current context. Some components of the model may be irrelevant to a particular client. If so, of course, those should be left out. **Personal details and examples should absolutely be woven in.** The wording used here is included to provide a generic frame but is obviously insufficient for a narrative case formulation and is not the language we would use talking to a client. Later in this chapter we provide examples of how to present your formulation to a client.

CHALLENGES THAT CAN ARISE WHEN DEVELOPING THE FORMULATION

Problems Not Accounted for by the Model

After we develop a case formulation, we review our client's presenting concerns to see which we have explained by the model and what problems may not be sufficiently addressed. The psychological processes described in ABBT don't fully (or even partially) account for all the kinds of problems clients bring to therapy. Some problems might be better explained by a range of factors such as biological mechanisms, external constraints or stressors, or skills deficits. We are careful not to wear "ABBT goggles" that blind us to these other potential contributing factors as we develop our case formulation.

For example, Cheyenne presented to treatment to learn about options for managing manic episodes. Through careful assessment, the therapist learned that Cheyenne inherited a biological predisposition for bipolar disorder from her father that impacted her brain circuitry and neurotransmitter functioning in such a way that she experiences periodic manic episodes. Given this conceptualization, the therapist recommended Cheyenne be evaluated by a psychiatrist to see if a trial of medication was indicated.

Jennifer came to therapy because she was struggling in school. The therapist learned that Jennifer was a first-generation college student who was never taught efficient and effective note-taking or study strategies. The assessment revealed a number of other obstacles that made it challenging for Jennifer to devote time to school. She was working 30 hours a week earning minimum wage and couldn't afford to buy textbooks, so she could only do assignments when she was on campus and had access to the library. The therapist determined Jennifer would benefit most from academic skills training and a referral to the first-generation student support program at Jennifer's university.

Based on the information provided, these problems seem to be caused and maintained by factors outside the ABBT model, and they are likely to respond to different types of intervention strategies. However, occasionally, as we get to know our clients better, we sometimes find that ABBT processes do in fact partially explain concerns that we may have originally thought were unrelated.

For example, although genetic factors were responsible for predisposing Cheyenne to bipolar disorder, and taking medication helped manage her symptoms, over time it became clear that when Cheyenne was particularly stressed, she was prone to manic episodes. Much of Cheyenne's stress seemed to come from her desire to make those around her happy. But even when she tried her best to help her family, Cheyenne was often disappointed with the outcome, which intensified her stress and sometimes triggered a manic episode.

Similarly, although the therapist expected Jennifer's grades to improve after she received skills training and a scholarship that allowed her to cut back on her outside employment, Jennifer continued to struggle. As the therapist began to earn Jennifer's trust, she learned that Jennifer was afraid she didn't fit in at college and that she felt extremely uncomfortable when those painful thoughts and emotions arose. Jennifer's unwillingness to experience that fear and those painful associated thoughts led her to procrastinate on assignments. Although she tried to complete her work when there was a looming deadline, she often found herself entangled in thoughts that she was a failure, which made it understandably difficult to concentrate.

When situations like these arise, therapists can expand their original conceptualization to include any newly acquired information, share the revised conceptualization with the client, and, if they agree, broaden therapy to include supplemental ABBT strategies that may also help to target presenting concerns and improve quality of life.

Difficulties Identifying Patterns of Relating to Experience That May Be Amplifying Distress

Sometimes clients present with considerable distress, but they don't seem to be particularly critical or judgmental about their responses, they don't seem entangled in their experience, and they deny using avoidance strategies. As we mentioned earlier, even though we are enthusiastic about the ways in which the ABBT model can often account for clients' concerns and inform successful treatment, we need to be cautious about trying to apply the model to distress that is better explained by other factors. It's a mistake to assume that all of the intense distress a client describes is a "symptom" produced by critical reactions and experiential avoidance. A client might be grieving a very recent loss or might be angry about being mistreated because of their ethnicity, religious affiliation, or gender identity. In these cases, it wouldn't make sense to use the ABBT model to account for these reactions or "treat" them; instead, the client could be offered resources or support and validation, and the therapist might focus instead on how to enhance the client's quality of life in the face of these injustices and understandable responses.

In other cases, there may be patterns of relating to experiences that do influence distress, but that are hard to detect. In Chapter 1 and the *Case Formulation Worksheet,* we touched on several qualities of values engagement that can interfere with our distress. Notably, we talked about the ways in which our desire to control elusive targets—like what other people think of us or how they behave, and whether or not something we fear might happen in the future—can interfere in values engagement and cause distress. These concepts are covered in more detail in Chapters 5 and 8, but we mention them here because when this is the central pattern contributing to a client's presenting concerns, it can sometimes be difficult to detect.

For example, Bertie came to therapy for help because she felt paralyzed by her fears about what might happen to her son, Dylan, when he left for college. Dylan was diagnosed with Crohn's disease, an illness characterized by long-lasting inflammation in the intestinal tract that has a waxing and waning course. Bertie was worried that flareups (i.e., periods of considerable abdominal pain, frequent watery diarrhea, and fatigue) would prevent Dylan from regularly attending class and negatively impact his grades. She also feared it would be impossible for Dylan to share a bathroom with all the other men living on the wing of his dorm without being harassed. Bertie wanted to advocate for Dylan by speaking to school administrators and his professors, but Dylan was opposed to her involvement, and since he was 19 years old, the college staff would not talk to Bertie without Dylan's permission.

It's easy to empathize with Bertie. She cares deeply for her son, and despite his age and independence, she is still his mother. And Dylan may very well have a challenging time in college which will be painful for Bertie. What then does the ABBT model offer in this case? As we'll discuss in Chapter 5, our emotional responses are absolutely influenced by people and events we care about and can't control, which is a painful part of being human. From an ABBT perspective, **struggling to accept this reality** can intensify our distress and prevent us from engaging in valued action (in Bertie's case, Dylan threatened to stop speaking to her when he left for college).

Difficulties Identifying Historical Influences on Patterns of Responding

Some clients provide multiple examples of their critical, avoidant style of reacting to internal experiences, but they can't identify any historical factors that may have contributed to these learning styles. Yang was critical of herself whenever she felt nervous, and she tried to distract herself from her anxiety as a way to calm down. When asked about her family history, Yang described her parents as supportive and open to talking about emotions, leaving the therapist puzzled as to how and why Yang developed such a critical, avoidant stance toward anxiety.

One thing we need to keep in mind is that learning doesn't only happen in the context of early childhood. We are constantly adding to our learning history throughout our entire lives, so experiences we have during adulthood certainly influence patterns of responding. Moreover, family is not the only context in which we learn. Yang's relationship with her internal experiences was likely shaped by the larger society in which she lives. Yang lives in the United States where she is bombarded with messages suggesting that fear and worry are unwanted states that we should, and can, avoid (e.g., *don't worry, be happy, keep calm, and carry on*). The therapist might check with Yang to see if the hypothesis that living in such a society at least partially influenced her reactivity.

Concluding Thoughts on Case Formulation

We can never truly identify with scientific precision the factors that initially caused a particular response. Countless controlled experiments, with animals and humans, provide strong support for the principles of associative and operant learning. However, in the uncontrolled experiment of life, it is much more challenging to isolate which of the multitude of events and experiences a person encounters over the course of their lifetime impacts a particular behavior. Although we can form working hypotheses about causal factors, given the vast number of influences on any one individual over a lifetime, the complexities of interactions, and the limits of retrospective report, we can never draw firm conclusions (e.g., Hayes et al., 2012; Hayes, Strosahl, et al., 1999).

As an example, if Joe has an alcohol misuse disorder, as did his biological parents by whom he was raised, it is tempting to conclude that the disorder was caused by some combination of genetics and learning history. Yet, Joe may have a brother Jimmy, born and raised by the same parents, who does not drink at all. And we could provide a compelling rationale that Jimmy is abstinent because he observed the negative consequences of alcohol misuse, and so he learned to avoid alcohol. The fact that Joe and Jimmy shared the same general learning environment, but learned different things, doesn't discount the importance of learning history on behavior, but it does remind us that learning is much more complicated than our simple explanations of behavior suggest.

Even if our ability to explain specific behavior is imperfect, some clients still find it validating to consider their behavior from that perspective. Acknowledging that she grew up in a family who never openly discussed their emotional responses allowed Niamh to bring some self-compassion to the fact that she struggles to identify her emotions. For some clients, however, viewing their current struggles as a natural result of their history can actually be distressing and interfere with treatment (Hayes et al., 2012; Hayes, Strosahl, et al., 1999; Linehan, 1993). A client who was repeatedly sexually abused as a child, and who struggles with feelings of shame and thoughts that he is damaged, may feel imprisoned by the explanation that his current symptoms are caused by his past. When working with clients who express these types of concerns, it may be helpful to acknowledge that while we can't change the past, we can (and do) create new "histories" for ourselves on a daily basis as we experience and learn new things. Therapy can be described as an opportunity for this client to learn new ways of relating to his memories, emotions, and thoughts that could significantly improve his quality of life.

Although this explanation can be freeing for some clients, it may raise concerns for others. Teresa felt validated by the explanation that her troubling behavioral habits, like deliberate self-harm, were a natural consequence of the severe abuse she experienced as a child. When the therapist suggested that Teresa could make life-enhancing changes in therapy even though her challenging behaviors were likely caused by her early life experiences, Teresa felt guilty and invalidated. If she had the ability all along to change her behavior despite her past, she worried that she was responsible for the fact that she was struggling. We agree with Marsha Linehan's (1993) recommendation that therapy be aimed at both accepting the client as they are (e.g., "It makes perfect sense that you have an urge to use self-harm to soothe yourself in this moment because it worked so well in the past") *and* offering the possibility of change through therapy (you can learn new ways of self-soothing and stop self-harming).

Considering clients' histories when creating a case formulation can be fruitful, but therapists should be careful not to get stuck trying to find the precise cause of a particular behavioral pattern. Fortunately, the goal of ABBT is to help the client develop a new way of responding, so it's possible to begin that work without an airtight explanation of the cause. If there is a significant factor maintaining the behavior that is missing from the initial formulation, it will likely become more apparent as the client starts to try to make changes and the factor serves as an obstacle. At that point, both the formulation and treatment plan can be revised.

SHARING THE CASE FORMULATION WITH CLIENTS

The main points we share with a client when presenting an ABBT formulation are summarized in Table 3.1 along with some examples demonstrating how these points can be conveyed to clients. Given the considerable individual differences in how clients relate to their internal experiences (e.g., with avoidance or entanglement, by constantly monitoring their bodily sensations or by dissociating from their emotional experience) and the various patterns of values inaction (e.g., being extremely busy but disengaged vs. intentionally avoiding certain activities or situations), every formulation is individualized to emphasize the unique pattern of responding most relevant to the client. The

TABLE 3.1. Major Points to Convey When Sharing Case Conceptualizations with Clients

Important points	Sample statements
It makes sense that the client is having very natural and human responses to challenging events in their life and as a result of reduced engagement in valued activities.	"I can understand why you might be having these feelings of sadness since the break-up—sadness is the emotion we feel when we've lost something we care about." "Given that sharing your thoughts and feelings with others is something you really value, and you haven't had many opportunities to do so recently, it makes a lot of sense to me that you would feel sad and lonely."
Unfortunately, these natural responses that usually ebb and flow have recently intensified in severity and duration.	"Even though it's understandable that the breakup triggered feelings of sadness, it sounds like these feelings have increased in intensity and really pulled your attention away from other important aspects of your life." "Although we all feel fear when we face a new challenge, I understand you are concerned because your fear has become so strong you're considering turning down this job opportunity."
The client's patterns of reacting make sense given their learning history.	"When you notice feelings of sadness, you beat yourself up for having them, in the same way your father used to criticize you for crying when you were a child." "Everyone tells you to just get over the fact your girlfriend cheated on you, making it seem like all you need is willpower to shut off the feelings you have for her. It makes perfect sense that you would start to blame yourself or feel weak when those feelings of sadness continue to arise."
The client is using strategies to try to improve their situations that they learned should be helpful	"It sounds like taking a few breaths before talking to your boss sometimes helps you feel calm. And it's what your last therapist recommended."
Even though trying those strategies makes sense, they're not always effective, at times they intensify distress, and sometimes they cause new problems	"Unfortunately, it sounds like taking a few breaths doesn't always help, which is confusing and frustrating." "Having a few beers at the end of the day definitely helps you feel less stressed. But it sounds like those relaxed feelings don't last very long and you don't like feeling hungover the next morning." "One benefit of 'not dwelling' on your feelings is that you feel less sad, but it sounds like sometimes you get confused and frustrated when your partner wants you to share how you feel and you're not sure."

formulation should always be delivered in a clinically sensitive way, drawing specific examples from the client's described experience and using their own words.

REACHING A WORKING CONSENSUS

A case formulation is always hypothetical. We do our best to apply psychological theory and research to a client's specific, unique experience in order to explain how various challenges are being maintained and so that treatment can address the underlying mechanisms and help the client improve their quality of life. As further described in Chapter 4, we hold the perspective that the client is the expert in their experience, while the therapist brings knowledge of general principles of human behavior and adaptation, as well as their own experience. The formulation is presented to the client as one possible way to understand their struggles, and the client is invited to share their perspective on how well it matches or does not match their experience, fill in what might be missing, or raise alternative explanations.

Before treatment starts, the client and therapist should reach a consensus on the validity of the formulation and the acceptability of the treatment plan. It's not uncommon for clients to have some uncertainty about whether a treatment will be successful, and it's important to validate and normalize those concerns. We wouldn't expect a client who has been suffering for some time and is trying their best to solve their problems on their own to feel completely confident about the potential success of a therapy offered by someone they just met. As long as the client thinks the formulation and plan sound reasonable, and they are willing to try out the treatment, it's safe to move forward. Undoubtedly, as therapy progresses, the therapist will develop a more in-depth, nuanced understanding of the client. Clients may share private information they were not willing to disclose during the initial assessment. In both cases, this new information can be used to refine the formulation and treatment plan. Therapists should avoid assuming a treatment will be helpful without considering how it fits the client's experience and accounts for their presenting problems, settling on a formulation without client input, and developing treatment goals, such as reducing the client's attempts at experiential avoidance, without client buy-in.

Challenges That Can Arise When Sharing the Formulation

Clients don't always accept a formulation without feedback. It may be that the clinician left something out or forgot an important detail that needs to be included. Or, upon hearing the formulation, the client may realize they forgot to share something about their experience that should be woven in. Again, a revision should be able to address this problem.

What can be more complicated is when the client and clinician agree on the accuracy of the information in the formulation but disagree on how to understand or interpret it. It's essential that the therapist and client discuss their different viewpoints, consider their options, and make a collaborative decision about how to move forward. Discounting, downplaying, or avoiding differences of opinion will interfere with the working alliance and prevent progress in therapy.

Some clients question or reject a formulation because the therapist didn't sufficiently explain a key concept. It can be challenging to introduce concepts like the paradoxical effects of experiential avoidance without sufficient time to fully define and explore them. For instance, Juan saw himself as very emotionally expressive, and he thought the way he responded to his emotions by trying to tone them down would eventually work, if he could just stick with those strategies and not give in to his emotions. Not surprisingly, Juan couldn't understand why his therapist was suggesting that Juan give up trying to suppress his emotions.

Juan initiated treatment because he was worried about losing his partner, Antonio. Juan valued sharing his emotions with Antonio, but often Antonio withdrew from Juan after these interactions, saying that he needed space. In response, Juan felt sad and frightened, and he would often impulsively increase the intensity and frequency of his attempts to connect with Antonio (which were met with more withdrawal). Juan hoped therapy would help him learn to keep his emotions in check and reduce the conflict they caused in his relationship.

JUAN: I don't understand how you think trying to keep my emotions in check makes things worse. Me feeling and expressing my emotions is exactly what's driving Antonio away.

THERAPIST: It feels like your emotions compel you to behave in ways you'd rather not, so of course it seems like you should try and stop them.

JUAN: I just think I've indulged my feelings too much, and now they're intense and out of control.

THERAPIST: What makes the feelings seem out of control?

JUAN: The way I always go after Antonio when he leaves the room. I just panic and I can't help going after him. I feel intensely sad and alone, and I can't stand those feelings.

THERAPIST: So, the way you react when you feel sad—the fact that you pursue Antonio—leads you to judge the sadness as dangerous? That makes a lot of sense. Can you tell me more about your reactions when you get that feeling? You said you can't stand it.

JUAN: It's awful. I feel so weak and vulnerable. I just can't stand feeling that way for one more minute. So I just run after him and say or do something to try to feel safe and loved. And then it makes everything worse!

THERAPIST: That sounds like such a hard cycle to be caught in. When you feel sad, that feels really dangerous, so you try to push it away, but the sadness just grows in intensity. Then you feel compelled to do anything you can to make the pain stop. But the very thing you do to try to improve the situation strains the relationship more, leaving you feeling sadder and angrier at yourself. Does that sound right?

JUAN: Exactly. That's why I have to control my feelings better!

THERAPIST: I think I understand your perspective on this. And I also know you've tried really hard for a long time to push away your emotions in moments like those. During the assessment session, I was struck by all the things you've tried to stop feeling sad, even when something painful happens. You've also shared some pretty convincing evidence that the strategies you've tried have actually made things worse. I can't help wondering if it is exactly those ways you react to your sadness—your fear of it, your strong desire to push it away, your sense that it will overwhelm you and control your behavior—that might actually be increasing their intensity. That's what I mean when I talk about how control efforts often backfire. And I am thinking that strategies aimed at helping you to notice and eventually change those reactions might be helpful.

Plus, I think it is pretty human to feel sad when someone you love withdraws from you. And I want to be honest—I don't know how to prevent you from feeling sad when you perceive a loss.

JUAN: Are you saying you don't know how to help me? Or I'm a lost cause?

THERAPIST: Not at all. Here is what I think happens. When you notice those very human responses that come up when someone you care about pulls away—sadness—I think that triggers a cascade of learned responses that intensify your feelings. The intensity scares you, because you are afraid having intense emotions will drive Antonio away, and so in those moments, you respond instinctively the only way you think might help—you reach out even more to Antonio hoping he will make you feel more comfortable.

> We provide guidance on how to respond to Juan's very important question below in the section "Questions and Concerns about the Treatment Plan."

JUAN: If that is what's happening, what is the solution besides trying to stop all that from happening?

DEVELOPING AND SHARING A TREATMENT PLAN

Once a shared formulation is reached, the ABBT therapist provides an overview of the treatment plan, highlighting how different strategies are aimed at targeting the mechanisms responsible for the client's presenting problems. On the one hand, the treatment needs to be described in enough detail for clients to provide informed consent. On the other, concepts like acceptance and values are challenging to convey without providing an overwhelming amount of information, particularly since these terms have specific meanings in ABBT that are different from their meaning outside of that context. Therapists should be intentional in the words they choose to describe ABBT at this early stage and frequently check in to ensure the client understands what the therapist is meaning to convey.

Below we provide an example of one way we might describe our general treatment plan. Again, it is essential that the treatment plan be individualized and tailored to address the specific concerns of each client and highlight the most relevant treatment strategies.

"Because of the role these patterns of reacting seem to play in intensifying your distress, I would suggest we start treatment by learning and practicing some skills in therapy and between sessions that will help you become more aware of when and how those patterns are triggered.

"Once you are able to notice and slow that process down, I can introduce you to some new ways of responding to your thoughts, feelings, images, and sensations that you can try out. Those new ways of responding include things like developing the ability to step back and observe your inner responses as individual thoughts, emotions, memories, and sensations, to notice that your responses actually come and go in response to different triggers, and that these inner experiences don't actually define you, even though they feel like they do. At the same time, you'll learn more about how our inner experiences work and the ways emotions can provide valuable information. And you'll learn and practice ways of responding to yourself with compassion that you can use in challenging moments.

"Because a lot of your daily stress and general dissatisfaction with your life arises from some certain behavioral habits you've developed, as we work to increase your awareness of inner experiences and willingness to allow all of your responses to be present, we will also start to look for opportunities to make some new behavioral choices. We can gradually shift your attention and energy away from efforts to avoid or escape pain and toward what you value. We'll spend some time considering what matters most to you in different domains of living and explore opportunities you can find or create to live in ways that are consistent with what is most personally meaningful to you. And you will learn and practice skills that can help you be more present and engaged when you are involved in activities that are meaningful to you.

"I know we talked about how your worry about your partner and children can be consuming, and about how frustrating it is not to be able to influence and protect them the way you want to. We will consider ways to reduce your worry and frustration, while also ensuring that you take actions consistent with the partner and parent you want to be.

"At the beginning of therapy, I will spend a good chunk of time teaching you some things psychologists have learned about how thoughts and emotions work and ways of responding that are more or less helpful and seeing if they fit with your experience. I will also ask you to practice things we do together in session out in your day-to-day life over the course of the week, and I'll ask you to record your observations and bring them to our next session so we can review what you noticed, what you found helpful, where you struggled, and what adjustments could be useful. This practice between sessions will help the things we do in therapy actually affect your life directly.

"We'll do some exercises together that help develop skills of noticing, stepping back from experiences in which you are often entangled, and responding to yourself with compassion. Those exercises are different forms of mindfulness practices and I'll ask you to try them out between sessions as well. What questions do you have for me about treatment?"

Mapping Client Treatment Goals onto the General Goals of ABBT

Although this example demonstrates how to share a general treatment plan, therapists will want to integrate the client's specific stated goals into this discussion. As discussed in Chapter 2, some of the initial treatment goals clients describe may not be a great fit with ABBT (e.g., "need a place to vent about my week") and may not actually be attainable (e.g., "completely get rid of anxiety"). As we demonstrated with Lucia in Chapter 2, careful questioning can often reveal underlying treatment goals that better align with ABBT and have the potential to improve clients' quality of life. In order to effectively connect a client's treatment goals with the general ABBT overall plan, it is helpful to first sort them into four categories—goals that are consistent with each of the three overarching goals in ABBT and goals that are inconsistent with ABBT, at least on the surface. In Table 3.2, we sort Lucia's goals into these four categories.

Categorizing goals in this way makes it easier to integrate them into the treatment plan. For example, when describing the first goal of therapy to Lucia, the therapist might say something like:

> "Because your patterns of *being hard on yourself, getting entangled in your worries, and ruminating about past events* seem to be intensifying your distress, I would suggest we start treatment by learning and practicing some skills in therapy and between sessions that will help you become more aware of when and how those patterns are triggered. Once you are able to notice and slow that process down, I can introduce you to some new ways of responding to your thoughts, feelings, images, and sensations that you can try out. *For example, when you notice the urge to respond to worries and thoughts of past events by engaging with them, you'll practice observing them for what they are—as individual thoughts, emotions, memories, and sensations that actually come and go in response to different triggers regardless of whether or not you engage with them.* At the same time, *in order to help with your pattern of being hard on yourself for having certain thoughts or emotions,* you'll learn more about how our inner experiences work and the ways emotions can provide valuable information. And you'll learn and practice ways of responding to yourself with compassion that you can use in challenging moments."

TABLE 3.2. Lucia's Goals for Treatment: Sorted into ABBT Overarching Goals

General goals of ABBT			
Cultivate expanded awareness and a compassionate, decentered stance toward internal experience	Increase acceptance/ willingness to have internal experiences	Mindful engagement in personally meaningful actions	Does not fit with ABBT goals
Stop being so hard on myself.	Procrastinate less.	Make choices based on what matters rather than impulsively.	Feel less anxious on a day-to-day basis.
Don't get so caught up in my worries.	Cut back on my drinking.	Improve my relationships; build more relationships.	Improve my self-confidence.
Let things go easier rather than ruminating about them.		Better self-care.	
Stop being so hard on myself.		Don't let anxiety stop me from doing things.	

When the therapist presented her treatment plan to Lucia, she addressed the two goals that did not seem to be a fit:

> "During the assessment, we talked about your goal of reducing your anxiety and broke it down a bit. As we've discussed, ABBT can definitely help you start to notice when worries are grabbing your attention and to develop skills that you can use to step back from your worries, allowing them to be there, but making space for you to attend to your music, friends, schoolwork, or whatever activity you are engaged in at that time. A main goal of ABBT will be to help you respond to anxiety in ways that will absolutely free you up so that you can choose which classes you want to take or how you want to spend your free time rather than always feeling like you have to pick the least anxiety-producing option. The other two parts of that overarching goal—to feel less anxious on a day-to-day basis and improve your self-confidence—are tricky, so I want to be sure we are on the same page.
>
> "Earlier we talked about those well-worn habits you've developed of 'coaching yourself' when you're worried you might get anxious, trying really hard to stay calm, getting more anxious, 'beating up on yourself,' and then feeling a lot worse. That process involves trying to be less anxious and trying to exert some control over the thoughts that are in your mind and, based on what you've told me, you have a lot of experience that suggests you can't really do that and trying often makes things worse. I think those are great observations, because it seems logical that you could get control over anxiety, most people believe it's true, yet you know it's not. Your observations match what we see in research—when people try not to think about something or feel something, although it sometimes works short-term, long term it makes those experiences more intense and frequent.
>
> "So, I want to be clear I won't be able to teach you any skills in ABBT that you can use when you feel anxious that will absolutely make you no longer anxious. And unfortunately, the same holds for thoughts. I don't know of any strategy that can make a human always feel confident. On the other hand, since we do know what makes anxiety worse, I think that learning to notice when you do that and to try a different way of responding will reduce the amount you currently struggle with anxiety and the impact of anxiety on your overall life. Does that make sense? And although I can't help you always feel confident, we can explore ways of taking risks and facing challenges even when you're scared or have doubts, and some ways of responding to that fear and doubt that will probably make them seem less bothersome."

Questions and Concerns about the Treatment Plan

Clients often have questions that tap into some of the complexities and nuances in this approach. We try to address common client concerns throughout the book as we delve into different aspects of the treatment, so here we only touch on a few examples of how we address concerns that arise when describing the treatment plan. We start by returning to the conversation between Juan and his therapist. They already discussed the formulation, and the therapist tried to clarify why she was recommending Juan try a different way of responding to his sadness. Like many clients, Juan expresses some doubts about whether treatment will be effective and some hesitancy about agreeing to the plan.

THERAPIST: I think learning to notice when that pattern of reacting to your sadness happens in the moment, slowing down the process, and trying out some new ways to respond in those really difficult moments could actually lead to a different outcome. I wonder if you'd be willing to try something new like that— just to see if it makes any difference.

JUAN: I don't understand what you are suggesting I try.

THERAPIST: For example, I think there are some practices that could help you notice the sadness when it first starts to emerge, because it sounds like right now you aren't really aware of your emotions until they feel extremely intense. Once you learn to notice emotions earlier in the cycle, you can try out some new ways of responding to them that may be helpful. I would share with you some ways to bring some self-compassion to those moments—compassion for how painful it is when someone you love withdraws, and for how challenging it is when the fear, self-criticism, and impulse to push the sadness away show up, and how hard you are on yourself for feeling what anyone in that situation might feel. And we would consider a range of responses you could try to take care of yourself in those moments, given that trying to get Antonio to make you feel less sad isn't working. Something that you might find hard to imagine in this moment is that as part of treatment I would like to show you some ways that your sadness might actually be quite precious and useful. Being able to acknowledge and listen to sadness when it arises may help you to really attend to and deepen your connections.

In treatment we would also come up with a clear idea of the partner you want to be with Antonio and some specific actions you can take consistent with those values. So in that vulnerable moment when it seems like there is only one option, you would have a number of choices about how to respond.

JUAN: Well, I guess that all makes sense, but I can't imagine actually being able to do all of those things.

THERAPIST: I totally understand—much easier said than done. Just knowing about the kinds of things that could helpful is not enough to put them in place. To make changes like these requires a real commitment and some pretty regular practice between sessions. Our goal is really to develop some new habits— which is absolutely possible—but you're right, not the easiest thing to do. It takes practice, and also patience because your new habits won't develop right away, and your old habits are strong. But each time you practice a new response, you'll be strengthening the new habit and weakening the old one. And the more that happens, the easier it will get. Why don't you take some time over the next week to see if you have any more questions or if you think this sounds like something you want to try?

Questions Related to Previous Therapy

Making the Time for Treatment

ABBT can be time intensive, and so therapists should have a discussion with clients about the real time constraints in their life that can make it challenging to practice skills outside of therapy. Ways of doing this effectively that help build the therapeutic relationship are discussed in Chapter 4.

Both a client's previous experience with therapy and their cultural identity can impact their expectations about therapy and therapy roles. For example, clients who previously worked with therapists taking a nondirective humanistic approach may be comfortable with the similarly accepting and validating stance of their ABBT therapist. However, they may be surprised or turned off by the fact that ABBT is a behavioral approach that asks clients to actively participate in skill development, practice, and application outside of weekly sessions.

Miranda, a client who had previously been in supportive, nondirective psychotherapy, expressed some concerns upon hearing that her ABBT treatment plan would include some out-of-session practices. As a working single parent with a stressful and busy life, Miranda explained that she would find it hard enough to carve out the time in her week to actually attend weekly therapy appointments. She expressed doubt that she would be able to devote additional time to therapy.

The ABBT therapist was honest about the fact that regular "out-of-session" practice was also an integral part of ABBT, explaining how developing new habits and skills typically required more practice than could be integrated into their 50-minute sessions. The therapist also validated Miranda's frustration and stress, genuinely acknowledging that the many responsibilities on Miranda's plate left little time for self-care. With Miranda's help, the therapist brainstormed ways in which skills practice could be modified to better fit with the client's schedule. For example, they agreed to slow the pace of therapy and increase the number of sessions aimed at skills building. They discussed ways of adapting mindfulness practices to better fit with Miranda's schedule. The therapist also explained that, although most of the practices would require Miranda to intentionally think about and practice strategies learned in treatment, many of them simply involved trying out new ways of doing what Miranda was already doing in her everyday life. For example, Miranda currently spent about 20 hours each weekend watching television. Although this habit was driven by a desire

> Questions about outside-of-session practice are common both during treatment planning and throughout therapy. In Chapter 4, we further describe how to approach these conversations in a clinically sensitive way.

> See Chapter 6 for a detailed discussion of the kinds of modifications that can be made.

to engage in self-care, Miranda noticed she did not feel nurtured and refreshed as a result of this time commitment. As part of ABBT, Miranda and her therapist would work to generate ideas of alternative self-care activities that could replace some of Miranda's current television time.

We frequently work with clients who have previously been in CBT. Not surprisingly, since ABBT falls under the CBT umbrella, many of the clinical strategies that clients may have used in previous therapy are also part of ABBT, including self-monitoring, psychoeducation, skills development and practice, and promoting exposure to previously avoided situations, experiences, and activities. However, given the heterogeneity of different applications of CBT, there could also be some differences that deserve attention during treatment planning.

For example, both Layla and Elijah initially expressed some concern starting ABBT when they heard it was a type of CBT. Fortunately, during treatment planning, it became clear that ABBT offered some unique elements that the clients found appealing. Layla had previously participated in a course of CBT that emphasized cognitive restructuring and she struggled with the idea of changing the content of her thoughts. During treatment planning she expressed feeling more comfortable with the ABBT approach of taking a compassionate and allowing stance toward her thoughts. Elijah was relieved to hear that ABBT would include mindfulness practices that could teach him new ways of responding to feared emotions while taking valued actions. Although Elijah felt like he had started to make substantial changes during the first few sessions of his previous exposure-based CBT, he eventually dropped out of therapy due to struggles with his "fear of fear."

Unique challenges can arise when a client who previously benefited from cognitive restructuring in CBT seeks out ABBT. The client may be hesitant to try acceptance strategies after learning to challenge and change painful thoughts through cognitive restructuring. This was a concern for Carlos, a client who met with an ABBT therapist for help with his worry and anxiety. Carlos found CBT very helpful in the past, when he was struggling with social anxiety. The ABBT therapist emphasized the ways in which the self-monitoring strategies that Carlos found so useful in his previous therapy would be similar to the awareness and observing skills developed in ABBT through both self-monitoring and mindfulness practice. She also connected the practices in ABBT used to promote defusion with Carlos's previous practice of not always accepting thoughts as facts. Rather than suggesting that Carlos discard the skills he learned in his previous therapy and replace them with those from ABBT, the therapist asked Carlos whether he was willing to learn some new skills to add to his repertoire. Carlos and his therapist also agreed to revisit the possibility that attempts to change the content of his worries could be contributing to their intrusiveness later.

Questions Related to Mindfulness

As mindfulness, meditation, yoga, and other Eastern spiritual practices become more popular in Western culture, more clients present to treatment with some thoughts about what mindfulness is and often some personal experience practicing it. It's not uncommon for clients to have positive and negative misconceptions of what mindfulness is and how it may or may not be helpful. As noted in Chapter 2, previous exposure to and experience with mindfulness should always be assessed. Questions of concern can be addressed during treatment planning and revisited when mindfulness is introduced in therapy.

> Chapter 6 describes how mindfulness is used in ABBT and addresses common misconceptions).

Questions about Medication Use

Given that one out of every six people living in the United States takes a prescription medication for mental health issues (Moore & Mattison, 2017), it's not surprising that many of the clients we see in therapy are already taking medication. In fact, of all the medications people living in the United States take for medical and psychological conditions, antidepressants are the third most commonly prescribed (Pratt, Brody, & Gu, 2017).

Although taking medication to reduce psychological pain could be characterized as a form of experiential avoidance, many clients would be unwilling to engage in therapy if they were required to be medication-free. Moreover, in our experience, clients still experience a wide range of painful emotions while on medication. During treatment planning, we tell clients that we expect challenging emotions to become more frequent and intense at different points in therapy, particularly as clients turn toward experiences and engage in activities that have previously been avoided and we ask clients to talk with us before increasing the dose of, or changing, their medication. We explain that our goal is to provide clients with skills they can use when strong emotions arise, so it's important that they have the opportunity to develop and practice skills in emotionally challenging moments while in therapy. We also ask clients for permission to talk with their provider so that we can discuss the treatment plan. If, in the later stages of therapy, a client expresses an interest in tapering and then discontinuing medication use, we will work with them and their provider toward this goal.

It can be a bit more challenging when clients are taking antianxiety medications that are prescribed to be used on an as-needed basis. This actually comes up frequently, as this group of drugs is the second most commonly used prescription medication for psychological symptoms group, after antidepressants (Moore & Mattison, 2017). Taking a medication from this class (like a benzodiazepine) for the specific purpose of avoiding an emotion or reducing its intensity can strengthen the belief that emotions are dangerous. We suggest that clients ask their prescribers about either moving to a more stable dose or taking a break from their medication (and offer to consult with the provider as well), so that they can more directly examine their experience of distressing emotions and learn new responses to them, rather than immediately reaching for medication.

Finally, even if clients are not taking medication at the assessment, it can be useful to discuss the topic. Otherwise, clients may seek and receive a prescription during therapy, often from their primary care provider, without raising the issue in therapy or even the impact of medication use on therapy.

CULTURAL CONSIDERATIONS

Cultural identity influences a number of factors that are relevant to therapy including our patterns of communication, relationship with our emotions, exposure to bias, beliefs about emotional expression, attitudes about individualism, view of psychological problems, opinions on therapy, how acceptable we feel it is to share about our families, ideas about what makes one's life meaningful, and the best way to cope with psychological distress. Those differences emphasize how important it is to be culturally responsive as therapists. Integrating an assessment of cultural identity into the first session (as discussed in Chapter 2) is an important first step, as is considering cultural factors in the case formulation. Developing a strong therapeutic relationship within which discussions about culturally related experiences are welcomed is essential (this topic is detailed in Chapter 4).

Culturally sensitive adaptations to therapy, which can include alterations in the content, format, and delivery of treatment, enhance outcomes (e.g., Benish, Quintana, & Wampold, 2011; Griner & Smith, 2006; Hall, Ibaraki, Huang, Marti, & Stice, 2016). Fortunately, there is flexibility within ABBT to tailor content (e.g., focus of values work; choices of mindfulness exercise) and to make client-centered choices about which problems or challenges arising in the client's daily life will be addressed through skill development and practice.

Some of the defining characteristics of ABBT may enhance its acceptability to clients who are diverse across many aspects of identity. For example, ABBT acknowledges the influence of sociocultural contexts on clients' experiences and current psychological functioning. Psychological problems are not pathologized in the ABBT model; instead, the struggle clients have with their internal experiences and their inclination to avoid painful thoughts and emotions are seen as reflective of human nature, a perspective that can be helpful to clients who might otherwise feel stigmatized for seeking therapy. Finally, the focus on helping clients to live their lives in accordance with their own values acknowledges that the client's personal and cultural beliefs and preferences are central to their psychosocial functioning.

We conducted a small qualitative study (Fuchs et al., 2016) that involved interviewing clients with marginalized identities who received ABBT to hear their perspectives on the fit between this approach to treatment and their identity. A few key themes emerged that therapists should keep in mind when sharing the treatment plan and throughout the course of treatment. Providing a strong rationale for mindfulness practice and being explicit about the ways a particular practice is relevant to the client's presenting concerns and goals for treatment is essential. The study also highlighted the importance of acknowledging the real external barriers faced by many clients. These barriers can make it challenging to carve out the time and space to complete outside of session work and to engage in valued actions. Although most clients in our

> External barriers are discussed in greater depth in Chapter 10.

study were open to practicing mindfulness, even if they had a strong religious identity, ABBT therapists should be sensitive to any concerns clients may have about mindfulness and its fit with their cultural beliefs and practices.

BOX 3.2. WHEN TIME IS LIMITED:
Case Conceptualization

Therapists who only see clients for a few sessions are limited in the extent to which they can personalize and adapt the general ABBT into a client-specific case formulation. Fortunately, a number of studies have demonstrated that even a nontailored, single session ABBT-informed workshop can provide some benefits (e.g., Danitz & Orsillo, 2014; Danitz, Suvak, & Orsillo, 2016; Eustis, Williston, et al., 2017). In addition, below we provide some suggestions as to how one can develop a brief formulation and adapted treatment plan when working in brief therapy contexts.

- Consider whether one aspect of the conceptualization (problematic relationship with internal experiences; limited engagement in valued actions) seems particularly central and focus the formulation and treatment on that, with briefer attention to other parts of the model.

- Explore whether outside resources, like mindfulness or yoga classes, or self-help materials such as the ABBT workbook (*Worry Less, Live More;* Orsillo & Roemer, 2016) can be engaged to help with some skills development.

- Unless it is particularly relevant to the client's presenting concerns (e.g., client describes extremely high levels of self-criticism and shame over developing patterns of reactivity and avoidance), think about giving less attention to the specific events and experiences in the client's history that may account for how their problems developed

  ○ Don't ignore current contextual factors that are contributing to the client's concerns or that could interfere with treatment.

THERAPIST FORM 3.1. Case Formulation Worksheet

CLIENT'S PRIMARY PRESENTING CONCERNS: _____

ITEM 1A: CHALLENGING OR PAINFUL INNER EXPERIENCES AND CONTEXTUAL TRIGGERS

Emotion	Thoughts/Images	Physiological Responses

ITEM 1B: POTENTIAL TRIGGERS

Current Context	Past Experiences	Concerns about the Future

(continued)

Case Formulation Worksheet *(page 2 of 4)*

ITEM 2A: CLIENT'S REACTIONS TO PAINFUL INTERNAL EXPERIENCES AND ENTANGLED AND FUSED AWARENESS

Problematic Relationship with Internal Experiences	Examples	
Fear/distress		
Critical reactivity/judgment		
Fusion (*i.e., responses experienced as truth; self-defining*)		

ITEM 2B: PATTERNS OF ATTENTION

Patterns of Attention	Examples	
Attention is narrow and selective; focused toward threat or negativity		
Difficulty noticing internal experiences		
Confusion or misunderstanding of internal experiences		

(continued)

67

Case Formulation Worksheet *(page 3 of 4)*

ITEM 3: ATTEMPTS TO AVOID INTERNAL EXPERIENCES

Strategies Aimed at Experiential Avoidance	Examples	Consequences
Avoidance of situations and activities that elicit challenging internal responses (*this may also take the form of procrastination*)		
Clinically problematic behaviors (*e.g., substance use, self-injurious behaviors, overeating*)		
Other behaviors where the consequences are subtler (*e.g., spending an excessive amount of time on the Internet*) or problematic only in some circumstances/when rigidly adhered to (*e.g., need to exercise to "burn off" anxiety*)		

ITEM 4A: LIMITED ENGAGEMENT IN PERSONALLY MEANINGFUL ACTIONS

Domains	Clear Sense of Values	Satisfaction	Engagement
Relationships			
Work/school/household management			
Self-nourishment and community activities			

(continued)

Case Formulation Worksheet *(page 4 of 4)*

ITEM 4B: LIMITED ENGAGEMENT IN PERSONALLY MEANINGFUL ACTIONS

Domains	Struggle with Internal Experiences	Desire for Things to Be Other Than They Are	Attempts to Control People and Events Outside of Control
Relationships			
Work/school/household management			
Self-nourishment and community activities			

ITEM 5: CONTRIBUTING INFLUENCES FROM HISTORICAL OR CURRENT EXPERIENCES/CONTEXTS

Lesson Learned: *Way of responding to internal experiences and/or control strategies*	Examples	Contributing Influence: *Historical or current experiences/contexts*
Punished for expressing emotions		
Witnessed someone close model avoidant coping		
Was instructed by someone close to change or suppress internal experience		
Was labeled for experiencing or expressing certain emotions		
Was taught ruminating or worrying are effective problem-solving strategies		
Other lessons learned		
Other lessons learned		

THERAPIST FORM 3.2. Case Formulation Narrative Template

(This form refers to numbered "items," which are components of Therapy Form 3.1.)

Given what is known about the client's current context _____ (*potential current context triggers from Item 1B*) and the client's limited engagement in _____ (*include here any personally meaningful activities that are currently characterized by low engagement from Item 4A*), despite the importance of these activities to the client's sense of meaning and purpose, it is natural for them to experience (*emotions and associated thoughts and physiological responses associated with current context triggers from Item 1A; it's best to note clear emotions here*) (defined and described in Chapter 5). _____.

[*Alternatively, describe disruptions in awareness of internal experiences from 2B here, if the client isn't able to report on internal experiences yet.*]

Although it is understandable that these thoughts/emotions/painful memories/challenging sensations arise, some of the ways the client has learned to react to their responses may in fact be contributing to the client's distress and lowered quality of life.

In (*describe specific historical or current context in which client learned how to view and respond to emotions from Item 5*) _____ the client learned (*describe lessons learned from Item 5*). _____. Due to that learning, when the client experiences (*internal experience from Item 1A*) _____, they often react by (*include relevant habits from Item 2A and Item 3*) _____. Moreover, these behavioral patterns are reinforced because in the short term they reduce distress.

Unfortunately, these patterns also function to increase the frequency with which the client experiences (*emotions and associated thoughts and physiological responses associated with current context triggers from Item 1A; Muddy emotions described in Chapter 5 may be referenced here*) _____ and their associated distress. *If items are included in 2B, include:* Either due to these ways of reacting, or due to other aspects of the client's learning (*describe relevant history from Item 5*), the client's awareness of their internal experiences is further disrupted in that (*include relevant items from 2B*). *If there are clear consequences to experiential avoidance in Item 3, include:* Some of the strategies the client uses to reduce the frequency and intensity of their painful responses such as (*strategies from 3*) _____ have become problematic because (*include consequences from 3*) _____.

If the client avoids engaging in values actions as noted in Item 4A, include: In order to minimize contact with painful internal experiences like (*internal experience from Item 1A*) _____, the client avoids (*describe activities and situations avoided from Item 4A*). Although the client understandably avoids in this way, lack of engagement in this valued domain elicits feelings of (*internal experience from Item 1A*) _____.

If the client is engaging in values actions, but the quality of their experience during valued action is problematic as noted in Item 4B, include any of the relevant responses from 4B: Although the client regularly engages in (*valued activity from Item 4A*),

1. They are often distracted by their entanglement in their internal experiences and their efforts to change or suppress their responses, which erodes their sense of fulfillment and (if noted) interferes with their relationship quality/task performance.
2. The quality of the client's engagement in valued activities is often reduced by the client's understandable, but problematic, wish that things be different than they are. For example (*examples from column 2 in 4B*), _____.
3. Although the client highly values (*from 4A*) _____, they understandably feel that their experience in this life area would be improved if (*examples from column 3 in 4B*) _____. Unfortunately, despite their best efforts, they have limited control over (*examples from column 3 in 4B*) _____ and thus they experience (*internal experience from Item 1A; Muddy emotions described in Chapter 5 may be referenced here*) _____ related to that life domain.

PART II

Cultivating Acceptance-Based Skills and Clarifying Values

In Part II, we provide an in-depth exploration of the key elements of skill building and values clarification that we typically use in our work with a wide range of clients. Although we separate these elements out (i.e., therapeutic relationship, psychoeducation, mindfulness and other practices, self-compassion practices, values clarification), we intertwine them in the context of each session, and there are clear overlaps across categories. For instance, self-monitoring is used to highlight aspects of psychoeducation, such as clear versus muddy emotions, but it is also a mindfulness strategy (i.e., helps clients to turn toward and observe their internal experiences), and we use monitoring to help clients notice opportunities for values-based actions as well. Similarly, we provide many examples of psychoeducation in Chapter 5, but we review psychoeducation around mindfulness in Chapter 6 and as it pertains to values clarification in Chapter 8. As in Part I, we indicate when a topic we're addressing is covered in more depth in another chapter.

As we describe in the introduction, ABBT can be delivered in many forms. In our research, we delivered 16 sessions, with the first 7 focused on psychoeducation, values clarification, and skills acquisition and the latter 7 (plus 2 tapered relapse prevention sessions) focused on flexible application. Table II.1 provides a general overview of the structure of these sessions, which may be a useful guide for your own flexible adaptation of this approach to your practice. We indicate the chapters in which we most directly address the specific content noted in each entry. The chapters in Part II map most directly onto the first phase of therapy (psychoeducation, values exploration, and skills acquisition), although they are also relevant for the latter phase of therapy, which we will address most directly in Part III. Chapter 4, which focuses on the therapy relationship, provides guidance for the entire course of therapy, from assessment to termination.

TABLE II.1. A Summary of the Structure of Early and Later Sessions in ABBT

Early sessions	Later sessions

Session focus

Early sessions	Later sessions
The session is typically preplanned with an agenda. The main focus of the session is psychoeducation on one or more relevant topics, skill practice and development, and values exploration (Chapters 5–8).	The therapist may have some items for the agenda based on the previous session, but the main focus of the session is helping the client to choose and engage in valued actions and apply skills to work with challenges that arise in the client's daily life experiences (Chapters 9–11).

Transition into session

Early sessions	Later sessions
The therapist comes prepared to introduce a particular mindfulness practice (based on the individualized progression described in Chapter 6). The therapist and the client practice together, share observations, and draw connections between what was noticed and the client's presenting concerns (Chapter 6).	The client chooses a mindfulness practice to engage in with the therapist. The therapist and the client practice together, share observations, and draw connections between what was noticed and the client's presenting concerns (Chapter 6).

Body of the session

Early sessions	Later sessions
Review out-of-session practices with the client. Introduce and explore new concepts (Chapters 5, 6, 7, and 8).	Apply previously learned material and skills to whatever particular challenges arise in the client's daily life.
	If the client is struggling with muddy emotions: Revisit clear and muddy emotions (Chapter 5) and practice identifying and addressing factors that are maintaining the muddiness (Chapter 9).
	If the client is struggling to choose a response to a challenging situation: help the client to consider options and explore whether values can guide choices (Chapters 8–10)
	If the client wants to enhance sense of meaning and purpose: Engage in values clarification and identify potential valued actions to be taken (Chapters 8 and 9).
	If the client is struggling with internal and/or external obstacles to valued action: Use skills to work with obstacles (Chapters 9 and 10).

Closing

Early sessions	Later sessions
Develop a plan for the client to complete exercises and/or practice skills related to session content.	Develop a plan for the client to complete exercises and/or practice skills related to session content.

As we noted in Part I, we have found these general strategies to be beneficial, with a wide range of clients in a wide range of contexts. Therefore, we provide many examples and suggestions of monitoring, psychoeducation, mindfulness-based strategies, and values clarification methods in the hopes that some of them will apply to your clients. We encourage readers to focus on those examples and suggestions that are most relevant to their work, potentially revisiting other examples and suggestions when they find a client who doesn't fit as well with the parts they have been using most frequently.

CHAPTER 4 ❦❦❦❦❦❦❦❦❦❦❦

The Therapeutic Relationship

A CONTEXT AND A MECHANISM FOR CHANGE

Sometimes the extensive strategies and techniques used in ABBTs and other CBTs can give the false impression that handouts, exercises, and techniques are the only active ingredients in treatment and where all the attention should be. However, both research (see Box 4.1) and clinical observation clearly highlight the important role of the therapeutic relationship as a context for change (e.g., helping clients feel safe enough to engage in emotionally challenging exercises) and also as a mechanism of change (e.g., the experience of empathic validation directly giving clients a new experience with the expression of their painful internal experiences). In this chapter, we focus on exploring the ways that you can effectively work within the therapeutic relationship to maximize clients' engagement and meaningful change.

What you will learn

- ❧ How to develop a successful working alliance to promote meaningful change.
- ❧ How the therapeutic relationship addresses targets for therapy in ABBT.
- ❧ How to cultivate and communicate validation effectively.
- ❧ How to address challenges and ruptures in the working alliance.

A comprehensive discussion of the many ways that the relationship between a therapist and client can enhance, create, or impede therapeutic changes is beyond the scope of this chapter (see Jordan, 2010; Kazantzis, Dattilio, & Dobson, 2017; Norcross, 2011, for more extensive discussions). We focus here briefly on those aspects that characterize CBT therapeutic relationships in particular, and more in depth on the ways we use the therapeutic relationship to target aspects of the ABBT case conceptualization and how to address challenges that may arise, drawing from the broader literature on the therapeutic relationship as a vehicle of change.

BOX 4.1. A CLOSER LOOK:
Relationship as a Context for Change

A joint American Psychological Association Task Force (Division of Psychotherapy and Division of Clinical Psychology) on Evidence-Based Therapy Relationships critically reviewed the psychotherapy literature and identified that the alliance (bond and agreement on tasks and goals), empathy, and gathering client feedback were all demonstrably effective elements of the therapeutic relationships (*http://societyforpsychotherapy.org/evidence-based-therapy-relationships*). They also noted that adapting therapy for client characteristics such as preference and cultural background was demonstrably effective. In our own research, we have found that both client and therapist ratings of the working alliance (and subscale ratings of bond, agreement on goals, and agreement on tasks) early in ABBT treatment were associated with better outcomes (Calloway, Hayes-Skelton, Roemer, & Orsillo, 2017), indicating that alliance may be an important factor in ABBT specifically. More research is needed to determine the contribution of both general and ABBT-specific elements of the therapeutic relationship to positive outcomes.

DEVELOPING A COLLABORATIVE, TRANSPARENT THERAPEUTIC RELATIONSHIP

A central feature of an effective therapeutic relationship in CBT is its collaborative nature (Kazantzis et al., 2017). As we described in Chapter 3, CBT therapists work to develop a shared understanding of the client's presenting problems and how best to approach them in therapy. The therapist is seen as a general expert in behavioral principles and cognitive science, while the client is seen as the expert in their own unique experiences (Craske, 2010); the two work together to consistently refine their shared understanding and plan. In addition, the therapist is responsible for bringing general knowledge of a range of cultural values, beliefs, and traditions, as well as familial and systemic factors that may impact the client, while the client brings their own unique relationship to these modal tendencies and intersectional identities (see Hays, 2016, for more in-depth discussion).

In addition to establishing a shared conceptualization and treatment plan, as described in the previous chapter, an important early task in therapy is to develop realistic expectations of the nature and roles in therapy. A number of client-related variables, including cultural factors (e.g., ethnicity, race, gender, age, social class, religion and spirituality, nationality, immigration and refugee status, and generational level), past therapy experience, developmental history, and interpersonal style can dramatically influence the expectations clients have about the nature of their role in psychotherapy. Clients may expect therapists to be relatively silent observers, active advisors, or supportive friends. Therefore, explicitly sharing our own assumptions about the role of the therapist and the client in our approach to therapy, as well as assessing the client's expectations, are important elements of establishing a working alliance.

As with other CBTs, the establishment of a collaborative relationship between the client and therapist is essential in ABBT. While our overarching general theory suggests that avoidance is negatively impacting the client's life and offers several clinical methods for addressing this avoidance, it is the client's personal concerns and values that ultimately dictate the course of therapy. Therefore, we assume that clients are the experts on themselves. However, we also acknowledge that fusion, avoidance, and inattention to behaviors may at times interfere with clients' ability to accurately observe their own experience and to be aware of the contingencies guiding their behavior. Therefore, although we expect that clients may not immediately see the relevance of some of the concepts we discuss or may disagree that certain strategies might be useful to them, we ask clients to be open to the possibility that making changes in the way they view their internal experiences and choose their actions may be helpful. In other words, we ultimately defer to the client's view of the utility of certain approaches or strategies in enhancing quality of life, but we ask that clients consider taking some time to closely observe their behavior and to try some new methods of responding before they reach a conclusion. To describe this relationship to a client who is struggling with an anxiety disorder we might say:

> "Here are my views on each of our roles in therapy and how we can best work together: As a therapist, I have some knowledge of general principles of anxiety and worry, the role of environment and context in these experiences, the ways responses to anxiety and worry can limit people's lives, and methods to help people struggling with anxiety to lead more satisfying and fulfilling lives. But my knowledge is general, and you are the expert on your personal experience and how these general principles do or don't apply to you. So I will do my best to present all of this information to you, to share thoughts and ideas I have, and to offer my support, understanding, and guidance. However, I believe that you are the only expert on you and the context of your life. Only you can say what is really important to you and how you would like to live the rest of your life. You are the only one who can honestly observe your own personal experience to see if the things we talk about together that might be causing your struggles are accurate and to judge whether the changes we come up with are life enhancing. If we are to work together, I would like to ask you to consider some of the suggestions I make to you based on my general knowledge to see if they fit your experience. I am also going to ask you to try out some new ways of responding that initially may not seem logical or useful to you. Your own experience with these new approaches will help us determine whether in fact they might be helpful to you or not. I would like you to commit to considering some new approaches and I would like to commit to listening to and honoring your experiences with these approaches."

In addition to explicitly discussing roles and expectations for therapy, we also try to embody a collaborative spirit by demonstrating our interest in, and respect for, the client's experience and perception and our willingness to talk about aspects of our relationship in order to enhance our working alliance. The process of developing a mutually agreed upon conceptualization described earlier is one example of this approach—by directly asking the client for their understanding of their challenges and forming a shared understanding, we communicate the importance of their perspective. We also ask clients directly about their past experiences with therapy, their hopes and expectations for therapy, and also any thoughts they had prior to meeting about what their therapist might be like. We ask if they have any thoughts about how our age, race, gender, ethnicity, or other identities might impact our work together, in order to establish that we can have conversations about apparent similarities and differences that may play a role in developing a strong therapeutic alliance. Explicitly raising issues of potential cultural differences may be particularly important when therapists identify as White or with other dominant identities, as clients who hold marginalized identities may assume that a therapist won't discuss these issues and need an indication that it is safe to have these conversations (Hayes, 2016). When clients communicate any concerns that we may not understand some aspects of their experience (often due to apparent differences), we validate that as a reasonable concern. We share our commitment to knowing and learning general information about these aspects of their experience (e.g., the challenges that new parents face, even if we aren't parents, and racial discrimination and race-based systemic inequities, even if we identify as White), and our openness to hearing when we are missing something important about their specific experiences. We acknowledge our inability to fully, experientially understand the complex impact of experiences we haven't had, while also communicating our commitment to being empathically attuned to experiences that differ from our own.

Following a meta-analysis of culturally adapted interventions (which indicated that cultural adaptions were effective), Smith, Domenech Rodriguez, and Bernal (2011) concluded that therapists' attempts to be culturally responsive likely enhance the therapeutic alliance.[1] They emphasize the importance of explicitly working to establish a strong alliance and understanding of the client across cultural differences. They note the importance of clear communication and continual feedback and agreement on indications of therapeutic progress, as well as use of cultural expressions and metaphors and values-congruent therapeutic strategies as a means to maintain a positive therapeutic alliance. The therapist responding to misunderstandings nondefensively and demonstrating a genuine willingness to take responsibility for independent learning relevant to aspects of the client's background to more accurately understand their context can help to repair any ruptures in the therapeutic alliance that occur (e.g., Jordan, 2010).

Although therapists cannot fully understand the particular lived experiences of a client and therefore must learn from their clients, therapists can and should inform themselves of general considerations and modal experiences of clients from similar racial, socioeconomic, sexual orientation, gender identity, immigration status, religious, disability status, national and geographic backgrounds (e.g., Hays, 2016; Sue & Sue, 2015). In addition to reading scholarly and first-hand accounts to expand our understanding of specific cultural and contextual experiences, we can consult with professional and personal experts to enhance our foundational knowledge. Nonetheless, we must always remember that identity is complex and multifaceted and that understanding modal experiences of a given group, or even a given intersectional identity, does not mean we will understand our client's specific relationship to all aspects of their identity and background. This is why establishing a strong alliance, open communication about the relationship, and a space in which misunderstandings can be heard and repaired is so important.

Our early discussions about therapy also include our sharing some specifics about what therapy will be like with us, such as that we will be presenting some ideas and principles that we think are relevant to their experience (i.e., psychoeducation). We will

---

[1] Hall and colleagues' (2016) more recent meta-analysis similarly concludes that cultural adaptations are more effective than nonadapted versions of treatments.

be doing some exercises together in order to build new skills (e.g., mindfulness practices), and we will also be asking that they bring therapy into their own lives because that is our target for change. We acknowledge that they likely didn't come to see us because they felt they had extra time in their lives, and we assure them that we will help them problem-solve how to fit these activities into their lives. As discussed in Chapter 3, because devoting time to therapy outside of a session is often identified as a particular challenge in ABBTs and other CBTs (e.g., Fuchs et al., 2016), we discuss this aspect of treatment frankly. We can fold this into the discussion of the model behind treatment; we can't change well-worn habits without repeated practice, so this requires time outside of session. At the same time, when we work with clients for whom extra time is a significant barrier, we adapt interventions accordingly to help them develop new skills in the midst of other activities, as we describe throughout the book. We sometimes use the metaphor of training for a long race or marathon to suggest that clients think about the time they're in therapy as a time of intensive training for the changes they want to make. Making meaningful changes takes some devoted time to practice new things, and so it can be useful to think about how to carve out a little bit of extra time each day to engage in the new practice so that repetition can make new habits stronger more rapidly. At the same time, not everyone has time to train for a marathon, and so sometimes we work more slowly, with practices that are paired to daily activities, when clients really don't have extra time for practice.

> See Chapter 10 for an in-depth discussion of how to help clients assess what they're spending time on so that they can potentially make more time for actions that matter to them, including the work of therapy.

COMMON FACTORS IN HOW THE THERAPEUTIC RELATIONSHIP LEADS TO CHANGE

Consistent with other therapeutic approaches, the therapeutic relationship in ABBT is an important context for promoting positive expectancies and hope, which are associated with positive outcomes (Norcross, 2011). Through conveying understanding of the client's presenting problems and suggestions of an approach that will lead to meaningful changes that enhance their lives, the therapist helps to engender hope in the client. By sharing a rich conceptualization that incorporates cultural and contextual factors and by eliciting feedback from the client, the therapist demonstrates an understanding of the complexity of the client's experiences, while still conveying a sense of a clear path toward meaningful change. This positive expectancy provides an important context to help the client engage in the tasks of therapy. We also often offer some coping strategies early on. For instance, we usually practice diaphragmatic breathing mindfully in a first or early session, suggesting that this may or may not be beneficial (so that unreasonable expectancies don't lead to disappointment). Early positive responses to concrete suggestions like diaphragmatic breathing can help build positive expectancies and may help build credibility and confidence in the therapist and further motivation to engage in therapeutic tasks.

ABBT therapists strive to develop an accurate empathic and nonjudgmental view of the client and to display this empathy, warmth, and acceptance genuinely and consistently in session (Rogers, 1961). This empathy and warmth provide a context that encourages disclosure and enhances clients' ability to turn toward painful material, which has numerous specific benefits related to the ABBT model described in more detail below. The ABBT model is an important foundation for the development of this foundational empathy and acceptance. Within this model, the basic processes (a critical fused relation with internal experiences, rigid, habitual experiential avoidance, behavioral avoidance, and constriction) that underlie the challenges a client is experiencing are universal, fundamental aspects of being human that are naturally shaped by learning experiences, contexts, and environments. This means that our clients are not fundamentally flawed in some way and that we also struggle with these processes, perhaps in different ways, in our own lives. Grounding ourselves in this understanding helps us develop empathy and understanding for our clients, which is an important first step to conveying this empathy genuinely in session.

HOW THE THERAPEUTIC RELATIONSHIP DIRECTLY TARGETS CHANGE FROM AN ABBT PERSPECTIVE

When we conducted our therapy trials for ABBT for GAD, we spent a lot of time developing a number of materials—monitoring forms, psychoeducational handouts, mindfulness exercises, values clarification strategies, valued action monitoring—to directly target the elements we thought were perpetuating clients' difficulties and to help them engage in new learning. We continue to think these materials are beneficial (and we include many of them in this edition of the book). However, through our own sessions and through observing countless hours of therapy conducted by therapists on our grants or in other supervision contexts, we have developed a renewed appreciation for the degree to which meaningful changes that are consistent with the ABBT model happen directly within the therapeutic relationship. Although there are many ways to develop effective therapeutic relationships and these vary by style of therapist and client, we share some general principles here as to how we think the therapeutic relationship can create change to serve as a guide in your own work.

Altering the Client's Relationship with Internal Experiences

Communicating That Challenges Are Shared Human Experiences

Each time the therapist communicates that a client's reactions, behaviors, and challenges make sense (from a learning, experiential avoidance, or systemic perspective) and are natural and human, this is counterevidence to the common, critical, judgmental response that clients have to their own experiences. This happens naturally within the process of developing a shared conceptualization, but we also convey this by acknowledging that we ourselves engage in human, habitual responses like experiential avoidance. For example, we often use an adapted version of the "two-mountain metaphor" (Hayes, Batten, et al., 1999) drawn from ACT to explicitly illustrate to our clients the universality of their struggles and to acknowledge that we are not immune to these forces. We have adapted this metaphor to also acknowledge that we may not see some things more clearly than they do.

"As your therapist, I will sometimes offer some observations about your struggle and make some suggestions about possible options in response to those struggles. It may seem as if I am on the top of a mountain, with the mountain representing the barriers that you face as you work toward climbing the mountain and obtaining a life that is fulfilling and satisfying. It may seem that from my perch on the mountain I can more clearly see the things that contribute to your struggle, because I have already succeeded with the climb. But that is not my view of therapy. I believe that many of the struggles that you are experiencing are common to all human beings and that therapists are not immune to those struggles. In fact, therapists are just like other human beings in that we are all on our own mountain, each with our own personal struggles and obstacles. But, as your therapist, I may at times be able to offer some perspective on your struggle because I have some distance, and a unique perspective, from my perch over here on my own mountain. At the same time, there may be some aspects of your experience that I can't see quite as well from my mountain, while you see them very well from close up, so I hope you will point those things out to me when they come up."

We often use the language of "we" when describing general processes like critical entanglement or experiential avoidance as another way of communicating that these are human challenges, not something problematic in the client, as they often imagine. Similarly, we intentionally disclose examples of the types of thoughts and feelings we personally experience in difficult situations when it is therapeutically appropriate. For instance, a therapist might share his thoughts of inadequacy that are elicited by an invitation to present at a scientific conference. Or a therapist might describe her urge to withdraw from a conflictual situation. We have found these disclosures to be particularly useful when a client is uncomfortable reporting on their own internal experiences. For example, a client who presented with major depressive disorder and who highly valued her role as a parent was initially unwilling to explore the ways in which her problems may have been interfering with her relationship to her children. Her therapist shared that being an available, connected parent was a value for her as well. However, the therapist admitted that while her behavior was typically consistent with that value, she found that when she was feeling significant pressure at work she noticed herself being more critical toward, and detached from, her children Following the therapist's honest, forthright disclosure about herself, the client was willing to provide examples of times that she was feeling sad and worthless and withdrew from her children. While these types of disclosures can be powerful, they should be carefully chosen and guided by the intention of providing a model of the universality of these struggles, rather than processing one's own difficulties.

The Use of Validation

The therapist's explicit and implicit validation of the client and their behaviors are an essential aspect of ABBTs (see Linehan, 1997, for an in-depth discussion of validation in DBT that significantly influences our work in this area). Linehan (1993, p. 222) notes, "The essence of validation is this: The therapist communicates to the client that her responses make sense and are understandable within her *current* life context or situation." This communication that the client's responses make sense is in direct oppo-sition to the habitual self-critical responses that clients typically bring to therapy. The therapist's consistent validation serves as a model for self-validation and cultivation of self-compassion, which in turn alter the client's habitual ways of responding critically to their own responses.

Validation occurs explicitly, such as when therapists communicate that they:

- Hear what the client is saying,
- Recognize and comment on a reaction the client isn't directly communicating,
- Share why a particular reaction makes sense historically, or
- Communicate why a reaction makes sense in a given context.

For example:

GEORGE: My new neighbor was sitting on her steps, and I wanted to introduce myself, but I was anxious.

THERAPIST: That makes a lot of sense. Humans are social beings who want to be accepted by others. And it's also the case that sometimes others can judge or reject us. So, reaching out to someone new is taking a risk. And taking risks raises our anxiety.

While this type of validation may reduce the client's self-criticism of this under-standable anxious response, the client may still go on to report on the self-criticism and judgment that he experiences when he gets anxious. Therapists can validate the humanness of these secondary reactions and still be careful not to suggest that it's rea-sonable to be ashamed of this kind of response.

GEORGE: It was just so stupid and ridiculous that I couldn't even say hello. Other people just say hello to people all the time. I got so angry at myself and felt really humiliated when I just walked back inside like an idiot.

THERAPIST: It sounds like a lot of critical reactions come up for you when you expe-rience that kind of anxiety. I can really understand that, given what you've told me about how your father would yell at you whenever you expressed anxiety of any sort. Are words like *stupid* and *idiot* words that he used when he yelled at you?

GEORGE: Yeah, I guess they were.

THERAPIST: It makes sense that that kind of reaction got really ingrained for you and now it just happens so automatically. And so maybe before when I said your anxiety was understandable it kind of sparked that pushback that he would have had to an idea like that?

GEORGE: Yeah, I think that's true. But I think I also think it's ridiculous. I don't want to be like this anymore.

THERAPIST: Of course you don't. It's so human to wish that you could just push that anxiety away and not have it get in your way. But, like we talked about

BOX 4.2. TRY THIS:
How Do You Validate Clients?

Validation is often the first thing we learn as developing therapists, and so it can seem like a novice technique. However, validation is actually a very powerful, complex intervention that is often worth revisiting to refine our skills in delivering it and the challenges we face. If you haven't thought a lot about validation in your therapeutic work or if you want to reconsider it, take out a piece of paper and jot down your responses to the following questions so that you can reflect on your own practice and development while you read the rest of this chapter.

- How do you typically validate your clients?
- What are you trying to accomplish when you use validation?
- Do you use validation for different reasons? What are they?
- What gets in your way when you try to validate your clients? When is it harder to do this? How do you address these challenges?
- Are there times that you think validation can be problematic? If so, what are they?

before, even though it's really understandable to be critical of our reactions and wish they were different, that doesn't really help us change them. And it might make it even harder for us to do the things we want to do, like talk to a neighbor. So maybe you're kind of caught in a cycle and maybe it's worth trying to change that by seeing if you can let in the possibility that your anxious response, which you have a lot of thoughts and feelings about, is understandable and doesn't have to mean you're stupid or ridiculous?

Here the therapist is careful to validate the initial reaction the client had, but also to validate the client's wish that he not have this reaction in the first place. In this way, we maintain the dialectic of validating that the client is understandable, human, and fundamentally okay as he is, while also simultaneously validating his desire to change. This validation can then bridge to sharing suggestions of potential different responses, in place of the self-criticism, judgment, and experiential avoidance that hasn't been working, as we explore in subsequent chapters.

An in-depth exploration of the different levels and types of validation that therapists can use is beyond the scope of this chapter (see Linehan, 1997, for a comprehensive discussion). The following principles and examples can guide the use of validation to help clients relate differently to their experiences:

- We want to specifically validate what is valid, not what is invalid.
  - For example: When the therapist above says, "It sounds like a lot of critical reactions come up for you when you experience that kind of anxiety," she is validating the humanness of the reactions but is not validating that the client "walked back inside like an idiot." This begins to establish some separation between a client's reaction and the truth, as we explore more fully below.
- One powerful level of validation is communicating that reactions (thoughts,

feelings, sensations, behaviors) happen for a reason, even those that the client may want to change (here the therapist balances validating the reactions as they occur with validating the desire for change)

- *Historical antecedents.* We often note that clients' reactions make sense given their past experiences, even if they don't make sense in their given context. In the example above, George feels humiliated and like an "idiot" when he experiences anxiety because his father used to yell at him for feeling that way. So, although we want to help him feel less ashamed of these responses moving forward, we can validate that it makes sense he has that reaction now, which helps to reduce one level of self-blame (when he is angry at himself for feeling humiliated).

- *Short-term versus long-term consequences.* Often the client's behaviors make sense in the short term. Leaving an uncomfortable situation does lead to immediate relief, so we can validate that natural reaction, while also suggesting that it may be worthwhile to consider remaining in that situation the next time, given longer-term goals and values.

- *Varied contexts.* Clients often respond rigidly to contexts, so their response may make sense or be useful in one context but they are responding the same way in a different context. Again, we can communicate why it makes sense that they are responding in a way that makes sense with one person in their lives, while still introducing the possibility that a different response might be worth trying with this new person, to see how it goes.

- Validation can focus on actions, cognitions, sensations, and emotions. In this way, validation also helps clients to begin to differentiate aspects of their experiences, as we explore more fully below.

Functional validation is also an important part of the therapeutic relationship that leads to change (Linehan, 1997). When we act as though the client's behavior is valid, we provide a corrective experience for clients whose behaviors have been chronically invalidated, and we also provide natural contingencies for their behavioral expressions (Tsai et al., 2009), which helps to promote their own awareness of their reactions and to treat them as information worth attending to. This can be particularly important when a client has habitually denied or discounted their emotional responses. For example, instead of thanking a client for expressing their frustration when they feel like we misunderstood something they said, which is not something that people in their lives are likely to do, we can redirect our attention and listen carefully to try to understand better. Just listening attentively, nonverbally expressing compassion or care, or asking about aspects of their experience, are simple ways that we functionally validate the client's experience, which helps them to attend more closely to their experience and relate differently to it.

Responses That Encourage Decentering/Defusion

We also both explicitly and implicitly encourage decentering or defusion from thoughts, emotions, and sensations in the context of the therapeutic relationship. Drawing from ACT, we make careful choices in the language we use to describe the client's experiences: we use precise, descriptive, nonpathological terms, and eventually we encourage clients to do the same. Even before we have introduced the concept of defusion/decentering, we make these language choices in order to cultivate new way of relating to internal experiences. In the following example, the therapist introduces this language change explicitly, while also implicitly making some language changes that also have a therapeutic goal.

IJEOMA: I had plans to go out to dinner with my friends on Friday night, but I couldn't because of my depression.

THERAPIST: I understand that you have been diagnosed with major depressive disorder and that sometimes you use the word *depression* as shorthand for many different thoughts, emotions, and physical sensations that you are experiencing. But in order for us both to really understand your moment-to-moment experience, I am going to ask you to try to be more specific when talking about your experiences. Is it okay with you if we try that? (*Client nods.*) So, what emotions did you notice were present on Friday night?

IJEOMA: I felt depressed.

THERAPIST: Would you say that you were feeling sadness?

IJEOMA: Yes, I definitely felt sad.

THERAPIST: Any other emotions?

IJEOMA: No, just sad.

THERAPIST: How did you feel physically? Did you notice anything going on in your body?

IJEOMA: My body felt very heavy. Like I was a block of lead.

THERAPIST: How about any thoughts? Did you notice yourself thinking or saying anything to yourself?

IJEOMA: Just the usual. I felt useless, like a loser.

THERAPIST: So you had the thought "I am useless, I am a loser." [The therapist shifts the language from describing thoughts as a feeling to labeling them as thoughts.]

IJEOMA: That's right.

THERAPIST: Often emotions are linked up with what we call action tendencies. In other words, certain emotions urge us to behave in certain ways. Like when we feel anxious, we have the urge to run away or fight against whatever is making us scared. Did you notice some sort of behavioral urge that arose when you felt sad?

IJEOMA: Sure, I felt like going back to bed. I just wanted to avoid my friends, jump back into bed and pull the covers over my head.

THERAPIST: Okay, one last thing. What did you choose to do in that situation? [Here the therapist is subtly distinguishing urges from chosen actions, which opens a possibility of choosing other actions, without fully exploring that possibility at this early point in therapy.]

IJEOMA: I stayed in bed. I didn't answer the phone when my friend called.

THERAPIST: Okay, so let me see if I understand what your experience was like on Friday night. You noticed feelings of sadness, your body felt heavy, you had the thought that you were useless, and you felt the urge to go back to bed and avoid your friends. In the end, you chose to go back to bed rather than to go to dinner. Does that capture your experience?

IJEOMA: Yup.

THERAPIST: If you are willing, I am going to ask you to try to talk about your experience in that very specific way, rather than using the shortcut term *depression*. Is that okay with you?

IJEOMA: Okay, I can try. But it is not how I am used to talking.

Therapist: I completely understand that. I am going to ask you to try a lot of new things that might seem strange and different at first. [Here the therapist validates that this feels unusual and strange to the client, while also discounting the potential implication that that makes it a bad idea. Instead the therapist suggests that therapeutic changes may feel new, strange, and different at first.]

In response to a client who stated, "I self-medicated my PTSD flashback," the therapist might explore the elements of that statement, encouraging the client to notice that he had experienced an image of a painful past event, along with feelings of sadness and fear and that he noticed thoughts such as, "I cannot cope with this," felt an urge to drink, and opted to drink a pint of whiskey with the hope that the painful images, thoughts, and feelings would go away.

Sometimes, the therapist models this way of relating to experiences more implicitly, with less explicit description of the process.

WINONA: Wednesday was a terrible day. I woke up knowing that it was a "fat" day.

THERAPIST: So as soon as you woke up you noticed the thought "I feel fat today."

WINONA: That's right. I couldn't stand the thought of putting on my jeans and going to class. I knew I had to go to the gym and work out for an extra session.

THERAPIST: So, that thought was followed by the urge to go to the gym and skip class. It sounds like the urge felt very powerful.

WINONA: I was just disgusted with myself. I had to go to the gym.

THERAPIST: Those emotions can be so intense and powerful. It sounds like you really felt a strong urge to exercise. What did you choose to do next?

WINONA: I went to the gym and then I hated myself for missing class again.

THERAPIST: So it sounds like you felt compelled to act on those very strong urges to exercise, and then it sounds like some other thoughts and feelings came up for you. Did they come up right away?

WINONA: Oh, well, actually first I just felt a lot of relief while I was on the treadmill. And then I started thinking about class and what I was missing.

THERAPIST: Oh, I see—that's helpful to know. So first you felt good for taking an action consistent with that very strong urge. And then some thoughts started to come up about the impact of that choice. And then you had some negative thoughts about yourself and maybe some negative sensations and emotions as well.

WINONA: Yes, exactly. When I first woke up, all I could think about was how fat I was and how much I had to go to the gym. It wasn't until I was on the treadmill that I thought about class.

THERAPIST: Well, that seems like a useful pattern to notice—of course, you followed the urge when you couldn't really think of anything other than the relief that you usually get when you have similar thoughts and feelings and you go to the gym. Your attention was narrowly focused on what seemed most important in that moment—to relieve those distressing feelings—so you didn't notice the consequences of that choice in that moment. [Here the therapist opens the door for potential changes in responding, after separating experiences into thoughts, feelings, urges, and behaviors.]

The language of naming responses precisely can seem cumbersome and unnatural to therapists and may feel like it isn't a genuine way of responding at first. However, with practice, therapists (just like clients) will start to find it more natural. And the habits of language do shape the way we perceive our own reactions as well as those of our clients, so they can be very useful to cultivate in order to get a more separated, distinct, disentangled sense of these experiences as they rise and fall. Another aspect of this reflection and modeling involves specifying the temporal unfolding of reactions, an informal version of chain analyses in DBT (determining the "links," such as situation, thoughts, feelings, sensations, and memories, that led to a problematic behavior). In addition to promoting decentering, this also helps to illustrate the ways reactions are understandable (validation) and sets up the realization that there are choice points when the client might do something different.

Enhancing Acceptance and Willingness to Have Internal Experiences

Developing a new, nonjudgmental, compassionate, decentered awareness of internal experiences through observations, modeling, and validation from the therapist will naturally reduce clients' urges to experientially avoid because internal experiences will be less aversive and intense. In addition, the therapeutic relationship provides a powerful context for encouraging turning toward, rather than away from, internal experiences. This is likely a common factor across different theoretical orientations, as therapists naturally create an accepting environment for reactions that can be punished and criticized in other contexts. ABBT therapists can enhance this aspect of the therapeutic relationship through their own practice of mindfulness and acceptance.

Some ABBTs, like mindfulness-based stress reduction, have explicit guidelines for the form and frequency of mindfulness practices that therapists need to engage in. To date, research has not established exactly what practice is necessary, and it is challenging to determine parameters when it is probably the impact, function, and application of practice that matters more than specific forms and frequencies. For this reason, we have taken a more flexible approach in terms of requirements. Nonetheless, our observations certainly support that experiential practice of mindfulness and acceptance is an important part of training for ABBT therapists.

For example, we encourage some form of mindfulness practice prior to and within sessions. Regular mindfulness practice can strengthen one's capacity for genuine and sustained attention toward clients, decreasing the probability that the therapist will "tune out" or become restless or bored in session with an emotionally disengaged client (Fulton, 2013). Similarly, a mindful, accepting stance in therapy allows us to remain engaged in the therapeutic process even when painful emotions emerge in our clients and in ourselves. In our experience, when we are being mindful, it is easier to notice our urge to alleviate distress in our clients and in ourselves and to be able to override that urge and stay with the moment, to behave in accordance with our long-term values as a therapist rather than seeking the short-term alleviation of distress. For example, if we feel uncomfortable and have thoughts of our own incompetency as a therapist when our client expresses increased distress, we might choose clinical strategies on the basis of their ability to reduce the client's immediate distress rather than on the basis of their longer-term impact. Noticing these reactions arise and accepting our feelings of discomfort and distress will allow us to make more effective choices for our client rather than being guided by these reactions. In turn, this will model for the client a willingness to be present with their distress, which can increase the client's acceptance of this response as well.

Our own practice of mindfulness and acceptance also makes it easier for us to disentangle our own reactions from our client's reaction in the moment, so that we can provide more accurate reflections and help them to recognize their own reactions. For instance, if a client with a disability expresses intense anger at the lack of accessibility in a therapist's waiting room, the therapist may immediately feel shame about not noticing this barrier themselves, accompanied by a lot of self-critical thoughts. These reactions can take up a lot of attention and might lead the therapist to redirect the conversation quickly, or jump immediately to reflecting the pain underneath the anger in a way that might be invalidating and discourage the client's genuine expression of their feelings of anger. If the therapist can notice the shame and self-critical thoughts as they arise and make room for them to be there, no matter how uncomfortable they are, then they will be more able to respond skillfully to the client. This might include accurately reflecting the anger being communicated, as well as expressing their regret at their error, and then exploring the client's response more comprehensively without trying to make themselves feel better.

Within the context of the therapeutic relationship, clients regularly express vulnerable emotions, thoughts, sensations, and memories. When they subtly or obviously avoid sharing these experiences, therapists ask about them, or point out the apparent avoidance, gently encouraging them to approach these avoided experiences. This may be as simple as noticing a facial expression and asking about it, or commenting that it seems like the client is feeling something or having a reaction. Encouraging clients to experience their inner responses in session can be conceptualized as a kind of exposure, which leads to inhibitory learning (Craske, Treanor, Conway, Zbozinek, & Vervliet, 2014), or new learning that "inhibits" the old learned response. Each time a client experiences and expresses their painful emotions, thoughts, and sensations and notices that they can be present with pain, that the therapist is willing to sit and be present with them as they express pain, and that the pain doesn't last forever or disrupt their lives, that new learning helps to inhibit escape and avoidance responses. As reviewed in Chapter 5, we explicitly describe the functional nature of our emotions as part of psychoeducation and work to generalize this learning in the context of values-based actions (as discussed in Chapter 9), but it's also important to recognize ongoing opportunities for new learning through the relational experience of therapy, so that we can intentionally maximize this learning.

Promoting Values-Based Actions

The therapeutic relationship plays an important role in promoting values-based actions because stating an intention to take certain actions provides a social incentive to follow through on the intention prior to the next session. The therapist conveys the dialectic of acceptance and change related to valued actions by validating the difficulties in behavior change and all the potential obstacles, and still encouraging the client to select meaningful actions for the coming week (see Chapters 9 and 10 for detailed descriptions of this). In reviewing the previous week, the therapist conveys compassion for challenges faced and socially reinforces actions taken.

In addition, some values-based actions occur within the therapeutic relationship, and these can be highlighted for clients. Often, attending sessions or engaging in between-session exercises are actions that are important and meaningful to the client but bring up challenging emotions. Clients' willingness and commitment to engaging in these aspects of therapy nonetheless provide early examples of their ability to take action even if challenging thoughts and emotions arise. Further, clients often have relational values that involve genuine expression of their thoughts and feelings, or being vulnerable or asserting themselves in the context of relationships. These valued actions

---

 BOX 4.3. TO SUMMARIZE:
How the Therapeutic Relationship Addresses ABBT Goals

Altering clients' relationship with internal experiences

- Treating reactions, behaviors, challenges as natural, human, "making sense."
- Conveying that therapists also face challenging thoughts, emotions, behaviors, habits.
- Validating responses decreases self-criticism, enhances self-compassion.
  - Validate historical antecedents.
  - Validate short-term versus long-term consequences.
- Naming aspects of responses precisely (thoughts, feelings, urges, actions).
- Highlighting the temporal process of responses.

Enhancing acceptance and willingness

- Therapist models this through their own practice.
- Turning toward experiences in therapy provides new inhibitory learning.

Promoting values-based actions

- Therapist provides social reinforcement, validation, and cheerleading for planned actions.
- Values-based actions can occur within the therapeutic relationship.

may first occur in the context of the therapeutic relationship. They can be reinforced in this context and then generalized to meaningful relationships in their lives. See Box 4.3 for a summary of how the therapeutic relationship addresses ABBT goals.

HOW TO ADDRESS CHALLENGES THAT OCCUR WITHIN THE THERAPEUTIC RELATIONSHIP

Failing to Attend to the Therapeutic Relationship

See Chapter 11 for a discussion of how to address challenges in the therapeutic relationship that lead to stuckness in therapy.

Because CBTs and ABBTs often include numerous techniques, strategies, and handouts, there's a real risk that therapists will get distracted by the elements of the treatment and fail to attend to the nature of the relationship. This is another reason to practice mindfulness prior to and during sessions—the more we can come back to this moment and attend to the person across from us, the lower the risk that we get distracted by tasks and lose our attention to the person. Conversely, there's also a risk of attending so much to the person that we fail to introduce strategies that we really believe will be useful to them, so this is a challenging dialectic that requires attention.

Not Understanding or Empathizing with the Client

Most of us found our way to being therapists because of a tendency to care for and empathize with the suffering of others. Nonetheless, we can naturally find ourselves reacting negatively to a client, or having trouble making sense of the choices they make, or finding it hard to be kind and caring toward them. This can happen for numerous reasons, and it is often one of the most upsetting parts of our work because we have come to rely so much on the empathy that usually comes more easily. That makes these reactions particularly important for us to attend to and address.

An essential first step is self-compassion and understanding. It is natural for critical, judgmental thoughts to arise when we do not feel compassionate toward a client; however, entanglement with these secondary reactions can exacerbate the disconnection between our client and us. Using our skills to recognize these reactions as natural, human, and transient will help us to effectively address them so that we can work well with the client. Being able to see our reactions clearly, without the muddiness of our judgment, shame, or efforts to suppress them, will help us to determine their source so that we can address them.

Often these negative reactions are useful information because they provide us with a sense of how others experience interactions with our client. Jack's therapist found that she often felt irritated by the way he discounted her observations and suggestions, asserting that there was no way that he could try her suggestions. When she noticed the urge to refute his points, she recalled Jack describing his coworkers, partner, and boss frequently responding to him in that way, and she remembered how poignantly he described feeling invalidated, isolated, and unappreciated in response. Considering that these other people were as frustrated with Jack as she was and remembering Jack's distress about those relationships led the therapist to have a flicker of empathy—that was a hard way to be going through the world. And it helped her to see the function of his response—he felt discounted so readily that he wanted to assert his views strongly to be heard. Unfortunately, Jack struggled with the skills needed to genuinely convey how vulnerable he felt in the moment when others disagreed with or discounted his perspective and instead usually responded with a defensive style that helped him to feel powerful and protected in the short term, but that led others to further discount him, which kept him stuck in a vicious cycle. This realization helped the therapist connect with Jack's pain, and she was able to try to validate his experience and join with him instead: "It sounds like it's really hard to imagine that anything could work at this point or that I could really understand what's happening for you. I can hear how hard you've been trying to make things different, so it's not surprising that you feel so hopeless. I wonder though, if it might be worth trying something out together, even if those thoughts that it isn't going to work still arise."

In general, failures in empathy can best be addressed by revisiting our case conceptualization and enhancing our understanding of why our client is the way they are. The more we can truly connect to the path that has led the client to where they are, the more we will find ourselves feeling compassionate toward them. With some clients, we may need to explicitly revisit this conceptualization before each session so that we can hold that frame as we interact with them to reduce our reactivity and enhance our empathy and alliance. This is another reason that practicing mindfulness (broadly defined—anything that enhances and expands our nonjudgmental awareness) is beneficial—the more clearly we can see our reactions arising, the more effectively and efficiently we can balance them with understanding. Consultation may also be indicated if we are having trouble making sense of our client in a way that allows for empathy.

Sometimes our failure to empathize has more to do with our own reactivity. A client may remind us of someone who has been difficult in our lives, or we may be feeling worn out, with depleted emotional resources. Again, mindfulness practice can help us to notice this is happening as we observe thoughts, feelings, sensations, and memories that are arising with compassion and curiosity. In those cases, we need to explore these reactions on our own, in our own therapy, or in consultation, so that we can separate our reactions from the client. We may need to attend to self-care more explicitly in our lives, so that we can be optimally engaged in therapy.[2]

In the process of attending to these issues, or sorting through our understanding of the client, we can continue to intentionally convey empathy and understanding even if we are not feeling it. It's important to remember that we don't have to actually feel a certain way to act in ways that are personally meaningful to us. Sometimes it is those actions that actually change our internal experience. So, for instance, Jack's therapist may have been able to genuinely communicate her validation based on her intellectual understanding even if she also still felt annoyed by him. And if she is effective in conveying validation, Jack may actually feel less compelled to argue (and become a bit less annoying), which may change her experience as well. Again, acting consistent with our values as a therapist, even while we are struggling with our reactions, is easier to do when we are aware of, and disentangled from, our reactions.

---

[2]This is also an important consideration more generally in promoting a beneficial therapeutic alliance. Therapists can use mindfulness and other awareness practices to observe and detect their own reactivity and attend to it so that it doesn't negatively affect the therapeutic relationship.

Of course, as in the case of Jack, when our response to a client is a clear emotion in response to a client's behavior that is related to the client's presenting concern, once the therapist has clarity about their own response, and in the context of a strong therapeutic relationship, it may be valuable to genuinely communicate this reaction. For instance, Jack's therapist may simultaneously validate Jack's pain and also share the reaction she has to having her suggestions dismissed or cut off. This feedback might help Jack to better understand his actions and their consequences, act more skillfully in other relationships, and potentially address some of his relational challenges.

Failing to Validate Sufficiently or Precisely

Difficulties empathizing with clients naturally lead to challenges in validation; although we can convey validation even if we are feeling other things, as just described. However, sometimes we feel empathically attuned and clients still do not experience us as validating, which can lead to challenges in the therapeutic relationship. An inherent challenge in ABBTs is maintaining a dialectic stance (Linehan, 1993). We simultaneously validate the struggle the client is experiencing, while suggesting areas for growth and change. Clients differ in the optimal balance of acceptance- and change-based communication. This balance is likely to shift over time, with more validation needed early on to establish a working alliance, while a greater change focus can make sense at a later stage of therapy. And during times of, or on topics associated with, a particularly high level of stress and difficulty, more validation may again be needed. It can be easy to slip into suggesting change too quickly. When clients become more emotionally distant or protected, or more dismissive of suggestions we make, one of our first hypotheses is that we haven't sufficiently communicated validation. Cycling back to statements that validate how painful or hard something is can often help clients become more openly engaged in therapy and willing to consider new options in responding.

For example, Steff came into therapy visibly upset and began describing an interaction with her daughter. She described how her daughter came home from college, dropped off all of her laundry, and left immediately to see her friends. Steff responded by sending a series of angry texts. Because Steff and her therapist, Corrine, had been working together for a few months, and most recently had been working on Steff's tendency to act in anger without considering what was important to her, Corrine responded by asking questions designed to help Steff consider the strategies she could have used to choose a valued action in that situation. Steff responded to Corrine's questions with increased distress, raising her voice, stating that she hadn't done anything she regretted, and listing all the ways that her daughter's behavior was disrespectful. Corrine realized that she had jumped too quickly into change strategies and failed to express understanding of Steff's pain. To correct this imbalance, Corrine asked Steff to share more about how she had felt when her daughter first came home and then when she left abruptly. As Steff slowed down to share these parts of her experience, she began to cry, and Corrine validated how sad and disappointed Steff must have been after she had been so excited about her daughter coming home. After Corrine made room for Steff's painful emotions, as well as her anger, Steff was more willing to talk about other options of responding to her daughter that were aligned with her parenting values.

One way to think about the balance we are trying to achieve is that we want to be (metaphorically) sitting next to the client, seeing what they see, and then pointing to new roads to potentially travel, rather than sitting across from them and trying to pull them in a particular direction. Validation communicates that we can clearly see where they currently stand. Koerner (2011) refers to this as validating a client's *location perspective,* or clearly communicating that we understand how the client views their situation so that the client can trust that our solutions are appropriate or adequate. Koerner uses the metaphor of getting directions from someone and points out that we can't trust someone's directions if we don't believe that they know where we are starting from (e.g., if they tell us to travel south when we know we are already south of our intended destination).

As we noted earlier, effective validation also needs to be precise. We don't want to validate potentially problematic beliefs or behaviors, although we may want to validate that these beliefs or behaviors make sense and are reasonable, even though they aren't effective. So, rather than saying, "Of course you responded to your partner that way after he provoked you!" when a client is describing anger that led to a shouting match, we might say, "It makes so much sense that really intense anger arose for you after he said that, particularly given your history together. It sounds like the urge to yell was pretty intense, and it was challenging to respond in the way you would have preferred to."

Clients also differ in the kinds of communication they experience as validating. So we may need to personalize the way we convey validation so that it can be received and felt by our client. Asking clients about their familial history of emotional communication and reinforcement can be helpful, as can direct questions about what is happening in a moment when we sense a disconnection between our intent to validate and the client's response. These kinds of conversations also convey that we care about the client's experience (which is inherently validating), and that we can talk directly about our communication in order to make it clearer. Using this interpersonal skill may be beneficial in the client's other relationships as well. These conversations may also help to identify some beliefs about emotions and emotional expression that we want to address through psychoeducation.

We also need to be sensitive to cultural differences in styles of communication (e.g., Hays, 2016; Sue & Sue, 2016). Often experiences of invalidation stem from a cultural mismatch. For instance, a therapist may fail to show respect, or *respeto,* which may be experienced as invalidating or may lead to a relationship rupture (described in more depth below). Or a therapist may tend to talk over a client, which may be experienced as invalidating, even if it is culturally typical for the therapist. Nonverbal communications, directness, word choice, and use or absence of silence all vary culturally and may be important dimensions to attend to when communications meant to be validating are not being received as such (Hays, 2016).

Validation in the Absence of Attention to Change

Therapists can also find themselves so focused on validating their client's distress that they fail to identify and examine opportunities for change. In our work with clients who present with generalized anxiety disorder, we often find that we or the therapists we are supervising can get immersed in listening carefully to and validating the distress associated with a range of expressed worries, particularly at the start of therapy. While this response can help a client feel heard and cared for, it can also leave them feeling helpless and hopeless about the possibility of change. Again, attending to the dialectic of validation and change is important here. A therapist might say "It sounds like there are so many things going on for you and your mind is really busy with all the ways that things might go wrong. I find myself wondering if it might be helpful to step back from the specifics of these worries and look at the process a bit to see if we can find some ways that you might respond to the worries that are more consistent with how you want to be in your life. How does that sound?"

Repairing Ruptures or Disconnections in the Therapeutic Alliance

Any of the challenges we have described might lead to "tension or breakdown in the collaborative relationship" (Safran, Muran, & Eubanks-Carter, 2011, p. 80) between therapist and client (i.e., the therapeutic alliance, which consists of the bond, tasks, and goals) if they are not addressed. Emotional reactions, such as anger or disappointment, may challenge the therapeutic bond. In addition, clients and therapists may disagree about tasks and goals (as with Jack and his therapist in the example of failed empathy). Research suggests that these ruptures are a natural occurrence in the course of therapy and that their repair can be therapeutic (Safran et al., 2011). Following a review of the available literature on rupture repair, Safran and colleagues highlight the importance of the therapist attending to the possibility of (and in fact likelihood of at least minor) therapeutic ruptures, helping clients to express any negative feelings that arise, and responding nondefensively and empathically.[3] Depending on the context and nature of the therapeutic relationships, therapists may choose different types of interventions. These are provided in Table 4.1, with some examples to illustrate how these might be applied by ABBT therapists.

Some ruptures arise because therapists don't understand aspects of the client's experience. This can make it more difficult to develop a shared case conceptualization and goals for therapy, as well as agreement on tasks to reach goals. These gaps in understanding can also interfere with the therapeutic bond as clients may not feel truly understood. In addition, when these failures in understanding happen across privileged and marginalized identities, with the therapist holding a privileged identity, these gaps in understanding can reenact experiences of marginalization that contribute to the client's stress. They can be particularly damaging to the therapeutic relationship and the work of therapy. As described earlier, having open, honest conversations about aspects of identity and disparate experiences provides an important context for addressing these ruptures and enhancing therapists' understanding. However, in addition to these conversations, therapists should engage in consultation and their own research to better understand aspects of experiences that they are less familiar with, so that they can approach these conversations with knowledge and sensitivity, conveying their commitment to understanding their client fully.

---

[3] Relational cultural therapy (e.g., Jordan, 2010) also describes the ways that disconnections are inevitable and that relational repair is an important part of healing and growth.

TABLE 4.1. Common Interventions to Repair Ruptures

Type of intervention	Example
Repeating the therapeutic rationale	Jack's therapist in the example above could have reminded Jack why she was making the intervention suggestions she was by linking each suggestion to the therapeutic rationale, for instance, reminding him that she was suggesting the repeated practice of mindfulness because practice helps to change habits and he had described challenges in directing his attention intentionally.
Changing tasks or goals	The therapist might recognize that tasks such as shared regular mindfulness practice in session are interfering with the client's desire to fully share the real challenges of his week and so decide instead to change to a mindful listening/speaking practice so that the client can share some specific details of the week, while also practicing with intentional attention.
Clarifying misunderstandings at a surface level	In exploring an apparent rupture, the therapist may learn that the client felt judged by the therapist. The therapist can nondefensively express understanding and regret that the client experienced the therapist's response that way.
Exploring relational themes associated with the rupture/ linking the alliance rupture to common patterns in a client's life	If the relational pattern continues with Jack, his therapist might make a connection between the pattern emerging between them and his patterns with other people in his life, if she wanted to begin to directly target these patterns in therapy.
New relational experience	This is the intervention Jack's therapist chose by deciding to validate him, instead of reacting to his criticism, as people in his life commonly did. This can lead to a new relational pattern, although sometimes explicit discussion of the pattern is needed for that change to occur.

Note. Based on Safran et al. (2011).

Therapists (and eventually clients) can use all the ABBT skills they've been developing to address challenges in the therapeutic relationship:

- Being aware of reactions (in themselves and each other),
- Noticing reactions as they arise and defusing/disentangling from them,
- Having compassion for these reactions (in place of judgment that intensifies reactivity) and accepting them as they arise, and
- Connecting to one's values within the therapeutic relationship.

All these skills help in being able to skillfully address and repair ruptures.
Further,

- Turning toward challenging experiences, such as being emotionally vulnerable and nondefensive, facilitates helpful communication about misunderstandings and ruptures that have occurred and promotes resolution.
- Therapists may also notice nonverbal evidence of ruptures or disconnection and ask about them in order to directly address these barriers to therapeutic progress.

BOX 4.4. WHEN TIME IS LIMITED:
The Therapeutic Relationship

When we work with clients in shorter-term contexts, we can't invest the same amount of time into developing and repairing a working alliance. Nonetheless, we can still enact several key principles in order to use our working relationship as a context and mechanism for therapeutic change.

- Convey the understandable, human nature of the client's challenges.
- Use "we" and personal examples to acknowledge our own humanness.
- Validate, often more briefly, prior to suggesting change.
- Use our own mindfulness practice, particularly in the moment, to maintain genuine engagement with the client during a brief time, deepening connection, and to attend to our own reactions or resource depletion.
- Acknowledge contextual, systemic, and cultural factors, even if unable to fully explore them.

CHAPTER 5

Psychoeducation to Cultivate Acceptance

Experiential exercises designed to cultivate compassionate, decentered awareness (described in Chapters 6 and 7) promote the learning that allows clients to change their relationship with their internal experiences and make meaningful, sustainable changes in their lives. Psychoeducation, the focus of the current chapter, sets the stage for this new learning to occur. Integrating psychoeducation into the early stages of treatment also deepens clients' understanding of the ABBT model and clarifies why particular treatment strategies are recommended. Finally, psychoeducation also allows clients to "own" ABBT and truly integrate the spirit of this approach into their lives between sessions and after termination so that they can draw from their knowledge and experience when encountering new contexts or facing unexpected challenges. Thus, we spend considerable time early in treatment describing the psychological mechanisms and processes contributing to their difficulties and helping clients to notice these processes in their daily lives.

What you will learn

- ๛ Guiding principles to keep in mind when conveying psychoeducational material in ABBT.
- ๛ Specific topics of psychoeducation that are used in ABBT to help clients cultivate an aware, curious, compassionate, and acceptance stance toward internal experiences.
- ๛ Self-monitoring practices to support learning.
- ๛ Obstacles that can arise when using psychoeducation and self-monitoring.

GUIDING PRINCIPLES THAT INFORM PRESENTING PSYCHOEDUCATIONAL INFORMATION

We emphasize psychoeducational elements in the early sessions of treatment and then we revisit them through therapy. In early sessions (and in this chapter of the book), we strive to briefly introduce each topic, allow clients to reflect on the relevance of topics to their experience using in-session discussion and experiential exercises, and recommend monitoring activities between sessions that are designed to highlight the centrality of topics to clients' presenting concerns and support learning. We also may provide handouts of supplemental reading (and encourage the use of a folder or binder) so that clients can mull over and revisit the concepts we discuss in therapy on their own. If clients' presenting concerns include anxiety, worry, and related difficulties, we encourage them to work through chapters in *Worry Less, Live More: The Mindful Way through Anxiety Workbook* (WLLM; Orsillo & Roemer, 2016) as we cover those topics in session.

Much of the psychoeducation we provide early in treatment is aimed at helping clients to identify the problematic relationship they have with their internal experiences; become aware of both learned habits of responding and intentionally employed "coping" strategies that may inadvertently contribute to their distress; and normalize both processes. This chapter provides a comprehensive overview of psychoeducational information on these subjects. However, the topics we choose to focus on with a particular client, the amount of time devoted to each topic, and the monitoring practices we recommend are always informed by our conceptualization, the needs of the client, and any treatment setting constraints.

> Psychoeducation focused on concepts introduced later in treatment are described in subsequent chapters. Specifically, psychoeducation on mindfulness is provided in Chapter 6, psychoeducation related to self-compassion is provided in Chapter 7, and psychoeducation related to values in Chapter 8.

Some clients are already reasonably knowledgeable about certain topics (e.g., the nature and function of anxiety), and thus we may move through that material quickly. Some clients may find a particular topic confusing and need more than one session devoted to its coverage. Although our goal is to simply touch on psychoeducation early in treatment and revisit complicated nuances as they naturally arise once clients are working to integrate skills into their daily lives, we sometimes find it necessary to delve more deeply into a topic during the early stages of treatment.

The brief introduction we provide at the start of therapy (and in this chapter) does not sufficiently capture the full complexity of the psychological constructs that are central to the ABBT model. There are many nuances and caveats that are deeply explored and experientially encountered throughout therapy. In most cases, it makes sense to present the psychoeducational material simply and concisely without delving into all of the complexities. Yet, there are exceptions to this general rule. For example, a client whose struggle involves challenging thoughts and emotions cued by ongoing racism could understandably feel invalidated by psychoeducation on the benefits of accepting painful, internal responses. If we're concerned that a client may feel invalidated by our usual way of describing a concept based on what we know about the client's experiences, we may share some nuances we think are important, even at this early stage of treatment. For example, we will spend time acknowledging the injustices of the context (e.g., racism, poverty, terminal illness) and provide some information distinguishing adaptive emotion regulation strategies from potentially harmful control efforts.

> See the section "Differentiating Experiential Avoidance from Emotion Regulation" later in this chapter for more information.

The ABBT Therapists' Stance in Psychoeducation

Delivering psychoeducational material may seem like a straightforward task, but in practice it requires considerable skill. ABBT therapists should keep in mind the ways in which client-specific presenting concerns and cultural identity may influence the relevance of different concepts and the manner in which they are presented. Clients may completely relate to some ideas and express skepticism over or vehemently disagree with others. And these responses may be direct or subtle. Therapists should closely attend to facial expressions, body language, and behavior (e.g., canceling or failing to show for a therapy appointment) that could be communicating a sense of invalidation or feeling misunderstood. It's essential to remain mindful of how easy it is to get hooked by the desire to "convince" clients early on that a concept is important or relevant and refrain from engaging in these persuasion efforts. Uncertainty and skepticism are very understandable responses at this stage of treatment that should be invited, genuinely heard, and validated.

The most effective method of minimizing a sense of disconnect between a topic of psychoeducation and the client's experience is to introduce the topic using specific examples drawn from the assessment. For example, a therapist might say:

> "Sometimes people develop habits of responding to difficult emotions that help in the short term, but also take them away from what matters most to them. I was thinking that this concept might relate to that story you told me about the time you skipped your family reunion because you expected people to ask why you and Imola broke up and you thought that would make you feel uncomfortable. I remember you mentioned how you felt a huge sense of relief when you RSVP'd, but that you were deeply saddened about missing the opportunity to connect with your relatives."

ABBT therapists strive to provide a context in which clients can respond to psychoeducation with skepticism and describe the ways a topic seems irrelevant to their experience. We listen closely to our clients, remaining open to the real possibility that certain ABBT concepts aren't applicable and that our case conceptualization should be altered. Yet, there can be other explanations that account for a client's dismissal of psychoeducation that are also worth considering. Clients might feel blamed for, defensive about, or insulted by information about how we sometimes unintentionally fall into habits that maintain our suffering (e.g., sometimes people worry to reduce distress). In these situations, it can be helpful to defuse any sense of pathologizing the client might be concerned about by sharing a personal example of how the concept is relevant to our own experiences as therapists. For example, a therapist might say:

> "When my friend was awaiting the results of a medical test for a potentially serious illness, I found myself scouring the Internet for information, caught up in a cycle of worry. At the time, I found the whole thing incredibly stressful, but looking back now, I realize that in some way, worrying and rumination over that information seemed to reduce my feelings of grief and I also felt less helplessness—like I was doing something to improve the situation—even though I really wasn't. Have you ever noticed an experience like that?"

Integrating Research into Psychoeducation

Many of our clients appreciate it when we integrate research findings into our psycho-education. Sharing research that highlights the universality of certain psychological processes can help destigmatize natural ways of responding. For example, we often cite Dan Wegner's paradoxical finding that trying not to think about a white bear increases the frequency of such thoughts. With our anxious clients, we like to illustrate how people can learn to associate people and experiences with fear without being aware of the initial pairing of a stimulus with a threat. For example, we sometimes share the story, described in LeDoux (1998), of the French doctor Edouard Claparede, who pricked the hand of a patient with anterograde amnesia when shaking her hand in greeting. The next time they met, the patient refused to shake the doctor's hand even though she didn't recall having met the doctor previously and couldn't explain why she was reluctant to shake his hand, demonstrating her learned fear. Sharing examples like this can help clients build compassion for the challenges that humans face.

PSYCHOEDUCATION TOPICS AND THE SELF-MONITORING PRACTICES THAT SUPPORT LEARNING

Principles of Learning

We view clinical problems as emerging from learned habits of responding that are maintained by the consequences of those responses and share this basic assumption with clients. Although this idea is often covered when we share our conceptualization and treatment plan with a client (see Chapter 3), depending on the client, we may revisit learning as a psychoeducational topic in therapy. As an example of some points we try to convey (although our approach would be more conversational, and we would integrate personal examples from what the client has told us so far), we might say something like:

> "Human beings naturally learn from past experiences. We learn to associate things that have occurred together in the past—for instance, we might come to associate threat or comfort with a particular sound, smell, or situation. We also come to expect certain consequences for our actions based on our past experiences, like someone who learns to avoid eating nuts after an allergic reaction, or someone who avoids crying in front of others because as a boy he was ridiculed for being 'too sensitive.' We learn from our own experiences, from observing others, and even from the messages we receive from our immediate and extended family, peers, teachers, social media, culture, and larger society.
>
> "Our ability to learn ways of keeping safe is definitely adaptive in some ways, but it's challenging in others. For example, we can *overlearn certain associations and responses,* especially if the lessons were part of our upbringing or the consequences were significant. Our responses might become so automatic and habitual that we don't even notice that our response isn't uniformly helpful across situations, or that the consequences are mixed. For example, smoking might relieve stress in the short term but increase risk for cancer in the long term. Avoiding conflict might make

us less anxious, but also more frustrated if the situation goes unresolved. Turning down a date might make us both less anxious and lonelier.

"Another challenge about the way we learn is that sometimes what we *believe* is helpful prevents us from actually *noticing* what is helpful. For example, many people believe that watching television all evening is good self-care after a stressful day but miss subtle signs that doing so leaves them feeling more lethargic. Or someone might firmly believe that 'putting one's best foot forward' is the most effective way to kindle a relationship and not notice how hiding parts of oneself can fuel feelings of insecurity.

"Given these human patterns of responding, we've found it can be helpful to provide clients with strategies that help them to start noticing their habits and responses and closely observe what's working and what isn't. Fortunately, there are a lot of different strategies we'll try out in treatment that work together to strengthen the skills of awareness and observation. Changing habits is really hard though, so it will take practice, patience, and time!"

Chapter One in *WLLM* is an example of the type of psychoeducational materials we might share with clients to supplement in-session learning. Client Handout 5.1, *Fear Is Learned* summarizes many of these points.

Emotions

From an ABBT perspective, many psychological problems are assumed to arise from our critical, judgmental responses to emotions and our attempts to change, suppress, and otherwise control them. A compassionate and genuine therapeutic relationship (as described in Chapter 4), mindfulness practice (as described in Chapter 6, as well as the self-compassion exercises in Chapter 7), and psychoeducation aimed at teaching clients about the nature and value of emotions are all methods used in ABBT to help clients develop a new relationship with their internal experience.

We often start this work by describing the paradox humans face with regard to painful emotions. On the one hand, it stands to reason that reducing our contact with situations and activities that elicit painful emotions would enhance our quality of life. On the other, to live a full, meaningful life, we often intentionally approach situations that inevitably evoke painful emotions like fear and sadness. We ask clients to consider how many of the most rewarding aspects of life—developing new relationships, initiating an intimate relationship, trying out a new activity, accepting a promotion at work—require us to be open to a range of emotions. It's impossible to take risks, without feeling vulnerable and scared. We might try to cook a gourmet meal for friends and instead produce an unappetizing mess. We might text someone an invitation and receive no response. At the same time, our attempts at cooking might help us discover a new passion, and reaching out to others may help us forge a new connection. Loving someone—a friend, child, parent, or partner—is a deeply meaningful, transformational experience. And losing a loved one to separation, breakup, or death is incredibly painful. Since emotions are an inherent part of being human, it's important to find a way to work with them.

Understanding the Nature of Emotions

With clients who present with an undifferentiated sense of their own emotional experience (i.e., an experience of "distress" or "upset" without a clear sense of specific cues and emotions and their correlates), we start by describing the multiple components of emotions (physical sensations, thoughts, and behaviors) and exploring the client's experience of whichever emotion (or emotions) is most closely linked with their presenting concern. We use emotion-specific handouts (such as Client Handout 5.2, *What Are Fear and Anxiety Made Up Of?*, adapted from *WLLM* for clients with anxiety; or the *Ways to Describe Emotions* handout from the *DBT Skills Training Manual* [Linehan, 2015]) to introduce the topic and ask clients to imaginally recall a significant episode of their presenting problem, describing the thoughts, feelings, and sensations they notice so that they can begin to differentiate the components of their emotional responses and see the reciprocal relationship among elements.

Although some clients' presenting concerns point to a struggle with a particular emotion (sadness in depression; fear in panic disorder), others present with a set of problematic behaviors like substance use or extreme dieting without much focus on the painful emotions associated with these habits. In most cases, the assessment process highlights the ways in which these behaviors function to control painful emotions, which sets the stage for this component of psychoeducation. If that's not the case, we might start by monitoring situations that elicit these behaviors, as well as the thoughts, emotions, and sensations that accompany the behaviors, as a way of learning more about which internal sensations might be most challenging.

After discussing the nature of emotions, we might recommend a monitoring form like Client Form 5.1, *Monitoring Your Fear and Anxiety*, to help clients turn toward their emotions (rather than trying to avoid them) and observe each component with curiosity (which can facilitate decentering).

The Function of Emotions

After exploring the nature of emotions, we turn to their function. We suggest to clients that, although we often want to control and change our emotional experiences, these efforts aren't always successful because each of the emotions we are hard-wired to experience serves a useful function.

CLEAR EMOTIONS

We define *clear emotions* as universal emotional responses we have to particular types of trigger events and ask clients to consider what function they think emotions serve. Through this discussion, we emphasize two key functions of clear emotions:

1. They communicate important information to us and to others (e.g., we feel guilt when we've taken an action that could cause harm or that is inconsistent with our moral standards or the moral standards of our community; Amodio, Devine, & Harmon-Jones, 2007).
2. They make suggestions about actions we may want to take or prepare us to act in a particular way.

We often will use the example of how fear (in addition to excitement) about an upcoming competition can motivate an athlete to maintain a challenging and time-consuming practice schedule or compel a student to prepare for an exam. Or say, for example:

> "Imagine Roy feels sadness and disappointment because his current job isn't fulfill-ing. Those feelings are uncomfortable, so he naturally wants to ignore or get rid of them. He might start staying out late at night spending time with friends and hanging out at bars so he doesn't feel the full impact of the sadness that some-times arises when he is at home alone. He might also find reasons to miss work or spend time when he is at work surfing the web or checking his phone to try and stave off those painful feelings. These actions may distract him from his sadness in the moment, but none of them resolves the problem, and they may create new problems if he isn't getting enough sleep or he is constantly reprimanded for his lackluster performance at work. Turning toward his pain and understanding its message can be the first step Roy takes toward making a life change."

We also underscore the fact that, although emotions can prepare us physiologically for action and increase the probability that we will choose a particular behavior, our actions are not caused by emotional responses. So, although we may be physiologically and behaviorally prepared to avoid or escape when we feel afraid, we can choose to approach or remain in a feared situation. Some examples of clear emotions and their associated features can be found in Client Handout 5.3, *Clear Emotions*, adapted from *WLLM*. After presenting some information about the function of clear emotions, we ask clients if they can think of examples of times when their emotional response gave them useful information or prepared them to take an action.

The idea that it is adaptive or useful that our emotions communicate important information *to others* can be challenging for many clients (and therapists) to accept. It conflicts with common beliefs many of us hold about the benefits of concealing our true feelings from others. Most clients can easily generate examples of times they were advised to suppress their emotions. Many of us have been told to act disinterested if we want to attract the attention of a potential dating partner, to hide the fact an adversary is "pushing our buttons," and to avoid crying tears of sadness or anger at work. There is a grain of truth to this advice. Excessive or inappropriate expressions, behaviors, and actions fueled by *muddy emotions*—complex, intense responses that don't always have an identifiable present-moment trigger and that tend to persist for long periods—can cause interpersonal problems (muddy emotions are described in more detail later in this chapter). And in certain contexts, it may be unsafe or considered culturally unac-ceptable to express one's emotions. On the other hand, there can also be some real costs to concealing our clear emotions.

I (SMO) often use the example of my son Sam, when he was a very young boy involved in youth sports, to demonstrate how our desire to hide our emotions in inter-personal situations can sometimes backfire. Despite having an ABBT therapist for a mother, like many boys, Sam was socialized by society to believe that expressing sad-ness is a sign of weakness. With that message in mind, any time Sam struck out in base-ball or let up a goal in hockey instead of showing his disappointment, he would actually smile or sometimes even laugh! As his mother, I knew he both felt sad and believed he

BOX 5.1. A CLOSER LOOK:
Suppression of Emotions

Over 40 research studies have shown that suppression of emotion is associated with poorer social well-being, lower social support, and poorer romantic relationship quality (Chervonsky & Hunt, 2017). For example, researchers Bonnie Le and Emily Impett found that when parents regulated their emotional expressions during caretaking in ways that were incongruent with their true feelings, they experienced lower authenticity, emotional well-being, relationship quality, and responsiveness to their children's needs (Le & Impett, 2016). On the other hand, therapists should also keep in mind the ways in which the potential costs of emotion expression suppression can be moderated by factors such as cultural identity and context. For example, the negative impact of emotion expression suppression on peer relationship quality that exists for European American teens is not evident among Vietnamese American adolescents (Tsai et al., 2017). Moreover, although suppression has negative consequences in some contexts, there may be others in which it is considered adaptive. For example, a victim of domestic abuse might refrain from expressing frustration for fear that it might provoke the aggressor to become physically assaultive. Research has shown that the negative effects of emotion suppression on well-being are lessened in contexts where one is lower on the social hierarchy (Catterson, Eldesouky, & John, 2017). However, although the intentional strategic use of suppression in specific situations may be helpful, chronic use of this strategy across situations can make interpersonal interactions less effective.

should hide those feelings. Not surprisingly, Sam's coaches were more likely to literally take his responses at "face value." Assuming he was not taking the game seriously or trying hard enough, they would respond with a reprimand. Ironically, the very emotion expression rules that Sam followed to "protect" himself from being criticized actually drew criticism. Research findings, including those presented in Box 5.1, can bolster the impact of sharing this piece of psychoeducation.

MUDDY EMOTIONS

Clients may understand and accept the general principle that emotions hold some value; yet their lived experience may be that their own emotional responses are rarely helpful. This discrepancy may be due to the fact that their emotional state is often dominated by *muddy emotions*. Muddy emotions are complex, intense responses that don't always have an identifiable present moment trigger and that tend to persist for long periods. They are experienced as distressing and increase the likelihood that we engage in emotion-driven habits such as experiential avoidance, behavioral avoidance, procrastination, and impulsive responses (see Client Handout 5.4, *Differentiating Clear and Muddy Emotions*). We review the major factors that contribute to muddy emotions described in Client Handout 5.5, *Factors That Contribute to Muddy Emotions,* with our clients. Specifically, our current emotional state can be complicated by emotions from imagined past or future events, and our clear emotions are amplified by our reactions to them, including critical, judgmental responses, fusion, and attempts to control, and by poor self-care.

Given this introduction to clear and muddy emotions, it may seem like our emotional responses are *either* clear *or* muddy. Yet, sometimes a situation will elicit the expected emotion (suggesting the presence of a clear emotion), but the intensity is much stronger and/or the duration considerably longer than might be otherwise expected (suggesting the emotion is muddy). For example, Peggy's mother, who has dementia, becomes agitated and challenging to care for when the neighbor plays loud music after midnight. Clearly, Peggy's rights are being violated by her neighbor and a natural (or clear) response to that situation is to feel angry. If Peggy becomes enraged when this happens and she stays furious for days after, that suggests that certain factors might be muddying her clear emotion and amplifying its intensity (i.e., exhaustion from caring for her mother with little support, guilt for feeling angry at her neighbors who are often kind to her).

Several monitoring forms can support psychoeducation about emotions, depending on the clients' needs and the pace at which we move through the material. For example, if a client is struggling with the concepts and we have sufficient time to devote to exploring them, we might have them complete all the forms described here over multiple weeks. With other clients, we may work through some of the forms together in session and recommend more advanced monitoring between sessions. A relatively straightforward monitoring practice that involves noticing emotions as they arise and then considering their potential function is Client Form 5.2, *Monitoring Emotions,* which asks clients to monitor when emotions arise, note their intensity, consider the situation that may have elicited them, and any possible message the emotion may have been communicating. Client Form 5.3, *Clarifying Emotions Reflection,* adapted from *WLLM,* is an expanded monitoring activity aimed at helping clients walk through the multiple steps involved in sorting through emotions, including (1) identifying a range of emotions that might be present in a given moment, (2) considering if any emotions are clear and whether they may be sending a message or providing information (and if so, what the message or information might be), (3) reflecting on the potential presence of each of the factors known to produce muddy emotions, and (4) identifying emotions and distinguishing between clear and muddy responses. This is a practice we continue to use with clients throughout therapy, particularly when trying to untangle complex emotional reactions.

> In Chapter 6, we describe mindfulness practices that can help clients become more aware of the full range of their emotions and practice decentering from them. These practices also help clients to notice when their attention has been pulled into the past or future and to guide it back to the present moment. Chapter 7 recommends strategies that clients can use to cultivate self-compassion when critical and judgmental thoughts are present, or poor self-care is muddying their experience. Finally, in Chapter 9, we discuss how clients can use their understanding and awareness of clear and muddy emotions, along with mindfulness practice, to work through muddy emotions.

Mental Content and Processes

Our abilities to imagine, create, and problem-solve have advanced humankind in unimaginable ways, but these cognitive abilities can also contribute to habits that increase self-doubt and criticism, depression, anxiety, rumination, and worry. Clients often come to treatment believing that their thinking processes and content reflect some basic pathological flaw in their character. They are locked in an ongoing battle

BOX 5.2. TRY THIS:
Clarifying Muddy Emotions

In order to gain a deeper understanding of the process of working through clear and muddy emotions, we recommend that therapists try to complete some of the monitoring forms on their own. See if you can bring to mind a recent session that elicited some challenging emotions in you. Perhaps you felt frustrated with a client who seemed to be pushing back on every suggestion you made. Or you felt anxious when a client who expressed anger about treatment not being helpful. Or you were disappointed when a client who seemed to be making great progress in therapy failed to show for his appointment and left a message saying he was quitting therapy.

If you are willing, sit quietly for a moment, focusing on your breath for a few breaths and then try to bring that experience to mind as vividly as you can. Allow your attention to widen so that you can notice any physiological sensations that are present, as well as your thoughts and emotions. Stay with the image for a few moments and see if you can notice the full range of emotions that arise. Observe their intensity for a few moments and when you are ready, open your eyes and complete Client Form 5.3.

with thoughts and mental images that impairs their concentration, interferes with their sleep, and overshadows their experience. Psychoeducation about how minds work is one of many strategies we use in ABBT to improve the relationship clients have with their thoughts. We also recommend Chapter 2 in *WLLM* as a helpful adjunct to this in-session work.

We start psychoeducation on this topic by considering the way minds work. We acknowledge the unique ability humans have to imagine innumerable future possibilities and revisit earlier experiences with vivid realism. We compare our minds to a movie theater that never closes—we can repeatedly imagine our most feared threats and relive our most painful encounters—and relate this concept back to how emotions can become muddy. We also consider how content ends up getting stored in our minds. Clients often feel personally responsible for their inner material and believe that their doubts, worries, and traumatic memories reflect some inner flaw. Revisiting basic learning principles, such as the way our life events and experiences establish learned associations, the fact that associations are never unlearned and new associations are constantly created, can be beneficial in responding to these beliefs.

As an example, Mariana was a recent graduate from a prestigious college who had majored in accounting with a nearly perfect GPA. She came to therapy because she had scheduled and canceled an appointment to take the Certified Public Accountant exam multiple times in response to fears about failing. Whenever Mariana sat down to prepare for the exam, she recalled a time she overheard her seventh-grade math teacher talking to another teacher about Mariana's performance on a standardized math placement test. The teacher made a number of racist and sexist comments about Mariana, referring to her "insurmountable educational deficits" and opining that she would end up working as a "cleaning lady." Mariana described a cascade of different painful emotions that accompanied this memory, but she was most bothered by thoughts that she was an imposter. Mariana described being frustrated with herself that she continued to question her own abilities despite all the evidence that the teacher's comment was racist and invalid. After validating Mariana's experience, the therapist described how preparing for a standardized test would naturally elicit thoughts associated through learning with previous academic and testing contexts. While acknowledging that those learned thoughts and memories would never "go away," the therapist explained how skills learned in ABBT, such as self-compassion and decentering, could help Mariana broaden her attention such that the thoughts from the past would become only one small part of her experience and hopefully have less impact on her daily life.

The nature and function of thinking processes such as rumination and worry are also topics of psychoeducation in ABBT. Rumination involves repeatedly focusing on past, painful experiences and considering their potential causes, meanings, and consequences through a self-focused lens (Nolen-Hoeksema, 1991). It's experienced as highly unpleasant, repetitive, and uncontrollable and is often associated with a sense of not having control over situations (Kircanski, Thompson, Sorenson, Sherdell, & Gotlib, 2015). Worry is defined as a future-oriented cognitive response to anticipated threat (e.g., Borkovec et al., 2004). Both of these perseverative processes are learned ways of responding, often triggered outside of awareness, that can produce considerable distress.

In addition to reviewing the ways we form associations and considering how thoughts and memories are elicited by internal and external cues, we also explore the function of "thinking." In other words, we ask clients to consider the reasons we so commonly turn toward and become entangled with worrisome thoughts and troubling memories. We also share the common reasons for worrying and ruminating noted in Table 5.1 and contained in Client Handout 5.6, *Common Reasons We Turn Our Attention to the Future (Worry) and Past (Rumination)*. If it seems like it could be beneficial, we may also share some of the research described in Box 5.3.

Although these reasons for, and beliefs about, worry and rumination are commonly endorsed by participants in research studies, not all clients connect with these ideas. Most notably, some clients may feel invalidated when a therapist talks about the perceived benefits of these cognitive processes, as it might seem like the therapist believes the client is intentionally choosing to worry or ruminate. Teaching clients how to recognize and change habitual patterns of responding can be a powerful therapeutic strategy, but it can also unintentionally strengthen the beliefs some clients hold that they are to blame for their current psychological distress. Highlighting the differences between factors that *contribute to the development* of behavioral patterns (and associated distress), those that *maintain* responses, and *strategies that can elicit change*, particularly in the context of a validating and accepting therapeutic relationship, can help with this challenge.

Confusion over the differences between worry, rumination, and problem solving is common with the clients we see, so we often spend a bit more time on this topic and recommend self-monitoring assignments to support learning. Again, we normalize the appearance of worrisome thoughts and troubling memories in our mind and the fact that our attention is drawn to these targets. Although a habitual response is to unintentionally or intentionally (with the hope of problem solving) remain with these thoughts and images until a resolution is reached, we propose monitoring activities aimed at practicing:

- Noticing when one begins to engage in intensive cognitive activity that could be worry, rumination, or problem solving,
- Noticing what cues these cognitive processes,
- Trying to discern the difference between worry, rumination, and problem solving, and
- Noticing when we switch between different processes.

Although problem solving does require a person to notice a problem and intentionally allocate attention to it, the key to resolving a problem is generating and selecting a solution. Both worry and rumination involve the first part of the problem-solving process (orientation toward the problem), but neither leads to a final, effective solution (Lyubomirsky, Tucker, Caldwell, & Berg, 1999; Szabo & Lovibond, 2002).

Worry and rumination (as compared to problem solving) are often triggered by attempts to control the uncontrollable. For example, it's possible to take some steps to solve a "problem" like figuring out what food one needs to buy at the supermarket. One might look at the family calendar to determine who will be home for dinner which nights, consult the school lunch menu to see whether the kids will be bringing or buying their lunches, choose a few recipes to cook for dinner, and make a list of needed ingredients. On the other hand, it is harder to solve the kinds of "problems" we tend to worry about, or ruminate over, and care deeply about, like whether a parent will

TABLE 5.1. Common Reasons We Turn Our Attention to the Future (Worry) and Past (Rumination)

Reasons	Worry	Rumination
Preparation	It seems like imagining what it will be like to face a threat could be a good way to prepare for it.	It seems like focusing on past mistakes will prepare for future successes.
Motivation	It seems like focusing on the potentially negative consequences of a feared future event will motivate us to prepare.	It seems like engaging in self-judgment and criticism of past mistakes will motivate us to improve.
Superstition	It feels like worrying about a potential threat will make it less likely to happen.	It feels like remembering how badly something went will make it less likely to happen again.
Avoidance	It seems like worrying will help us figure out how to avoid feared future outcomes.	It seems like going over past mistakes will help us avoid making them again.
Problem solving	It seems like focusing on a potential future problem is a first step to solving it.	It seems like identifying what went wrong in the past is a first step to avoiding a poor outcome in the future.
Distraction from more emotional topics	Worrying about minor matters often takes our minds off more distressing and serious concerns.	Focusing our attention on figuring out what happened in the past to contribute to our current distress is one way to avoid taking risks in the present.

BOX 5.3. A CLOSER LOOK:
Positive Beliefs about Worry and Rumination

Research shows that people with clinical levels of worry hold more positive beliefs about worry, such as the belief that worry reflects a desirable personality trait (i.e., conscientiousness), enhances motivation, reduces the likelihood of negative outcomes, protects against feelings like sadness and disappointment in the event of a negative outcome, and facilitates problem solving (e.g., Davey, Tallis, & Capuzzo, 1996; Hebert, Dugas, Tulloch, & Holowka, 2014; Ladouceur, Blais, Freeston, & Dugas, 1998; Laugesen, Dugas, & Bukowski, 2003). There is some evidence that these types of beliefs actually moderate the relationship between exposure to stressful life events and worry such that the impact of stressful events on subsequent worry is higher in those holding more positive beliefs about worry (Iijima & Tanno, 2013).

Similarly, research has found that positive beliefs about rumination, like the belief that repeatedly thinking about a painful experience is beneficial and may increase understanding and eventually reduce distress, are associated with more chronic rumination and depression in nonclinical samples, clinically depressed individuals (Huntley & Fisher, 2016; Papageorgiou & Wells, 2009), and those who recovered from a previous major depressive episode (Watkins & Moulds, 2005). A study that used ecological momentary assessment to look at this process as it occurs in daily life found that positive beliefs about rumination were significantly associated with both episodes of ruminative thinking and negative affect (Kubiak, Zahn, Siewert, Jonas, & Weber, 2014).

It's also important, however, to recognize the influence of *negative* beliefs about worry on our clients' functioning. Research suggests that negative beliefs about worry, such as the belief that worry is uncontrollable and dangerous, actually mediate the relationship between trait worry and GAD symptom severity (Penney, Mazmanian, & Rudanycz, 2013). Similarly, although positive beliefs about rumination predict the frequency of rumination, at least one study found that negative beliefs about rumination predicted depressive symptoms (Matsumoto & Mochizuki, 2018).

become ill, why our last relationship ended, or how to be happier. A lot of problems that we reflect on, think about, and plan for involve an interconnected web of things we can and can't control.

If worry and/or rumination are major components of a client presentation, monitoring episodes and working to discern the differences between these processes and problem solving remain a focus throughout therapy. We suggest to clients that when they begin to notice they are engaged in a mental activity that could be worry, rumination, or problem solving, they should pause and consider their responses using Client Handout 5.7, *Am I Problem Solving, Worrying, or Ruminating?* Clients who worry can be provided with Client Form 5.4, *Worry or Problem Solving?*, as a method of self-monitoring that might support this psychoeducation. An example of how a client might complete the form can be found in Figure 5.1.

The Challenges Associated with Control Efforts

Most of us struggle to accept that we have a limited ability to control fundamental parts of our inner and outer experiences. Yet for some, this struggle becomes a factor that maintains psychological distress and diminishes quality of life. Earlier in this

When you notice that your focus is pulled toward a possible future event, use the questions below to sort through whether intentionally spending time on this topic is worry or problem solving.

Questions	Future-Focused Topic 1	Future-Focused Topic 2
Description of the future-focused topic.	I am worried about being ready for the dinner party I planned for Saturday.	I am having my partner's family over for dinner Saturday night and I am worried they won't like me or the food and they will have a miserable time.
Is this experience likely to happen?	Yes.	Not sure.
Is there a specific action or actions I can take to prepare for it (or prevent it from happening)?	Yes, I need to finalize my menu and make a food shopping list.	Not really. I wish I had a bigger apartment and nicer things, but I can't change that by Saturday.
Will spending more time with these thoughts likely solve my problem?	Yes.	No, it's making me more stressed.
Am I focused on solving a problem or reducing uncomfortable thoughts and feelings of uncertainty?	Solving a problem.	I am trying to reduce my stress by thinking of ways to make things go better, but I don't think this is helping.
Is spending time with these thoughts moving me closer toward something I care about? Or is it getting in my way?	Moving toward. I love my partner, and I know family is important to her. I want to take this action because I care about these things.	Getting in the way. The more I think about how they might judge my place, the food, etc., the more I just want to cancel.
If I do think of an action I could take, will it add meaning to my life?	Yes—having them over for dinner is meaningful.	It would be a bad idea for me to go over my budget just to try and impress them—I can't afford it, and they might not even notice. Canceling would relieve stress but not add meaning.

FIGURE 5.1. Sample of Completed Client Form 5.4, *Worry or Problem Solving?*

110

chapter, we touched on the ways in which attempts to change, suppress, or otherwise control our emotional responses muddy emotions and trigger worry and rumination. Yet, given how widespread and automatic control efforts are, we tend to revisit and expand on the psychoeducation we provide on this topic. Chapter 4 in *WLLM* contains psychoeducational material and exercises that can supplement in-session work.

Control Efforts Aimed at Internal Experiences

Earlier in this chapter, we introduced the notion that attempts to control emotions can contribute to emotional muddiness by intensifying our responses. We draw from Dan Wegner's work on thought suppression (e.g., the "White Bear" studies; Wegner, 1989; Wegner & Schneider, 2003; see Box 5.4 for a closer look at this research) to supplement psychoeducation on this topic with an experiential exercise, and, if we think it would be helpful, a description of the research. For example, we might ask a client to bring to mind their favorite food and to vividly imagine it in their mind for a few moments.

BOX 5.4. A CLOSER LOOK:
Thought Suppression

Daniel Wegner's seminal work on thought suppression originated with a study showing that participants who were told to suppress thoughts of a white bear paradoxically experienced more white bear thoughts than those who were not provided with this instruction (Wegner, Schneider, Carter, & White, 1987). In addition to demonstrating an initial increase in the frequency of thoughts, this study and others have also demonstrated a "rebound effect." Specifically, compared to participants who were encouraged to think about the white bear throughout the entire experiment, participants who were first instructed to suppress white bear thoughts had many more occurrences of these thoughts when the restriction was lifted. Wegner and his colleagues concluded that instructing humans to suppress a thought actually enhances our preoccupation with it. A subsequent study found that experimental instructions to suppress a target led to increased responses of anxiety and depression to that target, regardless of the initial emotional valence of the target. This may indicate that a mechanism through the act of suppression increases the distress associated with the target of that suppression, paradoxically increasing its intrusiveness (Roemer & Borkovec, 1994).

Although the consequences of thought suppression appear to be ubiquitous, this process seems to play a central role in a broad range of clinical problems. Experimental studies suggest that attempts to suppress thoughts may contribute to trauma-related reexperiencing symptoms among those with PTSD (Shipherd & Beck, 2005), hyperaccessibility of alcohol-related thoughts among abstinent patients with a history of alcohol use disorder (Klein, 2007), and increased smoking behavior among smokers (Erskine, Georgiou, & Kvavilashvili, 2010). Although there is mixed evidence for the reoccurrence of suppressed thoughts during laboratory thought suppression paradigms among those diagnosed with obsessive–compulsive disorder (Magee, Harden, & Teachman, 2012), there is evidence that failures in suppression may increase discomfort with thoughts and negative mood in those with this disorder (Purdon, Rowa, & Antony, 2005). Research has also found that higher levels of self-reported trait thought suppression are linked to a range of difficulties, including binge eating (Nikčević, Marino, Caselli, & Spada, 2017) and increased urges to use opioids among chronic pain patients with symptoms of depression (Garland, Brown, & Howard, 2016).

Next, we ask them to sit for a few moments and think about anything but that object. Most clients have the experience that the image returns to their mind again and again.

We also sometimes adapt the *polygraph exercise* from ACT as an experiential method of helping clients to notice the paradoxical effects of control efforts. We might say:

> "Sometimes people feel like they should be able to just better manage or control their emotions or thoughts. That maybe if they tried harder or were more consistent with their efforts, they could stop anxious feelings or worry thoughts from coming up. Even though that sounds completely logical, ironically, it seems like the more we humans try to not feel an emotion or think a thought, the more intensely and frequently we experience it.
>
> "Imagine for a moment there was a machine, like a lie detector test, that was very accurate at picking up even the slightest change in someone's level of stress. Imagine this machine was extremely sensitive to small changes in our heart rate, the sweatiness of our palms, and any other physical sensation associated with stress, fear, and anxiety. Imagine that you were hooked up to this machine—I just taped some of the sensors onto different parts of your body to pick up your heart rate, pulse, etc., and I asked you to really concentrate—to use all your resources to focus on remaining calm and not letting the machine detect any change in your arousal. What do you think might happen?"

[If the client feels they could remain calm, continue on. If they feel strongly that they would fail at this task, but that others could do it, we might add—Okay, let's pick someone else to take your place. Who do you think is someone who would be really good keeping their cool even when they were hooked up to this machine?]

"Now imagine that I just remembered that there is a slight problem with this machine. I actually have to remove the sensors in just the right order or the machine could actually explode, causing both of us some serious physical harm. And unfortunately, I am not sure I remember the right order, and so I ask you/them to sit tight while we wait for someone to come and help us. Then imagine I added, oh and it's also really important that you remain calm, because there is a defect with this machine, and so if it senses any stress, fear, or anxiety at all, that will also cause it to explode. So please, whatever you do, just stay calm. What do you think would happen in this situation?"

This metaphor can also be useful to highlight the differences between trying to suppress the outward *expression* of our emotions and trying to actually *prevent the elicitation* of particular emotions. We often judge our own insides by others' outsides. That is to say, we are aware of our own anxiety in a frightening situation, but we might notice the person we are with doesn't appear anxious. It can be helpful to point out that without that mythical machine, we don't truly know the pain, anxiety, and anger others are feeling, unless they choose to share it.

Another way to help clients connect with the fact that we can't always change our feelings, even when it would be incredibly helpful to do so, is to talk about love or attraction. Most people can relate to the "I fell in love with the wrong person" story. For example, Kylie went out on a few dates with two women, Anna and Liv. Kylie, her friends, and family all agreed that Anna was a lovely person—caring, smart, and funny. Unfortunately, although Kylie truly enjoyed spending time with Anna and objectively found her physically attractive, Kylie did not experience any romantic feelings toward

Anna. On the other hand, Kylie found herself to be deeply attracted to Liv. Logically, Kylie knew that she did not want to be in a relationship with someone like Liv, who could be self-centered and mean. Liv often ignored Kylie's calls and texts and lied about her plans. Unfortunately, despite Kylie's wish that she could find some "chemistry" with Anna and push away her attraction to Liv, Kylie was unable to turn her feelings on and off.

When we present these types of stories to clients, we like to emphasize the fact that although it is often impossible to directly suppress our thoughts and sensations or change our emotions, often we do have control over our actions or behavioral choices. For example, with regard to the polygraph machine, if clapping one's hands could prevent the machine from exploding, it would probably be pretty easy for the client to keep us safe (at least until they became too tired to clap!). Similarly, although it would likely be challenging and painful, Kylie could choose to stop dating Liv even though she might continue to think about, and have strong feelings, for her.

If clients seem embarrassed by their control efforts or if they talk about how silly or ridiculous it is to keep trying to suppress their emotions given that it is not effective, it can be helpful to provide some psychoeducation about the reasons that control efforts are so common and so difficult to recognize and change. As described in Chapter 1, we are presented with multiple opportunities to learn that control efforts are desirable, from cultural messages we receive like "Don't worry, be happy" and "Keep calm and carry on" to advice about the importance of "getting over" a breakup and "thinking positively" when struggling with an illness. If it's relevant, we will connect the clients' persistence with control efforts to family messages they received that forbid and punish expressions of emotions. With some clients, we introduce the idea of intermittent reinforcement. If control efforts never worked, we probably would have given them up long ago. But emotion regulation can be successful in some situations, which can motivate us to try and regulate all our experiences (see our discussion in the section "Differentiating Experiential Avoidance from Emotion Regulation" later in this chapter). Most importantly, we share with clients that even those of us who write books about the paradoxical effects of control efforts still need to practice noticing our efforts and cultivating acceptance.

Although behaviors that may be serving as an experientially avoidant or control function are explored during the assessment (see Chapter 2), the range of strategies used for this function is often revisited during psychoeducation. We describe how habits develop when certain behaviors serve a function. For example, when Eve snags her fingernail on a piece of fabric and there is a crack at the edge of her nail, she might feel an uncomfortable sensation. If Eve feels relief after removing the ragged edge of her nail, that behavior has been negatively reinforced. The next day while having an uncomfortable conversation, Eve may automatically pick at her nail, and feel the same small measure of relief. As long as this habit continues to serve a function, Eve will likely keep doing it, often without being fully aware of the cycle. Even if Eve doesn't like how it looks when she picks at her nail, and she gets mad at herself for doing so, if the relief it brings is strong enough, the habit is likely to be maintained.

Similarly, many behaviors motivated by experiential avoidance can both bring some temporary relief and be frustrating, embarrassing, or otherwise troublesome. Some examples of habits that can dampen down, suppress, or change internal experiences and be associated with potential negative consequences are displayed in Table 5.2.

TABLE 5.2. Behaviors That Can Serve an Experiential Avoidant Function

Behavior	Possible functions	Potential negative consequences
Alcohol misuse	Reduce negative emotions, enhance sense of well-being, facilitate social interactions.	Relationship problems, health concerns, legal issues (e.g., DUI).
Smoking	Reduce stress, provide a break from monotony.	Impact on health, expensive to purchase cigarettes.
Overspending	Fun distraction, reduce feelings of self-deprivation.	Financial impact, guilt and shame, relationship issues if shared finances.
Procrastination	Delays activities that are boring, uncomfortable, or painful.	Impact on grades, work performance, household management.
Dissociation	Reduces the painful impact of a difficult event as it is occurring.	Challenging to be engaged in the present moment, may cause one to miss out on important information.
Self-injurious behaviors (e.g., cutting)	Reduce negative emotions, elicit concern and caring from peers.	Conflict with significant others, self-consciousness in public when scars are visible.

Differentiating Experiential Avoidance from Emotion Regulation

Sometimes clients (and therapists) assume that because control efforts often backfire or create additional life problems, according to ABBT people can never, and should never, try to alter their internal experiences in any way. We disagree. Our perspective is that all of us regularly engage in actions that have the potential to change how we feel and that emotion regulation can be both adaptive and successful. We also believe that it is essential to acknowledge this fact with clients as they themselves have certainly had successful regulation experiences. In fact, one reason changing avoidance habits can be so challenging is that they are intermittently reinforced. In other words, sometimes we are able to change how we feel, and that makes it even more likely that we will try again.

Typically, we acknowledge this challenge with clients during psychoeducation, and we wait until later to explore ways of engaging in regulation efforts in ways that promote, rather than constrain, functioning.[1] But depending on the client or context, we may delve into some of these nuances earlier. Below we provide some "advanced psychoeducation" about factors to consider when trying to discriminate between avoidance and skillful regulation. This psychoeducation can be provided to clients early in treatment if necessary, or it can be woven into later sessions as challenges in making this distinction in the client's daily experiences naturally arise. Table 5.3 provides some examples of actions we might consider serving an emotion regulation function.

---

[1]Extensive resources are available that explore the nature of emotion regulation (e.g., Gross, 2014) and approaches to promoting emotion regulation that are consistent with the model presented here (Linehan, 2015; Mennin & Fresco, 2014).

Several factors should be considered when trying to distinguish effective emotion regulation from problematic attempts to control internal experiences. First, effective regulation requires that we not be attached to the outcome of modulation efforts. For example, focusing on your breath before initiating a difficult conversation may slow your heart rate and quiet your mind a bit, allowing you to focus on your message more easily. Or it might not have any impact at all. Using this strategy while holding this stance is characteristic of effective regulation. Similarly, intentionally choosing to read a book after making a mistake at work and noticing that your mind keeps returning to the mistake might reduce the frequency and intensity of those thoughts. Or you might find that your mind continues to return to the event repeatedly. If we are able to allow for the possibility of *any* of these consequences of our behavior, there is no harm in engaging in actions that might modulate or alter our internal experiences. When they do, they might allow us to expand our awareness, gain additional perspectives, have new experiences, and increase flexibility. And when they don't, if we can accept that, we can continue living our lives with the internal experiences we were unable to alter. In contrast, if we strongly feel that our internal experience *must* change, our efforts are most likely to intensify our distress and to be unsuccessful.

One way rigid efforts at experiential avoidance become problematic is that they can become so automatic that we often aren't aware we are even avoiding. This can lead to disconnection from our experiences and make it harder to learn from our reactions. For example, if Monica continually ignores and suppresses the sadness and anger she feels adjusting to a recent loss of mobility, and instead acts cheerful around her husband, that might interfere with Monica's ability to acknowledge her loss and plan for the accommodations she needs to put into place. Monica may also miss out on an opportunity to receive her husband's emotional support and care if he doesn't know what she's feeling. On the other hand, if Monica regularly acknowledges her feelings and shares them with her husband, the occasional use of distraction as an emotion regulation strategy is unlikely to cause problems. For example, Monica may, on occasion, effectively redirect her attention away from the sadness she feels watching her husband play in the park

TABLE 5.3. Examples of Responses That Could Reflect Emotion Regulation Strategies

Challenging Internal Experiences	Response Aimed at Emotion Regulation
Kent notices he is ruminating over the fact that his coworker Steve can afford to buy a nice car and go on frequent vacations, while Kent is living from paycheck to paycheck and is worried about paying for his children's school supplies.	Kent broadens his attention to consider and appreciate the strong and supportive relationships he has with his husband, Jim, their children, and friends.
Molly, a recent widow, feels sad and lonely without her husband, Dan.	Molly calls her grandson to see if he is available to Skype with her.
Isabella feels harried and stressed from her busy day at school, and she worries about having the time and energy to complete her homework.	Isabella decides to take a break and go for a run.

with their granddaughter and toward the feeling of the sun on her face and the cool breeze on her skin. Similarly, after a week marked by too much exposure to insensitive and patronizing comments from her coworkers and too many encounters with barriers in spaces that are supposed to be accessible, Monica may recognize that she can't fully attend to all of the responses that arise when she receives a notice that they will be doing construction at her apartment building for the next month and her parking space may be blocked. Instead, Monica might intentionally engage in more self-soothing, regulatory strategies.

This awareness of choices may be particularly important when we are dealing with chronic stressors, such as illness, economic challenges, or discrimination. For example, people with marginalized identities often describe feeling a need to develop a kind of psychological "armor" to make their way through a world in which they repeatedly experience large and small acts of discrimination and belittlement. Noticing and responding to every instance may simply take too much energy and actually impair one's ability to thrive and live a meaningful life. At the same time, consistently ignoring external stressors and their potential psychological costs, and rigidly avoiding real experiences of pain, can have costly consequences. So, learning to notice when we engage in strategies designed to "shut out" our pain and hurt and monitoring the benefits and costs are important parts of using regulation strategies.

 See Chapter 10 for a more in-depth discussion of how engagement in values-based actions can help empower clients faced with external barriers that can lead to these types of emotional costs.

A final important distinction between successful and unsuccessful modulation is how we respond to ourselves and our experiences in the moment. We are much more likely to be effective at modulation, and, most importantly, less likely to feed problematic patterns of responding when we respond with compassion. Acknowledging that the situations we face are challenging, that emotions can be painful, that thoughts and images come to mind without our permission, and that many things are out of our control can help us more effectively modulate our responses (and accept when modulation efforts are unsuccessful). In contrast, chastising ourselves for being human only amplifies our distress. This also highlights an interaction between how we relate to internal experiences and problematic experiential avoidance. When we relate to our experiences in less critical, entangled ways, and instead bring curiosity and compassion to them, we may find that we don't need to try to modulate them so frequently. These characteristics are summarized in Box 5.5.

BOX 5.5. TO SUMMARIZE:
Characteristics of Effective Emotion Regulation Strategies

- Letting go of rigid attachment to the outcome of modulation efforts.
- Being aware of the choice to modulate/alter emotion.
- Cultivating kindness to self while modulating experiences.

Attempts to Control Others

One of the key challenges of being human is that many of the events and experiences that we encounter in our daily lives, particularly those that elicit the strongest emotional responses, happen outside of our control. For example, humans are innately social beings, and the perceived quality of our social network has a major influence on our lives, impacting everything from our mental health (Cacioppo, Hughes, Waite, Hawkley, & Thisted, 2006) to our cognitive abilities (Cacioppo & Hawkley, 2009) to our health and longevity (Hawkley & Cacioppo, 2007; Holt-Lunstad, Smith, & Layton, 2010). To illustrate the impact of our social environment on our emotional experience, we ask clients to think about the range and intensity of emotions that people in situations like these might experience: Leilani is in love with Amadio, but Amadio does not love her back; Trent's father "disowns" him after Trent discloses his transgender status; Lydia accuses her best friend Addie of disclosing a secret, and now Lydia refuses to speak with Addie; Tony's son was in a serious car accident, and his prognosis is uncertain. We also ask clients for examples of the ways in which the behavior and experience of other people in their lives are impacting their current emotional state.

Yet, at best, we only control half of every relationship we have. We can make choices about how to be in our relationships with our partners, family, friends, bosses, neighbors, and coworkers and what we want to bring to those relationships. And our words and actions can certainly *influence* what other people think and do. But we don't have *control over* the opinions, attitudes, emotions, or actions of the people who play a major role in our lives. If Nia wants to get promoted at work, she can put in a lot of effort and behave professionally in her interactions with her boss. It is very possible that these actions will positively impact her boss's decision. If Nia frequently calls in sick, arrives to work late, and is unprofessional and disrespectful in her interactions, there is an even greater chance that Nia can influence her boss's choice. However, Nia can't control the applicant pool, and it is absolutely possible that there is another candidate with more experience or a unique skill set. And Nia can't control her boss's preferences and implicit biases that could influence the selection process.

> The challenges that can arise when we try to control other people's emotions, thoughts, and/or behaviors are revisited in Chapter 8.

Attempts to Control Events and Circumstances

In addition to being deeply intertwined with, and impacted by, the thoughts, emotions, behaviors, and experiences of those we are closest with, our lives are also shaped by a broad range of events, and circumstances with even more remote causes. For example, strong emotions are likely to be elicited when Lee can no longer afford to stay in his apartment after his building is purchased by a large real estate management company; Yasmeen needs medical treatment, but the local clinic that accepts her insurance has a painfully long wait list; the Vargas family scrimps and saves for a beach vacation and it rains all week; Raoul regularly exercises, he has never been a smoker, he eats a healthy diet, and engages in good self-care to manage his stress, yet Raoul has a heart attack at the age of 50.

Because clients often feel alone in their failed attempts to control the thoughts and actions of others, certain circumstances, and the future, we provide psychoeducation that highlights the universality of this struggle, acknowledges how painful and frustrating it can be, and hopefully helps clients begin to cultivate some acceptance and self-compassion. We also try to begin to help clients notice the costs and benefits of different control strategies. Most notably, clients may get caught in an endless cycle of worry, feel frustrated and hopeless when their control efforts are unsuccessful, and by focusing on the uncontrollable, miss opportunities to take meaningful and impactful actions in valued domains. We delve deeper into this topic in Chapter 8.

ADDRESSING CHALLENGES THAT CAN ARISE WHEN USING PSYCHOEDUCATION AND SELF-MONITORING PRACTICES IN ABBT

Psychoeducation

Throughout the chapter, as we described our approach to psychoeducation and the main points we convey about each topic, we touched on the main challenges that can arise with this therapeutic strategy. Box 5.6 summarizes some of the best practices to follow when delivering psychoeducation.

Self-Monitoring

Monitoring experiences, behaviors, and responses outside of session is one of the most powerful ways clients can integrate what they learn in therapy into their lives. Yet it can also be a considerable burden. It's essential that therapists provide a strong rationale for every monitoring activity they suggest to clients. The goal of ABBT is to help clients become more aware of strongly established, automatically cued habits in the moment

---

 BOX 5.6. TO SUMMARIZE:
Best Practices for Delivering Psychoeducational Material

- Use client-generated examples from your assessment to personalize psychoeducation.
- Be willing to share (when appropriate and clinically indicated) the ways in which concepts fit with your experience.
- Balance didactic psychoeducation with a range of experiential exercises, including self-monitoring practices.
- Avoid efforts to convince clients that the concepts discussed in psychoeducation match the clients' lived experience. Instead, invite clients to consider observing their responses and experiences in new ways to notice how they may and may not be consistent with different concepts. Suggest trying this out for a couple of weeks and be willing to revisit the concept at that point in order to consider if, in fact, it doesn't fit.
- Consider your client's unique experiences and needs when deciding when to present broad overviews of psychoeducational topics and when to delve into the nuances.
- Be open to the possibility that some aspects truly do not fit the client. Listen to their experience and alter your conceptualization accordingly.

and try out new ways of responding. All the monitoring practices we share with clients are designed to help them meet those treatment goals. Early in treatment, monitoring is aimed at helping clients to notice patterns. Later activities help clients systematically apply the strategies learned in session to their experience during their most challenging moments. Self-monitoring forms allow clients to bring the therapy and the therapist into their moment-to-moment experience. Moreover, when clients self-monitor their failed attempts to use an ABBT skill introduced in a previous session, the material from the form can be used to walk through the client's application and help the therapist develop and provide tailored feedback for what the client can try next time.

Despite the widespread benefits of self-monitoring practices, many clients question their utility and find their completion burdensome. A number of therapist factors can contribute self-monitoring challenges. Some therapists "assign" self-monitoring as "homework," which may cue past memories of academic challenges, may be perceived as patronizing, or may overemphasize the power differential between the therapist and client. Therapists may also inadequately explain the relevance of a monitoring activity, simply suggesting that it is important for the client to complete without providing an individualized rationale related to session content and client goals. Occasionally, clients complete self-monitoring practices early in treatment, but their compliance tapers off over time. When this happens, it is usually because the therapist failed to sufficiently attend to the completed monitoring, suggesting the client's effort was wasted and missing an opportunity to reinforce and strengthen the frequency of monitoring behavior. Similarly, sometimes clients do not use self-monitoring practices as designed. Rather than responding to the specific instructions, clients may simply use monitoring forms to express their distress and conclude that the experience was not helpful. Both when introducing a new form and when reviewing monitoring, it is essential that the therapist carefully explain the importance of the different columns and ratings and demonstrate the benefits of filling out the form accurately.

Therapists sometimes underestimate the burden and distress associated with self-monitoring. We highly recommend that therapists practice any activity themselves before recommending it to clients; doing so provides us with a better sense of the experience which can inform our recommendation. For example, we make a point of predicting to clients that self-monitoring can actually increase their distress at first. For those clients who have been avoiding thinking about, or minimizing, the extent of their distress or the degree to which they have disengaged from parts of their lives, monitoring this distress or disengagement more closely can feel discouraging. We suggest to clients that, in order to make meaningful changes, we often need to clearly see and fully feel the impact of a problem. Thus, the distress they feel is conceptualized as an important aspect of the process of change. Here, again, research can be helpful. Process research suggests that change in psychotherapy is nonlinear, with spikes in symptoms (associated with exposure) predicting subsequent therapeutic gains (Hayes, Laurenceau, Feldman, Strauss, & Cardaciotto, 2007). This perspective on pain can keep clients from responding negatively to their own increase in distress and either prematurely terminating therapy or refraining from self-monitoring. It can also provide a behavioral example of choosing *not* to engage in experiential avoidance and instead continuing with a valued activity despite the distress associated with it. Box 5.7 provides some best practices therapists should adhere to in order to support their clients' engagement in self-monitoring.

BOX 5.7. TO SUMMARIZE:
Best Practices for Designing Self-Monitoring Practices

- Carefully choose language when talking about outside-of-session practices (e.g., avoid calling out-of-session work "homework").
- Provide an overall rationale for including monitoring practices in ABBT (as well as a rationale for each specific exercise), highlighting the ways in which the activities are aimed at meeting specific client-reported goals.
- Decide collaboratively which outside-of-session practices are worth practicing.
- Ensure and communicate to clients that self-monitoring activities are designed to benefit the client, not the therapist.
- Predict that self-monitoring can increase distress and help the client conceptualize the increased distress as a sign of change.
- Spend sufficient time reviewing completed activities and exploring their helpfulness.
- Make sure clients understand how to complete monitoring forms in advance, and address any confusion when reviewing forms.
- Alter assignments that do not seem to be particularly helpful.
- Take seriously client feedback regarding the burden versus the utility of self-monitoring.

A number of client factors, as well as contextual and situational constraints, can make it extremely challenging for clients to practice self-monitoring outside of session. Therapists need to be sensitive to the obstacles that clients may face and to be open to brainstorming workable solutions. For example, if a client frequently forgets to monitor, the therapist might suggest using Post-it Notes or programmed phone reminders. If they frequently don't have monitoring forms handy when a situation arises, the therapist might recommend making multiple copies to be kept at work, home, and in the car. Therapists can also suggest that clients use a journal, small notebook, the note feature on their phone, or some other app for monitoring. Some clients face challenges that make writing or typing difficult. One potential alternative is for them to use the voice recording feature available on most cell phones.

Sometimes clients are embarrassed to monitor in the moment or are unsure about how they can take the space they need to work through the process in the midst of a challenging interaction. Role-playing possible methods of asking for a few moments of privacy (e.g., excusing oneself to take a bathroom break or responding to a time-sensitive text) can be one solution. Alternatively, clients can try out "mental monitoring," or working through the self-monitoring process in their mind as the situation is unfolding and record it later for review. Some clients feel overwhelmed at the prospect of noticing and writing down every painful emotion or worry that arises, or they may experience situational constraints that may make it challenging to practice self-monitoring outside of session. In response, we emphasize the quality of monitoring a few key experiences that arise over the quantity of monitoring. Our goal in asking clients to self-monitor is to help them first develop and then refine skills that they can eventually deploy more naturally when challenging situations arise. In that spirit, we share our preference that clients complete a few self-monitoring examples thoughtfully, with awareness and intentionality instead of devoting their time to creating more frequent but less reflective entries.

BOX 5.8. WHEN TIME IS LIMITED:
Psychoeducation and Self-Monitoring

Time in session is extremely precious in therapy that is limited by the number of sessions, session duration, or both. In these contexts, it can be helpful to provide clients with psychoeducation material that can be reviewed out of session. That way, in-session time can be devoted to emphasizing the specific relevance of certain topics to the clients' therapy goals and addressing clients' questions and concerns. Throughout the chapter, we pointed to chapters in our self-help workbook that clients can be referred to for psychoeducation on the concepts of learning, emotions, thoughts, and the problem of control. Therapists might also consider adapting psychoeducational concepts into handouts that work best for the clients they serve. Although we covered a range of psychoeducational topics in this chapter, therapists working in brief therapy contexts might choose to focus on one or two themes that are more relevant to the client. Finally, in some settings, adjunctive group therapy that focuses on didactic presentations of psychoeducation may supplement individual therapy focused on personalized concerns and focused skill building.

If clients are willing to engage in self-monitoring activities between sessions, session time can be focused explicitly on the challenges that clients faced applying a particular skill in a particular context. Depending on the amount of preparation time available to the therapist and the availability of confidential methods of information transfer, therapists can request that clients submit their monitoring in advance of session so that therapists are prepared to hone in on specific topics and skill-building exercises.

CLIENT FORM 5.1. Monitoring Your Fear and Anxiety

The goal of this monitoring practice is for you to try noticing what comes along when you are feeling anxious or stressed. Simply observe and mark in the form below whatever physical sensations, thoughts, or behaviors you notice when anxiety or stress arises. You might notice some discomfort and/or critical thoughts as you observe your responses; there is no need to struggle with them and push them away. As best as you can, simply focus on observing and recording your experience just as it unfolds.

Date/Time	Current Situation	Physical Sensations	Thoughts	Behaviors

Reprinted with permission from *Worry Less, Live More* by Susan M. Orsillo and Lizabeth Roemer. Copyright © 2016 The Guilford Press.

CLIENT FORM 5.2. Monitoring Emotions

When you experience a strong emotion, note the following information on the form:

• When did the emotion arise (*i.e., day and time*)?
• What emotion(s) did you notice (*e.g., sadness, anger, fear*)?
• How intense was each emotion you felt (*i.e., 100 is the strongest emotional intensity you have ever experienced*)?
• Does it seem like the emotion was triggered in some way by a situation that is currently unfolding? (*If so, briefly describe the situation. If not, mark one of the following: P—past situation I am thinking about; F—future situation I am thinking about; DK—don't know.*)
• Please mark the message, if any, you think the emotion may have been communicating to you or others (e.g., "I am taking a risk, my rights have been violated").

Date/Time	Emotion(s)	Intensity 0–100	Situation That Elicited the Emotion (or P, F, or DK)	Possible Message the Emotion Was Communicating

When you notice an intense, long-lasting emotion that could be muddy, use the questions below to uncover factors that could be contributing.

A. Describe the current situation.

_____

_____

_____

_____

_____

_____

_____

_____

_____

_____

B. What emotions are you experiencing? How would you rate their intensity from 0 to 100?

Emotion: _____ Intensity: _____

Emotion: _____ Intensity: _____

Emotion: _____ Intensity: _____

Emotion: _____ Intensity: _____

Emotion: _____ Intensity: _____

Emotion: _____ Intensity: _____

C. For each emotion you described in section B, consider whether it seems to be a *clear* response to the current situation. Write in any emotions you think might be *clear* in the space below. Then, for each clear emotion, also describe the message you think the emotion might be trying to communicate to you about this situation.

Clear Emotion: _____ Message: _____

Clear Emotion: _____ Message: _____

Clear Emotion: _____ Message: _____

Clear Emotion: _____ Message: _____

Clear Emotion: _____ Message: _____

Clear Emotion: _____ Message: _____

(continued)

Adapted with permission from *Worry Less, Live More* by Susan M. Orsillo and Lizabeth Roemer © 2016 The Guilford Press.

D. Next, consider the following questions to see if any of the factors that can muddy emotions might be involved.

D1. Do you think any of the emotions might be linked to something that happened in your recent or distant past? It could be that your mind was on the present moment experience and also returning to some unrelated recent event. Or that this current experience reminds you of another challenging experience from the past. If so, describe how here.

_____

_____

_____

_____

D2. Are any of your emotions linked to anything you might be worried could happen in the future? This sometimes happens when something in the present triggers a fear we have about the future. If that is something you notice, describe that here.

_____

_____

_____

_____

D3. Do you notice your mind making any judgments about the presence of any particular emotions? Any thoughts that it is "bad" to feel a certain way? Any frustrations with yourself for having the emotional responses you have? Do you notice any self-critical thoughts? If so, describe them here.

_____

_____

_____

_____

D4. Does it seem as if you are tangled up in any of your emotions? Like any of these emotions are signaling something about you rather than something about the situation? Do you feel defined by any of your emotions? If so, describe that experience here.

_____

_____

_____

_____

D5. How has your self-care been recently? Are you getting enough rest and sleep, eating nutritious meals and snacks, getting exercise, making time for hobbies or socializing? If you have been neglecting yourself in some of these areas, describe how here.

_____

_____

_____

_____

CLIENT FORM 5.4. Worry or Problem Solving?

When you notice that your focus is pulled toward a possible future event, use the questions below to sort through whether intentionally spending time on this topic is worry or problem solving.

Questions	Future-Focused Topic 1	Future-Focused Topic 2
Describe the future-focused topic.		
Is this experience likely to happen?		
Is there a specific action or actions I can take to prepare for it (or prevent it from happening)?		
Will spending more time with these thoughts likely solve my problem?		
Am I focused on solving a problem or reducing uncomfortable thoughts and feelings of uncertainty?		
Is spending time with these thoughts moving me closer toward something I care about? Or getting in my way?		
If I do think of an action I could take, will it add meaning to my life?		

Adapted with permission from *Worry Less, Live More* by Susan M. Orsillo and Lizabeth Roemer. Copyright © 2016 The Guilford Press.

Fear Is Learned

- Fear helps us avoid real physical dangers.

  These are natural, human responses and are helpful to us.

- Fear is easy to learn.

  Our nervous system has evolved so that we can readily detect and learn danger, to keep us safe.

- Fear and anxiety can easily spread to other things.

  We easily learn to fear things that are similar to, or associated with, objects or situations that we perceive as threatening.

- Fear cannot be unlearned.

  The only way we come to be less afraid of an object or an activity is to have lots of experience with it that teaches us we are safe.

- Some fears are biologically inherited.

  We are more likely to fear things that threatened our ancestors' survival. We are "hard-wired" to very quickly learn to fear and avoid snakes and spiders.

Physical Sensations

- Rapid heart rate
- Sweating
- Dizziness or lightheadedness
- Shortness of breath
- Trembling or shaky feelings
- Blushing
- Dry mouth
- Stomach distress
- Tension or soreness in the neck, shoulders, or any other muscles
- Headaches
- Restlessness
- Fatigue

Thoughts/Cognitive Symptoms

- Worries about what might occur in the future
  - "No one will talk to me at the party."
  - "I will fail this test."
  - "My parents will become ill."
  - "My children will not be happy."
  - "I will end up alone."
  - "I will have a panic attack at the supermarket."
  - "I am going to get sick from the germs in this bathroom."
  - "People won't take me seriously at school."
- Ruminations about the past
  - "I can't believe I said that."
  - "My boss thought I did a terrible job."
  - "I wish I hadn't snapped at my partner that way."
  - "Having nothing to say in that conversation was so humiliating."
- Thoughts about being in danger
  - "I can't do this."
  - "I am having a heart attack."
  - "I am losing my mind."
- Narrowed attention toward threat or danger, inattention to evidence of safety

Other Emotions

- Sadness
- Anger
- Surprise
- Disgust
- Shame
- Hopelessness
- "Overwhelmed"
- "Numb"

(continued)

Reprinted with permission from *Worry Less, Live More* by Susan M. Orsillo and Lizabeth Roemer. Copyright © 2016 The Guilford Press.

Behaviors

- Repetitive behaviors or habits
  - Biting fingernails
  - Picking skin
  - Playing with hair
  - Tapping feet
- Avoidance or escape
  - Turning down a social invitation
  - Passing up a promotion
  - Calling in sick to work
  - Making an excuse to cancel a social engagement
  - Leaving an event early
  - Asking someone else to make a phone call for you
  - Taking an alternative route to avoid a bridge or tunnel
  - Using a ritual, security object, or lucky charm to get through an anxious experience
- Distraction techniques
  - Overeating
  - Smoking
  - Watching television
  - Having a few glasses of wine or a couple of beers
  - Sleeping excessively
  - Shopping
  - Putting excessive energy into work
  - Exercising vigorously to try to "tire out" your body
  - Coming up with a busy schedule to keep your mind off worries
- Doing what you "should" do
  - Taking care of every responsibility you have to avoid being judged negatively or criticized
- Checking and overpreparing
  - Asking others for reassurance
  - Reading every report that your colleague wrote before writing your own
  - Endlessly searching the Internet to find out how to prevent an accident from happening
- Attempts to gain power or protect oneself
  - Acting aggressively toward others
  - Using threatening language
  - Lashing out in anger

Clear Emotions

Clear Emotion	Message	Examples of Situations That Elicit the Emotion	Actions Suggested by the Emotion
Fear	We are taking a risk or facing a new challenge.	• Asking someone on a date • Getting laid off • Becoming a parent	Escape; Avoidance
Anger	Our rights, or the rights of others we care about, have been violated.	• Being constantly interrupted by others in a meeting • Earning less than others doing the same job • Hearing someone make a racial slur	Stand up for ourselves or others; fight back
Sadness	We've lost something or someone we care about.	• Moving to a new country and leaving your family and friends behind • The death of a close friend	Retreat; Self-soothe; seek care from others
Guilt	We've taken an action that could cause harm or that is inconsistent with our moral standards or the moral standards of our community.	• Telling an offensive joke • Gossiping about another congregant during a church supper • Being unfaithful to one's partner	Make amends
Disgust	We've encountered something that could sicken us (e.g., spoiled food) or that we find unacceptable (e.g., immoral behavior).	• Seeing feces smeared on a toilet seat in a public restroom • Watching a story on the news about someone who was tortured • Finding out that a trusted caregiver sexually abused the children in their care	Escape; Avoidance

Adapted with permission from *Worry Less, Live More* by Susan M. Orsillo and Lizabeth Roemer. Copyright © 2016 The Guilford Press.

Differentiating Clear and Muddy Emotions

Clear Emotions	Muddy Emotions
Seem to have a clear cause. • *Example:* Feeling nervous about an upcoming test.	Can sometimes seem like they came "out of the blue." • *Example:* Feeling nervous but not knowing why.
Seem to have a clear message. • *Example:* Fear is signaling that you are about to take a risk.	Don't provide you with useful information. • *Example:* You know you have been feeling keyed up and grouchy all day, but it is not clear why.
Seem like a response anyone might have. • *Example:* Most people would feel some fear before an audition for a play.	Seem like part of your personality. • *Example:* Feeling like you are an anxious person.
Seem to fit the event. • *Example:* Feeling nervous about giving a presentation. • *Example:* Getting a little frustrated when a driver cuts you off. • Example: Feeling anger and sadness when someone insults you.	Seem out of proportion to the event. • *Example:* Feeling terrified about giving a presentation. • *Example:* Becoming enraged when a driver cuts you off. • *Example:* Feeling self-hatred when someone insults you.
Seem to come and go. • *Example:* Feeling embarrassed for the first few minutes of a meeting because you arrived late.	Seem to linger on and on. • *Example:* Feeling embarrassed for the rest of the day because you arrived late to a meeting.

1. Current emotional state is complicated by emotions from imagined past or future events.	
a. Worries about future potential threats	*Example:* Afu is confused by the feelings of fear and dread that arise on a relatively quiet night at home with his wife. Although there are no threats in his current context, his mind is busy with worries about his parents' upcoming visit and fears that the wintry New England weather will worsen their already compromised health.
b. Rumination over events remembered from the past	*Example:* Afu is also remembering the last time his parents visited and the way they criticized his approach to parenting, the food he served, and his overall lifestyle.
2. Clear emotions are amplified by our reactions to them.	
a. Critical, judgmental responses	*Example:* Ash feels sad when their mother makes an insensitive comment, then angry and ashamed for feeling sad.
b. Fusion	*Example:* Jenny has the thought "I have nothing to contribute" during a meeting at work. She fears that having that thought shows she is weak and lacks the confidence needed to succeed in her job.
c. Attempts to control	*Example:* Marvin attempts to push away his feelings of sadness, embarrassment, and anger as he talks with the principal at his son Matt's school about Matt's behavior problems.
3. Poor self-care (e.g., not getting enough sleep, little engagement in activities aimed at nurturing the self) heightens emotions.	
	Example: Shirley feels distressed and cries easily on her way to work Monday morning after babysitting her grandchildren all weekend and getting little sleep on her daughter's couch.

Common Reasons We Turn Our Attention to the Future (Worry) and Past (Rumination)

Reasons	Worry	Rumination
Preparation	It seems like imagining what it will be like to face a threat could be a good way to prepare for it.	It seems like focusing on past mistakes will prepare for future successes.
Motivation	It seems like focusing on the potentially negative consequences of a feared future event will motivate us to prepare.	It seems like engaging in self-judgment and criticism of past mistakes will motivate us to improve.
Superstition	It feels like worrying about a potential threat will make it less likely to happen.	It feels like remembering how badly something went will make it less likely to happen again.
Avoidance	It seems like worrying will help us figure out how to avoid feared future outcomes.	It seems like going over past mistakes will help us avoid making them again.
Problem solving	It seems like focusing on a potential future problem is a first step to solving it.	It seems like identifying what went wrong in the past is a first step to avoiding a poor outcome in the future.
Distraction from more emotional topics	Worrying about minor matters often takes our minds off more distressing and serious concerns.	Focusing our attention on figuring out what happened in the past to contribute to our current distress is one way to avoid taking risks in the present.

Am I Problem Solving, Worrying, or Ruminating?

Problem Solving	Worrying	Ruminating
• Problem I am currently facing • Problem I am very likely to confront in the future	• Problem I may face in the future • Problem that I could (but probably won't) face	• Problem that I encountered in the past
• There are specific actions I can take now or soon to prepare for it, fix it, learn from it, and/or prevent it from happening in the future.	• The problem and solution are largely out of my control.	• The problem has passed, but I am struggling to let it go.
• There is a clear relationship between the time and effort I invest in this problem; the more I focus on it, the greater my changes of solving it.	• Investing time into thinking about this problem is not getting me any closer to solving it.	• My focus seems to be more on criticizing myself for what happened rather than considering actions I can take now and in the future.
• I am investing time and energy so that my solution is well developed and effective.	• I am investing time and energy in an attempt to feel more in control of the situation and less worried.	• I am investing time and energy considering how terrible it was and wishing that it never happened.
• Devoting time to thinking about how to solve this problem is meaningful to me; it's bringing me closer to the things that matter most to me.	• Devoting time to thinking about how to solve this problem is taking me away from things that are meaningful to me.	• Devoting time to thinking about how to solve this problem is taking me away from things that are meaningful to me.
• Problem I am currently facing • Problem I am very likely to confront in the future	• Problem I may face in the future • Problem that I could (but probably won't) face	• Problem that I encountered in the past.
• There are specific actions I can take now or soon to prepare for it, fix it, learn from it, and/or prevent it from happening in the future.	• The problem and solution are largely out of my control.	• The problem has passed, but I am struggling to let it go.
• There is a clear relationship between the time and effort I invest in this problem; the more I focus on it, the greater my changes of solving it.	• Investing time into thinking about this problem is not getting me any closer to solving it.	• My focus seems to be more on criticizing myself for what happened rather than considering actions I can take now and in the future.
• I am investing time and energy so that my solution is well developed and effective.	• I am investing time and energy in an attempt to feel more in control of the situation and less worried.	• I am investing time and energy considering how terrible it was and wishing that it never happened.
• Devoting time to thinking about how to solve this problem is meaningful to me; it's bringing me closer to the things that matter most to me.	• Devoting time to thinking about how to solve this problem is taking me away from things that are meaningful to me.	• Devoting time to thinking about how to solve this problem is taking me away from things that are meaningful to me.

CHAPTER 6 ∾∾∾∾∾∾∾∾∾∾∾∾∾∾

Mindfulness and Other Experiential Methods

Although both the therapeutic relationship and psychoeducation help clients to cultivate this new relationship with internal experiences that is more aware, curious, compassionate, and accepting, experiential practice is a central method for targeting this important goal in therapy. In our work, we consider a wide range of exercises in order to cultivate this new way of relating to thoughts, feelings, sensations, and memories. Broadly, these exercises cultivate *mindfulness,* or "an openhearted, moment-to-moment, non-judgmental awareness" (Kabat-Zinn, 2005, p. 24). In other words, we use practices that help clients develop their ability to pay attention, in the present moment, to whatever arises internally or externally, without becoming entangled or "hooked" by judging or by wishing things were otherwise. This cultivation of mindfulness is seen as therapeutic because it helps to promote acceptance of internal experience and to diminish avoidance. We use traditional formal mindfulness practices that appear in many mindfulness-based interventions, informal practices that involve applying the skills of mindfulness to daily activities, and self-monitoring practices that are a standard part of CBTs. In Appendix B, we provide a few scripts for the mindfulness practices we describe here and in subsequent chapters. We also provide audio recordings on the Guilford website (see the box at the end of the table of contents). Because so many sources provide extensive guidance in using mindfulness practices in therapy, we focus particularly in this chapter on the why and how of these practices, how they link to our case conceptualization, and how we address barriers that arise in practice. Although many of the strategies we present in this chapter also help to cultivate self-compassion, we provide a more in-depth exploration of this particular target in the following chapter in order to address the specific challenges that arise in helping clients to cultivate compassion for themselves.

What you will learn

- ❧ How a wide range of experiential exercises cultivate awareness, decentering, and acceptance.
- ❧ How to effectively balance experiential learning with psychoeducation and discussion.
- ❧ How to connect practices to the client's presenting problems and treatment goals.
- ❧ How goals for mindfulness practice evolve over time.
- ❧ How cognitive restructuring and relaxation relate to mindfulness and decentering.
- ❧ How to address barriers to mindfulness practice and acceptance.

Given the role of repeated, consistently strengthened habits of responding in the challenges that bring clients to therapy, a central method of therapy is to promote repeated practice of new responses in order to increase flexibility and promote more adaptive responding. For ABBT, problematic habits of responding include mindlessness (lack of awareness of the present moment), reactivity and judgment of responses, fusion and entanglement, and experiential and behavioral avoidance. We use a range of strategies to help clients directly practice responses that will weaken these habits, and enhance their flexibility in responding. In this chapter, we address three strategies that are integral to promoting this new learning: self-monitoring, formal mindfulness practice, and informal mindfulness practice. In our experience, clients vary in how they respond to

---

 BOX 6.1. A CLOSER LOOK:
Cultural Considerations in Integrating Mindfulness in Therapy

Mindfulness approaches to psychotherapy are secular approaches that draw heavily from the historical traditions of Buddhist and other Eastern religions. We honor the wisdom of these traditions and are influenced by Buddhist writers from both the East and West, as we adapt and apply these approaches to psychotherapy, separate from a religious context. At the same time, it is important to recognize the cultural lens of the therapy traditions we work in, which are largely developed in Eurocentric contexts (Harrell, 2018). Similarly, as mindfulness has become popularized in the United States and other countries, it is often presented in a narrow cultural context (e.g., thin White women calmly meditating on the cover of magazines) that may make a wide range of clients feel excluded from these practices (e.g., Harrell, 2018; Magee, 2016; Yang, 2017). Shelly Harrell (2018) provides a rich conceptual model of an approach she calls soulfulness that is instead grounded in diasporic African cultural influences and can help clinicians to broaden our lens and approach to incorporating mindfulness. Harrell's approach is an inspiring model of how the principles of these strategies can be synthesized with culturally resonant material to engage clients fully. We encourage clinicians to flexibly apply these principles in their own work with clients from a range of backgrounds, focusing on the intended function of the practice, rather than the form, which may not be accessible and inclusive.

each type of strategy and so we make a point of introducing and incorporating all three to start. Then we make idiographic decisions on how to apply or modify each one based on the client's circumstances. For instance, with a client facing a lot of challenges in developing a regular formal practice, we may focus more on informal practice for skill development.

SELF-MONITORING

The self-monitoring described in the previous chapter is one form of new practice that we consider a type of mindfulness practice.[1] When clients are asked to notice experiences as they arise, they

> See Chapter 5 for a discussion of challenges associated with self-monitoring.

are attending to their experiences, turning toward them rather than away from them, and observing them as they unfold. The act of writing down what they notice also gives them a little bit of distance from the experience and naturally involves a decentered response. This practice will also eventually serve to help identify choice points in which new responses can be tried, such as engaging in value-driven actions. In order to ensure that self-monitoring serves the function we intend, we make suggestions and give feedback to clients that promote this new learning:

- We emphasize the importance of monitoring in the moment so that they can learn to notice responses as they arise and respond differently.
- We ask them to use the columns in the monitoring forms so that they can separate out their experience in terms of aspects of responding (e.g., thoughts, feelings, sensations, actions), as well as the temporal unfolding (e.g., first reactions, second reactions).
- We take time to review at least some entries each session to reinforce their practice and help to shape their monitoring so that it is promoting decentered awareness.
- During this review, we may break down responses more by going moment by moment (e.g., "What happened next?"; "When you noticed that thought or feeling, how did you respond?").
- As described in Chapter 4, we use decentering/defusing language (e.g., "So you had the thought that . . .") to further promote these new habits of responding.
- If clients express judgments while reviewing their monitoring (e.g., "My responses are so ridiculous"), we validate their responses based on past history, habits, general principles, or context and explore the possibility of cultivating self-compassion when these judgments arise.

---

[1] As Hayes and Shenk (2004) note, one point of confusion in the literature has been whether the term *mindfulness* refers to a process (such as the self-regulation of attention toward immediate experience, with that attention having the quality of openness, curiosity, and acceptance; Bishop et al., 2004) or to practices, such as meditation, that are thought to evoke that process. We use the term *mindfulness* to refer to the process, and we use mindfulness or mindfulness-based practices to refer to those practices that can be used to evoke this process.

FORMAL PRACTICE

We incorporate specific, *formal* practices into each session to give clients an opportunity to develop the skills of awareness, observing with curiosity, decentering, and compassion through repeated practice. We guide them through these practices in session, discuss their observations and experiences, and then ask them to practice between sessions as well in order to build up new habits, as well as the ability to practice without us present. Our goal in formal practice is to help clients to develop these skills intentionally, at a set-aside time when they are only practicing the skill. This is similar to shooting or passing drills in basketball or soccer in which players practice these essential skills in a focused way so that they will be able to rely on them more easily during a game. Here we want to help clients be able to apply these skills in their lives as thoughts, feelings, sensations, and memories arise and they have critical reactions to these responses, becoming fused and entangled in their experience. We will also help them to apply these skills as they engage in valued actions, as we describe in Chapter 9.

Although we can teach people about mindfulness (defining it, reviewing the skills it cultivates, and explaining how to do it), actually engaging in practices promotes a more powerful, experiential learning. When clients are able to observe for themselves the ways that their thoughts can rise and fall, or change, or become less "sticky," it's more compelling than us telling them that this is the case. Also, our explanations can actually get in the way of clients' direct experiences, setting expectations about how mindfulness "should be." So in our use of mindfulness in ABBT, we try to limit psychoeducation, encourage practice, and use postpractice discussion as an opportunity for learning. Postpractice debriefing, which includes helping clients connect their experiences of mindfulness practice with their presenting concerns and goals for therapy, challenge misconceptions about mindfulness, and consolidate new learning, is an essential part of ABBT.

To be consistent with the way we conduct ABBT, we begin here by inviting you to engage in a brief, introductory practice (see Box 6.2).

General Principles and Procedures That Guide Formal Practice

Later in this section, we will describe some of the specific practices we often use, but first we describe the general principles we apply to our use of formal practice regardless of the specific practice. People can engage in formal practice in different positions (sitting on a cushion on the floor, in a chair, standing, lying down). We generally use regular chairs in the therapy context and encourage clients to find seated positions that work well for them at home. Although many people associate mindfulness with relaxation, it's actually used to promote a state of being awake, alert, and present. Thus, we invite clients to sit upright, as if they had a string attached to the top of their heads. Given the multitude of distractions that compete for our attention, we recommend that clients either close or lower their eyes during practice.

We typically begin practices with some instructions to notice (in order):

- How one is sitting.
- Where in the body one feels contact with the chair or the ground.
- Where in the body one notices in- and out-breaths.

BOX 6.2. TRY THIS:
Practicing Mindfulness

Something that we personally practice, and a strategy that we recommend to those therapists we train and consult with, is trying out self-monitoring, skill-building, and behavioral change strategies ourselves before using these approaches with clients. Mindfulness practice is no exception. Developing our own personal practice allows us to draw from our experiences and challenges with mindfulness when working with clients. It also helps us to be patient and empathic when our clients struggle with mindfulness and provides us with skills that make us more effective as therapists.

Before you read any further, we encourage you to take a few minutes to practice mindfulness yourself and reflect on your own experiences as you read the rest of this chapter. Even if you already practice on a regular basis and are tempted to skip this exercise, we invite you to still take a moment now to engage in this brief practice.

Please find a comfortable, upright way of sitting, with your feet even on the ground and your spine upright. Set a timer on your phone or computer for between 2 and 5 minutes. In a moment, either lower or close your eyes and just allow your attention to rest on wherever you feel your breath in your body. Each time your mind wanders, bring it back to that place again, just noticing whatever you notice. You may have thoughts, sensations, or feelings arise, you may lose focus again and again. Just notice each time where your focus is, and gently bring it back, until the timer goes off. If you'd like to use an audio recording, you can listen to "mindfulness of breath" on the Guilford website (see the box at the end of the table of contents). Each time you wonder if the time has passed, or the timer isn't working, just return to your breath again, until the timer goes off.

Next, depending on the practice, clients are often instructed to practice bringing awareness to the target (e.g., the breath, sounds, physical sensations), noticing when attention wanders from the target, and gently bringing attention back to the target, again and again. Practices may also involve expanding awareness to attend to one's whole experience.

Early in therapy, after we introduce a practice in session, we ask clients to try to practice it daily at home. As needed, we specifically problem-solve with clients to help them find a time and place for this practice. Unlike some other approaches, we do not generally require clients to engage in lengthy practices at home. This choice is based on the absence of evidence for optimal length of practice as well as our desire to deliver a flexible treatment that clients can easily incorporate into busy lives.[2] Instead we emphasize the importance of committing to some regular length of practice and trying to practice consistently, in order to develop new habits. We have clients complete a simple monitoring form of the practices

> We talk about how we address obstacles to regular practice later in this chapter.

_____

[2]Some clients take up longer practices on their own, which we certainly encourage. Clients may also choose movement-based mindfulness practices like yoga or tai chi outside of therapy. We incorporate their experiences of these practices in session just like any other out-of-session practice, connecting their observations to their presenting problems and treatment goals.

they engage in, so that we can discuss their between-session practice in the following session.

Mindfulness practices are often delivered in a slow-paced style that helps the listener follow instructions and bring awareness to their experience. However, altering one's voice can make some clients feel uncomfortable, particularly if they are skeptical about trying mindfulness. Harrell (2018) notes that the typical slow, whispered pace may be perceived as unfamiliar, "weird," impersonal, or inconsistent with a cultural value of authentic expressiveness for some individuals. Depending on the client, clinicians may consider following Segal, Williams, and Teasdale's (2013) suggestion to speak in a "matter-of-fact" voice, rather than changing one's tone when leading a mindfulness practice, to help demystify the experience. Pausing frequently during instruction is important; this allows the client to really engage the practice rather than solely listening to the therapist. We also follow Segal and colleagues' suggestion of using "ing" verbs (e.g., "noticing," "bringing awareness to") to highlight the continual process of mindfulness. Although we provide some scripts and recordings as a supplement to this book, we also encourage therapists to develop their own exercises and their own language (ideally reflecting language the client uses to describe their observations later in therapy) as you become more comfortable using these strategies.

We are intentional and client-centered in the way we select and plan which formal mindfulness practices to use in session. We start by building foundational skills using practices that are generally more accessible before moving to more challenging ones. For example, we typically introduce mindfulness of breath and physical sensations in the body before encouraging mindfulness of emotions or thoughts. However, with a client whose presenting concerns include reactivity to physiological cues, such as anxiety sensitivity or panic disorder, we might start with mindful eating or mindfulness of sounds and build up to the more challenging practice of noticing one's breath.

Connecting Formal Practice to Treatment Goals

We often hear clients and therapists express a disconnect between formal mindfulness practices and the changes they are trying to make in therapy. For us, connecting these two explicitly, both during treatment planning and repeatedly throughout treatment, is an essential part of successfully using mindfulness in therapy. Although there can be benefits that arise simply from practicing mindfulness, a client's willingness to engage in practice is often facilitated, and their learning more powerful and generalizable, when the client can see how observations and experiences during these practices relate to their presenting concerns and treatment goals. Drawing these connections in the moment requires the therapist to have a good working knowledge and understanding of mindfulness and a strong case conceptualization. We describe here how we draw these connections early in treatment, and then we revisit how we draw these connections later in the chapter after we've explored other mindfulness practices.

Early in treatment, we use mindfulness practices to help clients notice how minds work and cultivate the compassion (i.e., reduced judgment) that can arise when we recognize the challenges inherent in our human experience. After each practice, we ask

"What did you notice?"[3] Our responses to their observations are shaped by our goals of helping them to:

- Notice the nature of their experiences,
- Recognize the humanness and naturalness of these experiences,
- Cultivate compassion and understanding for their habits of responding, and
- Learn that mindfulness is a process.

Clients can notice a broad range of experiences during mindfulness practice. Sometimes they experience a reprieve from the challenging thoughts and emotions that brought them into therapy during a mindfulness practice. They may be pleased and excited that they experienced feelings of calmness or relaxation during the practice or that it seemed to help them clear their mind. Or clients may notice the presence of the very worries and painful feelings they constantly battle against and feel frustrated and conclude that mindfulness did not "work" for them. Sometimes clients are completely surprised by what they notice. They might observe that they are tired, sad, or angry when they hadn't been aware of those experiences. They may "blame" mindfulness practice for making them feel worse than they did before practicing.

Therapists will be most effective in responding to these observations if they remain focused on the intended function of mindfulness practice in ABBT. As described earlier in the book, our human nature and learning experiences expose us to a wide array of painful thoughts, emotions, and sensations. Some ways of responding to those internal experiences can intensify distress and reduce quality of life. Mindfulness will not rid us of thoughts and emotions, but it offers us a new way of responding to them. From this perspective, mindfulness practice is aimed at noticing what is present, whether it is the scent of a candle we find pleasing or the sound of an ambulance we find jarring. It involves noticing that our minds judge different scents and sounds in different ways. And if we are able to step back from the thoughts that typically entangle us and we let go of our struggle to control our feelings, we may at times feel centered and present.

In responding to clients' descriptions of mindfulness, we first validate their experience, whatever it may be. For example, if clients find mindfulness relaxing and are enthusiastic about continuing their practice, we validate this enthusiasm, reflecting that it is natural to enjoy a reprieve from challenging thoughts and emotions. If they are frustrated that their mind wandered, we normalize the busyness of minds and validate how challenging minds can be.

If clients' experience with mindfulness practice is similar to the experiences they have in their everyday lives, we make sure to draw those connections. For example, if clients notice they judge themselves for breathing the "wrong way" or for having attention that wanders, we might observe, "Those judgmental thoughts sound similar to the ones you have when you get angry at yourself for making a mistake at work."

In contrast, if clients are able to practice noticing and allowing experiences during mindfulness practice, we explore how that may be different from the client's typical way of relating to internal experiences. This is particularly important when clients

---

[3]"How was that?" encourages judgment, while "What did you notice?" encourages nonjudgmental observation.

experience mindfulness practice as calming and relaxing. We gently remind clients that mindfulness practice doesn't reliably elicit a particular set of thoughts or feelings. Just as every moment is different, every mindfulness practice, or observation of a moment is different. The relief and centered experience we sometimes have when practicing mindfulness comes from letting go of our struggle against our experience. We link this idea back to the goals of treatment—although we can't avoid having our memories or feeling our feelings, we can develop new ways of responding that may be less likely to deepen our pain and prolong our struggle (although we might still feel sad, frustrated, bored, or anxious while practicing mindfulness). Later, after we provide psychoeducation about the problems with control efforts, we may remind clients that even though it's natural to enjoy having a clear mind or feeling relaxed during mindfulness practice, becoming attached to wanting these outcomes can have paradoxical effects.

If clients report that the practice "didn't work" or they were "bad" at it, several lines of responding can be useful. As always, we validate the universality of those reactions. When they are first introduced to the practice, people often experience mindfulness as an attempt to achieve an outcome (i.e., successfully keep your attention on your breath without distraction). We take this opportunity to notice our minds' tendency to treat our experiences as tests of our abilities and sometimes of our worthiness. We remind clients that the practice is not staying with the breath; rather, it is returning to awareness again and again, no matter how many times our attention wanders. This line of responding can help emphasize mindfulness as a process.

Asking some variant of the question "What happened next?" can also be useful here. When clients "fail" to achieve their expected outcome (i.e., their mind wanders elsewhere), it's not uncommon for them to "give up" and stop practicing. Through this line of questioning, we hope to normalize attention-wandering, the appearance of judgmental thoughts, and the tendency to act on our thoughts, while also opening up possibilities they may not have considered (i.e., we can guide our attention back to our breath once more).

 BOX 6.3. TO SUMMARIZE:
Ways to Explore Mindfulness Practice Early in Therapy

- Ask questions like "What did you notice?" and "What happened next?"
- Validate all observations.
- Cultivate compassion for the challenge of internal experiences like busy minds.
- Connect experience and challenges with presenting concerns.
  - Identify judgments that arise.
- When clients experience a sense of being calm, relaxed, or centered, highlight ways of responding to internal experiences that may have been different from usual patterns and connect them to ongoing practice and treatment.
- When clients describe an inability to be mindful, try to identify moments of awareness and opportunities to return to practice.
- Underscore mindfulness as a process and suggest that it is possible to return to the practice at any point.

Finally, postpractice exploration sometimes reveals that clients had a moment of mindfulness without realizing it. If they say, for instance, "I couldn't focus on my breath at all," we might ask, "When did you first notice that you weren't focused on your breath?," emphasizing that the noticing itself is part of the practice. Sometimes clients are aware during their practice that their attention shifted, but they don't know how to respond, or they feel stuck. In those cases, we point out that noticing is a core feature of mindfulness, one that is a first step toward change. We also normalize how natural it is in those moments to feel discouraged and stuck and how reasonable it can be to want to stop practicing. Again, we connect their observations to their presenting challenges, noting that although they have come to recognize patterns that have been really bothering them, which is an important step toward change, that recognition in and of itself has been painful. And we validate how disheartening it can be, especially if we are not clear on what specifically we might do differently, or we struggle with establishing a new habit. In these instances, we review the skills to be practiced—noticing, recognizing the humanness of our responses, and practicing compassion—and remind clients that developing new skills takes patience and practice. Please see Box 6.3 for a brief summary of how to explore mindfulness early in therapy.

Psychoeducation about Mindfulness

After clients have engaged in one or two formal mindfulness practices (typically, mindfulness of breath and the raisin—or some other edible object—exercise), so that they have an experience of mindfulness, we typically introduce the concept of mindfulness more formally, focusing on the skills we are trying to cultivate with these practices.[4] We often send them home with a brief description (Client Handout 6.1). We then give a simpler handout with mindfulness skills listed (Client Handout 6.2) and review the skills of awareness, curiosity, acceptance, and self-compassion and care in session.

Sometimes clients respond to psychoeducation by explaining that they are already extremely aware of their internal experiences and in fact came to treatment to be less aware. We validate that perception, while also using examples from clients' assessment or ongoing self-monitoring to highlight the ways in which the *quality* of awareness in mindfulness practice is different. For example, we might choose an example of a time a client's awareness was narrowed on potential threats or failures and contrast that with the spacious awareness cultivated in mindfulness. In describing how bringing curiosity to their experiences may be different, we remind them of how their *observations* and *experiences* while eating mindfully (i.e., eating an object like a raisin or mint as if you've

---

[4] Alternatively, depending on context, therapists could avoid using the term *mindfulness* initially, or at all, and instead talk about cultivating skills of awareness, acceptance, and compassion. In *WLLM*, in order to reach the broadest audience, including people who might have a negative reaction to the concept of mindfulness, we introduced the concepts of awareness and acceptance, as well as many practices to cultivate these skills, before we turned to a discussion of mindfulness and connected it to those skills. In their brief intervention for racism-related stress, Martinez (in Martinez & Roemer, 2019) chose the term *compassionate awareness* to avoid negative connotations of mindfulness. On the other hand, as described earlier, Harrell (2018) proposes an approach specific to people of African descent that uses the term *soulfulness* and connects mindfulness principles to Afrocentric cultural principles. In a qualitative study (Watson-Singleton, Black, & Spivey, 2019), African American women suggested the terms *awareness, relaxation,* or *mindful* in place of *meditation.*

never seen it before—looking at, feeling, smelling, and tasting it as if for the first time; Segal et al., 2013) were different from their past eating experiences and their expectations of what eating would be like. We also describe what this skill might look like in their daily lives. For example, we often use the example of how easy it is for us to fall into the habit of not fully attending to a conversation with a familiar family member. It's natural to tune out a bit because we think we already know how the conversation will go based on our history with that person, but the experience can be very different if we attend to and hear each comment, seeing each subtle change in facial expression and tone as if for the first time. By intentionally bringing curiosity and a beginner's mind to these kinds of situations, we can be more open to what is actually happening in the moment and can have a more expanded experience rather than one dictated by our own reactions and expectations. Finally, we distinguish between the type of critical, judgmental awareness the client may currently have of their internal experience and the compassionate one we aim to cultivate. Developing a compassionate, instead of critical or judgmental response, is a particularly challenging mindfulness skill that we address in more detail in Chapter 7.

 BOX 6.4. A CLOSER LOOK:
How Mindfulness Is Related to Relaxation Training

Clients (and therapists) often wonder how mindfulness practices relate to various relaxation strategies. In theory, relaxation strategies and mindfulness practices have different goals in that relaxation is typically aimed at reducing anxiety and discomfort, while mindfulness is aimed at noticing things as they are. However, in practice, they can be more similar than they may seem. First, as noted earlier, clients often experience relaxation while they are practicing mindfulness (e.g., Spears et al., 2017). And similarly, clients using a relaxation strategy like progressive muscle relaxation (PMR; Jacobson, 1934), which involves noticing signs of tension as they arise, often report increased present-moment awareness and relating differently to their internal experiences (e.g., with curiosity or self-compassion; see Hayes-Skelton, Roemer, Orsillo, & Borkovec, 2013). In our randomized clinical trial comparing ABBT with applied relaxation, we found that, similar to clients receiving ABBT, clients receiving applied relaxation demonstrated significant increases in mindfulness skills over time. These increases were related to clinical outcomes (Eustis, Morgan, Hayes-Skelton, & Roemer, 2017).

As we describe in Chapter 5 regarding emotion regulation strategies more broadly, we recommend using slightly altered instructions for relaxation strategies in order to reduce the risk that efforts to reduce anxiety or quiet the mind might have paradoxical effects. Instead, we emphasize the process of observing one's experience while slowing one's breath (for diaphragmatic breathing) or tensing and releasing one's muscles (for PMR*) and allowing the process to unfold however it does. Sometimes clients may experience a reduction in anxiety, which can help with spacious awareness, and other mindfulness skills. Other times, clients may find their minds get busier or they feel more tension in their bodies. This can provide an opportunity to practice a different response to internal experiences—acceptance and self-compassion. As with any emotion regulation strategy, we emphasize the importance of not attaching to an outcome of reduction in distress, instead focusing on living a meaningful, engaged life regardless of the thoughts, feelings, and sensations that arise. Relaxation strategies may facilitate awareness and help clients to take intentional actions that matter to them.

*Recordings of our guidance in PMR are available on the Guilford website (see the box at the end of the table of contents).

Misunderstandings of Acceptance or Mindfulness

Clients often have misconceptions and misunderstandings about what we mean when we talk about acceptance during mindfulness practices, so we explicitly address this issue in psychoeducation (see Table 6.1).

A useful metaphor for explaining acceptance is the tug-of-war metaphor in ACT (Hayes et al., 2012). We tell clients that a natural response to any kind of distress is to try to change and alter it, but this can leave us engaged in a constant battle with distress. If we imagine our distress holding one end of a rope and us the other, our natural instinct would be to brace our feet and pull back to resist it. This pulling can seem like the only option we have to stop the monster from overtaking us, but it causes tension in our body and blisters on our hands, requires our full attention, and prevents us from doing anything else. Acceptance is dropping the rope. We don't have to keep battling with the distress monster. We can drop the fight, accept that these thoughts, feelings, sensations, and images are what's here right now, and then decide how we want to respond.

> Part III focuses on how we help clients choose their actions in the face of distress, after they've "dropped the rope."

ABBT therapists begin assessing clients' reactions to the idea of mindfulness during treatment planning and continue to elicit and address questions and concerns during psychoeducation. When clients have previous experience with mindfulness-based practices, we encourage them to draw from their past experiences while also attending to ways that their past use of mindfulness may differ from our intended use. This is particularly relevant when clients have used mindfulness as a way of taking a break

TABLE 6.1. Clarification of the Nature of Acceptance

Acceptance is *not* ...	Acceptance is ...
Liking things as they are.	Recognizing that things are as they are.
Resigning oneself to things always being this way.	Recognizing the way things are in this very moment and noticing subtle variability in our experiences.
	Recognizing that trying to fight thoughts, feelings, and sensations that arise often makes them worse.
Complacency.	Recognizing that our thoughts, emotions, and sensations don't dictate our behavior.
Passive.	A word that stems from the Middle English root *kap,* meaning to take, seize, or catch[a]—actively entering into the reality of what is.
Something we achieve.	A continually evolving process: the thoughts, memories, and judgments we have are learned and elicited automatically by internal and external cues. Our ways of responding to them are learned as well. Each moment offers a new opportunity to notice our experience and practice cultivating an accepting process. Engaging in the act of noticing and cultivation is the goal, not an end-state of ongoing acceptance.

[a]Sanderson and Linehan (1999; cited in Robins, Schmidt, & Linehan, 2004).

from their lives; we emphasize that our approach is to use mindfulness to more fully engage in lives instead.

Clients may also hold preconceived notions of what mindfulness is that make them hesitant to engage in practice. Sometimes clients are concerned about the connection between mindfulness and Buddhism, and they worry that practicing mindfulness could be inconsistent with their own religious traditions and beliefs. We discuss the role of mindfulness or awareness in different religious traditions as well as our use of mindfulness within a secular rather than a religious context. Clients are often able to find their own connections between aspects of their personal religious or spiritual practice and the principles of mindfulness relevant to ABBT.

As we noted earlier, we address the common misperception that mindfulness involves clearing the mind or relaxing, and we suggest that being aware in the moment has benefits even when it is also painful or challenging. Although it is important for clients to consider this possibility, raising it requires considerable clinical sensitivity particularly with clients facing major challenges such as chronic illness, exposure to trauma, or systemic discrimination or oppression. It's important to be clear that mindfulness can allow us to be more skillful and effective in response to these situations (e.g., King, 2018). Specifically, mindfulness can interrupt the cycles of self-judgment, criticism, and experiential avoidance that intensify reactions and make it harder to intentionally choose how to respond.

Early on and throughout treatment, we emphasize that mindfulness, like acceptance, is a process. Returning to our awareness is the action of mindfulness; it is irrelevant how many times our attention wanders, only that we again return. To illustrate this concept, we sometimes quote the traditional Zen saying, "fall down seven times, get up eight." Similarly, we return to compassion repeatedly rather than reaching some kind of steady state of compassion that never wavers. For each moment of judgment, we have the opportunity to practice nonjudgment. Thus, each perceived "failure" at mindfulness is simply an opportunity to practice again.

Progression of Specific Formal Practices[5]

As we noted earlier, consistent with many other mindfulness- and acceptance-based approaches, we typically introduce mindfulness practices following a standard progression. In these practices, clients begin with breathing and other sensory-based exercises, move on to the challenges of noticing emotions and thoughts, and then engage in practices that cultivate awareness of a transcendence of fusing the self with thoughts and feelings. Given that the function of the practices is more important than the form, to enhance our clients' autonomy and flexibility, we introduce them to multiple methods of cultivating mindfulness and encourage them to adopt the practices they find most relevant, effective, and feasible. We may adapt practices for the spaces clients inhabit (e.g., encouraging them to notice how different muscles tense and release to help you maintain balance on a subway train as it accelerates and slows down; Kaplan, 2010), using images that are more resonant in imaginal practice. For instance, urban instead of rural images are used for clients for whom those will be more accessible, and we

---

[5] As noted previously, audio recordings of these mindfulness exercises are available on the Guilford website (see the box at the end of the table of contents).

consider images and practices that involve families or other people rather than solitary images for those with more collectivist orientations (LaRoche, D'Angelo, Gualdron, & Leavell, 2006).

We try to choose initial practices that our clients will be willing to try. For example, in our research studies treating clients with GAD, one of our earliest mindfulness practices is a modified version of progressive muscle relaxation (PMR). We did *not* choose this practice with the goal of helping clients to achieve a particular level of calmness or to avoid distress. In fact, the mindful, nonjudgmental, nonavoidant experience of physical sensations and distressing thoughts and feelings is a central goal of these methods. However, similar to exposure exercises, mindfulness practices aren't helpful if clients aren't willing to use them. Whereas clients with GAD might find it initially intolerable to focus on their breath for 20 minutes, many are willing to tense and release different muscle groups while observing the sensations associated with those actions if they are guided through the experience with verbal prompts. Thus, choices about the nature and order of the practices are informed by general and client-specific hypotheses about how to keep clients fully engaged in practice and minimize distraction or premature termination.

Once clients complete the progression, we return to practices that represent particular challenges or develop new, individually tailored exercises to meet clients' specific needs. We also have clients select the exercises they want to focus on for a particular week or that they want to make part of their regular practice in order to encourage clients to develop their own mindfulness practices, which they will continue after the end of treatment (as discussed more fully in Chapter 11).

Mindfulness of Breath, Eating, and Sensations

As we noted earlier, we typically use a breath and an eating exercise as ways of experientially introducing clients to mindfulness practice. With anxious clients, we sometimes adapt diaphragmatic breathing, emphasizing the process of noticing and curiosity, rather than changing experience, just as we do with PMR. First, we have clients simply observe their breath, noticing whatever arises. Often clients will notice a tightness in their chests, shortness of breath, or anxious thoughts. We validate these observations as natural parts of the process, ask clients to gently shift their breath so that it starts lower down, in their diaphragm, and observe the effects of this shift.[6] Alternatively, we might simply guide clients through an awareness of breath exercise (see Appendix B for an example or listen to the recording on the Guilford website [see the box at the end of the table of contents]). Sometimes, early in practice, it can be helpful for clients to count

---

[6]This type of instruction is not typical of mindfulness/acceptance-based strategies. We are adapting relaxation instructions (Bernstein, Borkovec, & Hazlett-Stevens, 2000) with demonstrated efficacy, particularly with generally anxious clients, so that our clients can potentially benefit from this activation of the parasympathetic nervous system, while also noticing their responses and practicing a nonjudgmental response to them. We predict that they may actually experience increased anxiety or have difficulty following the instructions. In all cases, they are asked to practice allowing whatever is, while gently altering their breath. We feel this instruction in gentle change helps clients with high levels of anxious arousal or tension to more fully engage in awareness of breath (which otherwise can generate such heightened judgment and anxiety sensitivity that clients have difficulty complying with instructions).

their breaths, if they find that their minds are wandering a great deal. Again, alterations are particularly important in the early stages of treatment to enhance willingness and engagement.

We often use a mindful eating practice at this stage, helping clients bring a "beginner's mind" to the activity (Segal et al., 2013). Clients are guided through very slowly eating a familiar object (e.g., raisin, mint), as if they had never seen it before. They begin by looking at the object carefully, from all angles, and then they move on to touching it and smelling it. They next place the object in their mouths, noticing their responses and the urge to chew or swallow. Finally, they slowly chew and swallow the object, attending to all their sensations, thoughts, and reactions as they do so. After the exercise, we take time to review clients' experiences of this exercise afterward, which typically evolves into a discussion of how different it would be to do daily tasks (like washing the dishes, eating, brushing our teeth, or even facing challenges) with this type of awareness, curiosity, and "beginner's mind."

As discussed earlier, we use a modified version of progressive muscle relaxation (Bernstein et al., 2000) with our generally anxious clients. In these exercises, we emphasize drawing attention to the sensations associated with both tensing and releasing each muscle group and allowing whatever response to occur. Similar to our use of diaphragmatic breathing, this is a somewhat unusual mindfulness exercise because it includes an action that may actively change the client's experience (tensing and releasing muscles can relax muscles). However, we find that integration of this empirically supported strategy for generalized anxiety disorder helps our clients to broaden their experience (by introducing a more relaxed response into what is typically a rigid, habitual experience of tension), while also allowing whatever arises. We are careful not to suggest that the exercise will result in relaxation and to encourage clients to notice whatever occurs. The experience of noticing the sensations of tension and then "letting go" of tension can serve as a useful metaphor for how clients might start noticing and allowing thoughts, emotions, and sensations in their daily lives. However, we generally prefer to use the phrase "letting it be" when referring to the general practice of allowing challenging experiences to be present. We do so because "letting go" sometimes conveys the expectation that experiences will "leave" or change if we just stop struggling with them, which isn't always the case. We recommend that clients practice PMR at home between sessions, gradually reducing the number of muscle groups, so that it becomes a briefer and eventually an applied exercise. (Recordings of these exercises are available on the Guilford website [see the box at the end of the table of contents]). In mindfulness-based stress reduction (MBSR) and MBCT, practitioners use a body scan as a lengthy sensory practice.

Other useful sensory practices include mindfulness of sounds (Segal et al., 2013) and mindfulness of physical sensations. These practices guide clients through awareness of sounds and physical sensations just as they are, without judging them or trying to change them. In these practices, clients often notice how frequently we name and judge our experiences as soon as they register ("annoying truck" instead of "loud beeping sound," "irritating mosquito bite" instead of "prickly sensation"). This observation helps build understanding and compassion for our judging habit and makes it easier to notice judgments in other contexts.

Mindfulness of Emotions and Thoughts

Once clients have some practice in intentionally shifting their attention toward their sensations and senses, and coinciding with the delivery of psychoeducation about thoughts and emotions, we introduce some more challenging practices focused on emotions and thoughts. We frequently use an exercise that invites clients to recall an emotional event in their recent experience and practice an expansive awareness of their full range of emotional responses to this event. Clients are asked to notice where emotions are felt in their body, the ways emotions may change over time, and urges to change or get rid of the emotions.

Initially, we have clients choose a moderately distressing past experience as a means of maximizing the likelihood that they will be willing to remain aware of the emotions throughout the exercise. Over time, we practice in session with more emotionally evocative, recent events, and we encourage clients to practice on their own when events in their daily lives elicit strong emotional responses.

This practice can help clients to notice that their emotional responses are more varied and nuanced than they originally seemed. For instance, Sondra was aware of a high level of anxiety and worry for her daughter Julia's safety when Julia won an opportunity to go on a trip for a sports competition. During this exercise, Sondra noticed that she also felt pride and happiness at Julia's success. Although this observation didn't eliminate Sondra's fear, it reminded her why she might want Julia to go on the trip despite these fears. Sometimes clients learn that painful emotions that initially seem unrelenting actually come and go, rising and falling in intensity, an observation that may make them seem less frightening. Or clients may notice that a strong and painful emotion they thought was "intolerable" can in fact be tolerated or allowed. These experiences weaken learned avoidant and escape responses to emotional experience, opening up the possibility that one could engage in meaningful activities even if challenging emotions might be elicited. Linking these observations to clients' presenting problems helps them see how these skills would apply to their daily lives.

Clients can also practice mindfulness of emotions using the *Mindfulness of Current Emotions* handout from DBT (Linehan, 2015). This handout instructs clients to observe their emotion by stepping back and noticing it, experiencing it as a wave, coming and going, and imagine surfing it. They are encouraged not to block, suppress, or try to get rid of the emotion, and also not to try to keep it around, hold on to it, or amplify it. They are instructed to *remember* to not necessarily act on emotion and to remember times they have felt different. Finally, they can *practice* loving their emotion by not judging it, practicing willingness, and accepting it. The "Guest House" by Rumi (see Box 6.5) can also be used to practice a new way of relating to emotions.

In addition to using language conventions in session to promote decentering and defusion (as described in Chapter 4), various mindfulness practices can be shared with clients to help them have the experience of noticing thoughts without getting caught up with them. We've adapted the clouds exercise from DBT to help clients develop this skill (see Appendix B for the script and listen to the audio recording on the Guilford website [see the box at the end of the table of contents]). A similar exercise from ACT, "Leaves on a Stream," can also be used for this purpose. Other images like watching thoughts on a conveyor belt or traveling across a movie screen may be used if they have greater resonance with clients.

BOX 6.5. TRY THIS:
Relating Differently to Emotions

To give you some practice relating differently to your emotions, we encourage you to take a moment to practice mindfulness of emotions using the poem "The Guest House." We, along with many other mindfulness-based practitioners (e.g., Segal et al., 2013), use this poem in treatment to offer a different perspective on responding to emotional challenges. Take a moment now to first notice how you're sitting, and bring your awareness to your breath, and then slowly read the poem, noticing what it evokes for you.

> This being human is a guest house.
> Every morning a new arrival.
>
> A joy, a depression, a meanness,
> Some momentary awareness comes
> as an unexpected visitor.
>
> Welcome and entertain them all!
> Even if they're a crowd of sorrows,
> who violently sweep your house
> empty of its furniture,
>
> still treat each guest honorably.
> He may be clearing you out
> for some new delight.
>
> The dark thought, the shame, the malice.
> meet them at the door laughing,
> And invite them in.
>
> Be grateful for whoever comes,
> because each has been sent
> as a guide from beyond.
>
> —RUMI

Did you notice yourself initially reacting with surprise or reluctance when you were told to welcome experiences such as depression, shame, or malice? Did the opposite action of welcoming them, rather than pushing them away, lead to a moment of openness or relief? Often clients report these kinds of experiences and, after practicing repeatedly with the poem, say that they remember it during emotional times and that they use it as a reminder that they do not have to push experiences away and instead can allow and make room for them. This helps to promote a new response that can reduce reactivity, judgment, and struggling with emotions.

Note. Copyright © Coleman Barks. Reprinted by permission.

BOX 6.6. A CLOSER LOOK:
Mindfulness and Acceptance versus Cognitive Therapy

People often draw contrasts between cognitive therapy and mindfulness- and acceptance-based behavioral therapies, emphasizing that the former focus on changing the content of thoughts, while the latter focus on changing the way people relate to their thoughts. This is a useful way to think about what may be an important distinction between the two. However, in reality, these approaches do overlap, so noting their commonalities is beneficial. Both cognitive therapies and ABBTs promote *decentering* or seeing thoughts as thoughts (Safran & Segal, 1990), and evidence suggests that decentering is a mechanism of change in both traditional cognitive therapy and mindfulness-based cognitive therapy (e.g., Fresco, Segal, Buis, & Kennedy, 2007; Segal et al., 2019). (Interestingly, decentering emerges as a mechanism of change in both ABBT and applied relaxation for GAD as well; Hayes-Skelton et al., 2015). In both approaches, monitoring thoughts and identifying them as thoughts is one strategy to promote decentering. In cognitive therapy, other strategies like identifying cognitive errors and restructuring thoughts to be more realistic are an integral part of therapy, while in ABBT these strategies are not typically used. Instead, the emphasis is on acknowledging that our minds produce both factual and inaccurate thoughts due to our learning and life experiences and on encouraging meaningful actions even when our thoughts recommend avoidance. Nonetheless, clients who broaden their attention beyond threat cues or self-judgments through mindfulness practice may certainly come to make more realistic assessments. The process of labeling and challenging thoughts may be one path to learning that thoughts are just thoughts and not enduring truths. Therefore, similar to the ways that relaxation strategies might be adapted and used within an ABBT approach, some cognitive therapy strategies might be adapted to enhance decentering and engagement in valued action. Again, an internally consistent case conceptualization and the selection of strategies based on their function rather than form should guide treatment.

For clients who initially found mindfulness practices relaxing, mindfulness of emotions and thoughts can raise some new challenges. As always, experiences like maintaining awareness and reactivity to thoughts and emotions can be connected to presenting concerns and new ways of responding linked to treatment goals. These practices can be explicitly linked to observations that are emerging on monitoring forms, while monitoring may be facilitated by developing these skills through practice. This is also the point in treatment when we might begin to talk more explicitly about clients starting to use language that defuses their experiences such as "I'm having the thought that I can't succeed at anything" or "I noticed feelings of anger arising" (Hayes et al., 2012). We also introduce exercises explicitly focused on self-compassion, which we describe in Chapter 7.

Mindfulness Practices That Promote a Sense of the Transience of Experiences and Sense of Self

The final exercises in our typical progression bring the multiple aspects of mindfulness (awareness of the breath, sensations, thoughts, feelings) together, highlighting the overall transience of human experience. The *observer-self exercise* from ACT (Hayes et al.,

2012) systematically takes clients through each aspect of their experience, noticing the ways that no specific sensation, feeling, or thought is constant or defining. This exercise highlights the ways that some aspect of our personhood exists beyond the experiences we have in a given moment and labels it the observer self. Kabat-Zinn (1994) describes several meditation exercises that similarly evoke an experience of the transient nature of our experience. We often use the seated version, the *mountain meditation;* a standing and lying-down meditation (tree meditation and lake meditation) with similar themes are also available in Kabat-Zinn (1994). These meditations often allow clients to develop a vivid image that they can recall in difficult situations to remind them at an experiential level of the transience of their experience and their ability to transcend whatever distressing responses emerge for them.

Although many of our clients really connect to the mountain meditation and evoke the image of a mountain when they are distressed, finding an inner strength and stillness in the midst of external challenges and surface storms, other clients struggle to relate the image to their experience, and still others have found the meditation unhelpful. For example, some clients have shared with us their experience that embodying a mountain leaves them feeling stuck and immovable. As always, therapists should be culturally and clinically sensitive and responsive in their choice and adaptation of imaginal mindfulness practices.

One aspect of these practices that can be clinically useful is their illustration of how clients are not simply defined by their thoughts, reactions, feelings, or sensations. The observer-self exercise and mountain meditation both evoke a sense of transcendent observer of these experiences who is distinct from the content-driven self with which clients so often identify. This sense allows clients to disentangle from ideas of themselves that have developed over their lifetimes, such as "I am a nervous wreck" or "I always fail at things," and potentially act in ways that are inconsistent with these definitions of self. For instance, a client can have the thought that she is unassertive while she clearly communicates her needs to someone.

Connecting Practice to Goals of Therapy after Repeated Practice

As clients continue to engage in a range of mindfulness practices, what clients can learn from their experience and connect to their lives expands. The initial benefits (summarized in Box 6.7) remain.

> **BOX 6.7.** Early (and Ongoing) Lessons Learned from Mindfulness Practice
>
> Observing experiences while engaging in a range of mindfulness practices helps clients to:
>
> - Notice the nature of their experiences,
> - Recognize the humanness and naturalness of these experiences,
> - Cultivate compassion and understanding for their habits of responding, and
> - Learn that mindfulness is a process.

As practice deepens, clients will also learn that:

- The process of being aware in the moment can become more habitual after continual practice so that it is easier to bring awareness, even in the midst of challenging experiences.
- The process of being aware can be rewarding, even if the content of one's thoughts, emotions, or sensations is judged as "unpleasant." Even though we have a natural tendency to want to avoid unpleasant thoughts and feelings, turning toward and noticing them can actually feel like a relief. And when that content is an important part of our experience (e.g., noticing sadness when sitting with a family member who is terminally ill), being aware and present can honor the meaningfulness of that experience.
- When we observe our experiences with curiosity, we can see the transient, nondefining nature of these experiences and gradually become more decentered from them.
- The aspect of mindfulness that we experience as calming actually comes from dropping the struggle with our experience. Paradoxically, when we no longer fight against the stress we are experiencing, we can often discover a calmness. Of course, the trick is that we can't try to force this experience by falsely letting go of the struggle in order to make our distress go away. Instead, truly allowing our current experience often reduces the diffuse distress of that experience.[7]

This learning helps clients to develop a different relationship to their internal experiences, one that is more willing and accepting, and prepares them to be able to make intentional choices that are consistent with what matters to them and to notice the impact of these actions in order to evaluate whether they want to continue to act in these ways.

The following discussion between Betty and her therapist about Betty's experience with mindfulness of thoughts and emotions in session and in her home practice illustrates how a therapist can help clients to consolidate their experiential learning from practices and apply it to meeting their treatment goals. Betty presented for treatment with a lot of reactivity to her physical sensations, including catastrophizing that they might be signs of a serious illness. This pattern of responding led her to frequently worry about her health and spend time monitoring and reading health information on the Internet instead of engaging in activities that might be rewarding, leading to feelings of sadness and loneliness. Betty's goals were to increase her engagement in meaningful activities and to learn how to respond to her physical sensations and worries in ways that didn't escalate her distress as much. After she practiced mindfulness of clouds and sky in session, she and her therapist explored her experiences during this practice, her home practice, and how they related to her presenting problems.

THERAPIST: What did you notice?

BETTY: Well, the first thing I noticed was that it was easier to settle into the practice

---

[7]One way we think of this phenomenon is to recognize that letting go of the struggle reduces the muddiness of our emotions. Clear pain may remain, but it will be less intense and long-lasting because the struggle has been muddying our response and maintaining it.

and start to see my thoughts and feelings as being on clouds instead of defining me. I remember how hard that was for me at first. But after a few minutes I got a little lost. I think I stopped having thoughts.

THERAPIST: Sounds like you had a few different observations. Let's take them one at a time. So, you noticed this experience was different from other times you've tried this practice? Great observation. What else did you notice?

BETTY: It felt nice, kind of a sense of relief as I could see that thoughts like "My throat feels tight" were just thoughts and not an early sign of something terrible happening. And then I started to wonder why I can't always see that and why I sometimes get so wrapped up in my worries.

THERAPIST: Minds can be so predictable in that way—one minute we are observing and noticing thoughts and the next judgmental thoughts appear and start competing for our attention and drawing us in. It sounds like first you noticed some judgments that this was a good experience. And some wondering thoughts that were maybe judgments too? And some predictions about the future?

BETTY: I didn't really see my wondering as judgments or thoughts when they came up—I can see it now that you say it. There was definitely some self-criticism in my wondering.

THERAPIST: That makes sense—it's always a bit easier to see once we have some distance. Were there emotions and sensations noticeable to you?

BETTY: Yes, definitely. My throat got even tighter, and I felt a little anxious and sad.

THERAPIST: What happened next?

BETTY: Well, like I said, I didn't see those judgments as thoughts, so I definitely didn't place them on clouds. And once I started wondering, I lost my focus a bit, so I didn't put those sensations and feelings on clouds either.

THERAPIST: Of course, that makes sense.

BETTY: I did notice the sky was all clouds, and I remembered us talking about how we all have those moments when there's no sky to be seen and it's just a swirl of clouds of thoughts and feelings that we're tangled in. And, I actually was able to notice that, and I think I brought some compassion to myself in that moment. I think it helps that you're here because I remember how you always say how hard it is to be a human with this busy mind. And I could feel that—it's hard to have a mind that cycles so quickly.

THERAPIST: So, even though it was hard to see thoughts as thoughts in that moment, or to notice specific judgments, sensations, and emotions, you were able to notice some pain and to bring some self-compassion.

BETTY: Yes. It didn't make the pain go away, but it did feel like less of a struggle.

THERAPIST: It sounds like you were able to use a few different mindfulness skills here, which is really wonderful. And I think you are right—your ability to do that is definitely related to the fact that we have been practicing together for some time now and you've worked hard to learn a lot about your experience, habits, and options. It's nice to take a minute to really notice that. I want to ask a bit more about the observation you made about me being here. It sounds like you are having thoughts that practices are easier in session. How has your home practice been?

BETTY: It's mixed. I'm still struggling with making time to practice. But when I do practice, I have different experiences. Sometimes I'm really able to see the sky and the thoughts, sensations, and feelings I'm having seem less overwhelming or encompassing. And sometimes it's hard to stay focused on the practice, and I find myself focusing on sensations in my body, or my worries.

THERAPIST: I definitely understand the constraints on your time. Maybe we can revisit your schedule together and see if we can find some ways to weave practice into your daily life without putting too much more on your plate. I also want to say it's completely natural to have variability in your practice. Even therapists who write books about mindfulness struggle with busy, judging minds. Do you think it would be helpful for us to walk through a practice at home you found difficult?

BETTY: Sometimes I feel like I don't want to dwell on the negative. And I am proud of myself for the improvements I've made. So, I like to share those moments with you.

THERAPIST: Of course. I completely agree that recognizing the time you've put in and acknowledging the changes you've made is important. It's a helpful reminder that although life happens and we all experience a range of experiences and emotions, we aren't just passive recipients. There are choices we can make and actions we can choose that can have an impact. And it's nice to celebrate that.

BETTY: On the other hand, I did find talking through today's practice helpful. Even though my first reaction was that I was bummed we focused on what I did wrong (*catching self*) . . . wait, that's just a judgment. And it's also natural for me to feel a little sad when I reflect on how hard these habits of the mind can be.

THERAPIST: Nice work! So, what do you think about us making time to both recognize skills you've used in a particular week (and celebrate them) and to explore moments you struggled as opportunities to both practice self-compassion and brainstorm new responses you can try out.

BETTY: Sounds like a plan. Oh, I just remembered a moment I wanted to share.

THERAPIST: Great, tell me about it.

BETTY: I had this moment a couple of days ago when I was noticing the tightness in my throat, and I started to focus my attention on the sensations. I caught myself and decided to go visit with my neighbor instead. While we were drinking coffee, I noticed the weather on television and saw that the pollen count is high. That recognition made the sensations feel less scary.

THERAPIST: Interesting. So, broadening your attention changed the impact of the sensation?

BETTY: Yeah, it was kind of nice. But of course thoughts that I had throat cancer came back later.

THERAPIST: Of course, that's how minds work. That's why mindfulness is a practice we develop and not a goal we achieve.

BETTY: Exactly. I should make that a notification on my phone that pops up throughout my day.

THERAPIST: Great idea!

INFORMAL PRACTICE

In the last example, Betty's therapist mentions the potential usefulness of revisiting how Betty might integrate mindfulness into her daily life. This application of mindfulness skills into a client's everyday experience is an essential part of ABBT, and we are explicit with clients in our view that formal practices are all in the service of applying mindfulness to daily life.[8] We suggest that clients start this application by bringing mindfulness to neutral activities, like washing the dishes or taking a shower. In other words, they practice noticing the sensations that arise as they engage in the activity, noticing their minds wandering, and then gently bringing their awareness back to the task at hand. Initial practices could involve any number of activities such as:

- Washing dishes
- Shoveling snow
- Tending to a garden or farm
- Folding clothes
- Changing a light bulb
- Fixing something
- Brushing teeth
- Shaving

- Riding the bus or subway
- Waiting for the bus
- Walking
- Cooking
- Eating a meal
- Quilting
- Knitting
- Shelling peas[9]

Over time, we encourage clients to bring their awareness to more challenging daily activities, such as job interviews, challenging conversations with family members, or parenting situations. We also encourage clients to bring mindfulness to their valued actions as they engage in them. This is a particularly important application: sometimes clients have been engaging in things that matter to them, but they are distracted or are multitasking and so aren't fully experiencing them in the moment. For these clients, applications of mindfulness may be more important than behavior change. For those who have been avoiding engaging in meaningful actions, applied mindfulness helps to promote the new learning that emerges from trying new behaviors and allows them to determine which actions are satisfying and meaningful.

Informal practice is particularly important when clients struggle with finding time for formal practice because of busy lives (e.g., caring for small children or ill or aging family members, working and going to school, or working multiple jobs). We work

---

[8]This is similar to the approach in applied relaxation, in which we teach relaxation formally, but the eventual aim is to apply these strategies in anxious situations (e.g., Bernstein et al., 2000).

[9]The last three examples come from Woods-Giscombé and Gaylord (2014).

> **BOX 6.8. A CLOSER LOOK:**
> How Does Mindfulness Practice Relate to Outcomes?
>
> The research on the association between mindfulness practice and outcome across a range of acceptance and mindfulness approaches has yielded disparate outcomes. A systematic review of a broad range of mindfulness programs found that half of the studies revealed a significant relationship between formal practice and outcome, while half didn't (Vettese, Toneatto, Stea, Nguyen, & Wang, 2009). A recent meta-analysis of MBCT and MBSR studies did reveal a small to moderate association between (formal) home practice and outcome among trials with standard home practice assignments (which are considerably lengthier than what we assign in our approach), but they were unable to explore this association among trials with reduced recommended practice (Parsons, Crane, Parsons, Fjorback, & Kuyken, 2017). In our own trials of ABBT for GAD, we found that reports of informal, but not formal, practice were significantly associated with maintenance of clinical gains over a follow-up period (Morgan, Graham, Hayes-Skelton, Orsillo, & Roemer, 2014). A recent study of the broader construct of "therapy-acquired regulatory skills" across both MBCT and cognitive therapy found that practice of these skills (which included formal and informal practice in the MBCT group) during the follow-up period was indirectly associated with reduced risk of relapse/recurrence through the association of practice with increased decentering skills (Segal et al., 2019). Authors consistently note that quality of practice may be more important than quantity (e.g., Morgan et al., 2014; Parsons et al., 2017). Taken together, these findings suggest that encouraging informal practice when clients are not able to maintain a formal practice may still be beneficial, particularly when these practices cultivate skills such as decentering.

with clients to try to find potentially overlooked moments that can be used for formal practice (e.g., practicing mindfulness of breath during the subway ride to school), but we also acknowledge real external constraints and help clients to identify some daily activities during which skills can be practiced. (We have seen clients develop strong mindfulness skills through this kind of consistent informal practice and then be able to apply those skills to more challenging situations.)

OBSTACLES IN CULTIVATING MINDFULNESS AND ACCEPTANCE

Mindfulness Is Practiced as a Way to Avoid Distress

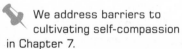

We address barriers to cultivating self-compassion in Chapter 7.

As we noted earlier, clients often find the practice of mindfulness pleasant or relaxing, and can begin to engage in these practices in order to alleviate their distress. We validate the inevitability of enjoying that consequence and highlight the cost of clinging to that outcome. We encourage clients to be present to whatever emerges from their practice, to notice when they begin to judge an outcome as more or less desirable, and to gently let go of that judgment and return to the experience itself. Clients will usually notice variability in their responses to their practice, providing an opportunity to observe the effects of wishing for one outcome when another occurs. This observation sometimes allows clients to see, and develop compassion for the fact, that our desire to reduce distress can actually escalate distress if we hold it too tightly. Instead, clients might consider "inviting" distress and their reactions to it to "sit next to" them, while they continue with their practice.

If clients are repeatedly experiencing mindfulness practice as pleasant, we will invite them to practice mindfulness in more distressing contexts in order to ensure that they also have experiences during the course of therapy in which mindfulness is difficult or challenging, rather than having these experiences emerge as obstacles following termination. Mindful emotion practice provides an excellent opportunity to practice with distressing responses, as does informal mindful practice as challenging emotional contexts arise during their lives. Also, when clients begin to engage in valued actions (as described in the next chapters), they often find that they experience increased distress and emotional arousal, leading to more challenging mindfulness practice.

Some clients begin to use mindfulness practice as another form of experiential avoidance. For example, Steve frequently retreated from challenging conversations with family, even though those relationships were personally meaningful to him, and so he sought out stress-free spaces in which he could listen to his favorite recording of a guided breathing exercise. Although his therapist recognized that this avoidance was problematic, her initial attempt to address this issue with Steve was unsuccessful, likely because she focused on efforts to "convince" him that mindfulness should sometimes be difficult. The most effective way to work with this issue is to draw out the clients' own observations to highlight the ways in which avoidance is only temporarily attenuating distress and also interfering with their quality of life. We may also remind clients that although getting a respite from their lives for a brief time can seem restorative, it doesn't produce the kinds of lasting changes they sought treatment to make.

Mindfulness Seems Invalidating

Some clients grappling with significant life stressors (e.g., parenting a child with a terminal illness, living in fear that one's family member will be deported, facing systemic discrimination) find the suggestion to try mindfulness practice or "listening to the birds sing" minimizing. This perception typically arises when clients perceive mindfulness practice as aimed at cultivating a pleasant state of detached relaxation. This is why assessing a client's perceptions of mindfulness at the beginning of therapy and revisiting understandings throughout therapy is so important. Doing so gives us an opportunity to validate this very understandable reaction. It also helps clarify our goal of using mindfulness practice as a way to develop skills that can be applied in the face of real stressors that elicit genuine pain and thereby help clients access some flexibility and choice in constraining, unjust contexts. We can repeatedly acknowledge that mindfulness won't eliminate real pain, yet it can help clarify that pain and provide some freedom and empowerment amid adversity.

Mindfulness Is Too Distressing

Some clients come to therapy because they recognize they want more out of their lives, even though their overall distress does not appear significant. If their emotions have been muted by ingrained avoidance habits, practicing acceptance and mindfulness can bring clients into contact with more distress than they expect. Clients who have restricted their lives significantly without noticing the full cost of that choice may feel deeply saddened when they begin to attend to their experience more openly. They may find the thoughts and feelings that arise during practice and during their daily lives surprising and upsetting, and subsequently they may well find reasons to avoid practice. Therapists can respond empathically to these experiences; if it were easy to open up to our experiences, we would all do it naturally and clearly we don't. It's human to want to shield ourselves from pain and distress, but unfortunately doing so comes at a cost. We often return to the tug-of-war metaphor and describe mindfulness practice as one way of "dropping the rope." With practice allowing their emotional experience to be present, clients often find that, although pain doesn't ever completely disappear, internal experiences do rise and fall and change over time and across contexts, which usually enhances their willingness to practice. This helps clients to have the secondary experience of "calmness" that comes from not struggling, rather than trying to remove or avoid distress.

Mindfulness Requires Too Much Time

As discussed earlier, there are a number of ways we can work with busy clients to help them find time to engage in formal practice and integrate informal practice into their daily lives. In Chapter 10, we describe an exercise we do to help clients identify the way they're spending their time—sometimes there are activities like surfing the web, gaming, or watching TV or Netflix that are taking up a great deal of time and may not be rewarding. We sometimes ask clients to try out truncating the time they spend on these activities in order to add in some mindfulness and then notice the impact of this change.

This obstacle can also emerge, particularly early in treatment, when clients aren't certain that investing time into mindfulness practice will be valuable for them. Understanding the factors contributing to infrequent practice informs the strategies used to facilitate practice. An exchange with Lila provides an example of how we work with this obstacle.

LILA: I just couldn't set aside any time for the practice this week. I have too much else going on.

THERAPIST: I know how challenging it can be to find extra time. Can you give me an example of a particular day and what happened when you tried to practice?

LILA: Well, the day after I saw you, I thought I would wake up in the morning and do the breathing practice. I got up and even sat in the chair where I was planning to practice. But then I started thinking about everything I had to do that day, and I just didn't see how sitting and doing nothing would help.

THERAPIST: I see; so part of what happened is that it didn't feel like practicing would be useful for you and, given everything you have going on, you didn't want to waste time on something unhelpful. Is that right?

LILA: Yeah, I guess so. I mean I understand what you said about how doing this would help me to see my emotions differently, but when I have so many things on my plate, I just don't feel like I can indulge myself in this way. People are counting on me to take care of things.

THERAPIST: I really understand that reaction. Sometimes I feel like spending time on mindfulness practice is the last thing I need to do when I have so much else on my plate. And it can feel selfish. And yet, sometimes I find that I can practice, even when my head is swirling with those thoughts, and often it actually helps me to be more focused and efficient with all the other tasks I need to get done. And I'm often able to be with other people, and meet their needs, better. That doesn't necessarily mean the next time I won't have the same thoughts about it being a waste, but over time I've learned those particular thoughts aren't very accurate or helpful for me. I've come to trust my experience more than my thoughts in this situation. But it's really hard to get started without those experiences. So, I guess in a way I'm asking you if you can take a leap of faith and try these practices, even if they feel like a waste of time, for just a couple of weeks. I promise, if after a few weeks of practicing, you haven't seen anything about them that seemed useful, we can move on to trying other things. I really want you to use your own experience with mindfulness practice to help you determine the role it might play in your life. But I think you have to work through this obstacle to gain the experience you need to make the best choice for you. Do you think it's worth trying, given how hard things have been for you and how the other things you've tried haven't seemed helpful?

LILA: Well, when you say it like that, I guess it's worth trying something instead of not trying at all.

THERAPIST: Great. Now, just to really help you get started, what about trying to practice for 5 minutes a day this coming week?

LILA: Really, is that enough time?

THERAPIST: I am not exactly sure how much time you need to spend practicing to see the benefit you are hoping for and to make the changes that matter to you. That's another thing I hope we learn about through experience. What I do know is that right now our most important goal is to see if you can establish enough of a mindfulness practice habit to evaluate its usefulness. And it's a hard habit to develop. It's much better to practice for 5 minutes regularly than to set your goals so high that you can't meet your expectations and you feel discouraged and give up. So let's pick a more reasonable goal to make it easier for you to feel like it's worth the sacrifice to start out. Then maybe we can increase the time if you find it useful.

LILA: Okay, I can definitely do 5 minutes.

THERAPIST: Okay. Now remember, you're still probably going to have the thought that it's a waste of time. And you might still have that thought after you practice. Practice might be boring, or anxiety-provoking, or you might feel bad at it, and then you'll be thinking, "Why did she recommend this to me?" Do you think you can stick with it even if all of those things happen?

LILA: Yeah, I can do anything for 5 minutes. I'll remember what we said and just do it anyway.

THERAPIST: And if you don't? And you skip three days in a row before you really notice what's happened, would you be willing to practice on the fourth day even with thoughts like, "I can't believe I didn't practice every day" and "Now, this is definitely a waste of time"?

LILA: Well, I'll be frustrated if that happens, but I can totally see that it could. Yes, I will.

THERAPIST: What do you think about putting a reminder to practice into your phone along with some of the points that you think might seem helpful to remember? Like, "I can practice even when my thoughts are giving me reasons not to, and I am just trying this for now—if it doesn't seem like its helping me make the changes I want to make in therapy, we will come up with other options."

LILA: That might be a good idea.

THERAPIST: Let's take a moment and do that now.

In this example, the therapist used several strategies to help the client make this initial commitment. First, she validated the feelings and thoughts related to mindfulness practice being a waste of time. She shared her own experiences with those reactions (which were genuine). She acknowledged that practicing initially involves a leap of faith. She also addressed the client's concern that practicing is selfish by describing her own experience of feeling more connected to and responsive to others when she's practicing. This is something that clients often notice on their own later in therapy, but suggesting that possibility before they have had the chance to experience it themselves can help increase willingness. Finally, the therapist reduced the assigned practice so that it would seem particularly manageable for the client and predicted difficulties keeping the commitment. We wouldn't necessarily do all of these in a single exchange, but they are all ways to address client concerns about practice being a poor use of their time.

In our experience, even early, brief mindfulness practices can provide clients with a deeper awareness of what they may be missing out on by not attending to the present moment. Detailed exploration of a client's experience with practice can address obstacles and emphasize benefits reinforcing continued practice. Further, clients often have at least some experience of mindfulness deepening their experience of life after some degree of practice, so a commitment to practice for a few weeks is usually enough to engage them in more consistent and sustained mindfulness practice. And later, when that practice lapses, as it often does, clients typically have their own experiences and observations to draw from regarding how regular practice improves their lives.

BOX 6.9. WHEN TIME IS LIMITED:
Integrating Mindfulness

Because mindfulness exercises are available in so many different forms outside the context of therapy, including through books, meditation groups, yoga classes, martial arts classes, online exercises, and apps, they can be a particularly useful strategy to introduce in a brief therapy context so that clients can use them on their own. The aspects that are probably most important to incorporate in an in-person context are:

- Presenting a rationale for how cultivating mindfulness skills (which the therapist should describe) can address the client's presenting problems.
- Providing some experiential practice and exploration of the experience of practicing, giving the therapist an opportunity to direct misconceptions that:
  - Mindfulness should clear the mind.
  - Mindfulness is a state that can be achieved (as opposed to an ongoing process and practice).
  - Mindfulness is always pleasant.
  - Having thoughts, sensations, or feelings is "failing" at mindfulness.
- Describing how mindfulness can be applied to aspects of daily life so that clients can make intentional, valued choices instead of reacting.
- Providing resources like websites and books that the client can use to support their ongoing practice (see *http://mindfulwaythroughanxiety.com/resources* for examples).
- Some problem solving about how to add mindfulness practice into their lives, including informal practice.

What Is Mindfulness?

In this treatment, we will talk about the role of *awareness* as a first step to helping us make changes in our lives. In particular, we will focus on a special kind of awareness called *mindfulness*. The term *mindfulness* comes from Eastern spiritual and religious traditions (like Zen Buddhism), but psychology has begun to recognize that, removed from the spiritual and religious context, it may be used to improve physical and emotional well-being. Although many of the ideas we suggest here will be consistent with Eastern philosophies and traditions, we will not be focusing on the religious or spiritual parts of mindfulness, and we believe this approach can be useful no matter what your religious or spiritual preference.

Mindfulness is nonjudgmental (or compassionate), present-moment awareness of what is going on inside of us and around us. We often live our lives focused on something other than what is happening in the moment—worrying about the future, ruminating about the past, focusing on what is coming next rather than what is right in front of us. It is useful that we can do a number of things without paying attention to them. We can walk without thinking about walking, which allows us to talk to the person we're walking with without having to think, "Now I should lift up this foot." However, this ability to do things automatically, without awareness, also allows us to lose touch with what is happening right in front of us. We can develop habits (such as avoiding conflict) that we aren't aware of and that may not be in line with our broader goals.

Sometimes we do pay close attention to what we are thinking and feeling, and we become very critical of our thoughts and feelings and either try to change them or to distract ourselves because judgmental awareness can be very painful. For example, we might notice while we are talking to someone new that our voice is wavering, or we aren't speaking clearly, and think, "I'm such an idiot! What is wrong with me? If I don't calm down, this person will never like me!"

Being mindful falls between these two extremes. We pay attention to what is happening inside and around us, we acknowledge events and experiences as what they are, and we allow things we cannot control to be as they are while we focus our attention on the task at hand. For example, when talking to someone new we might notice those same changes in our voice, take a moment to reflect, "This is how it is now. There go my thoughts again," and gently bring our attention back to the person and our conversation. This second part of mindfulness—letting go of the need to critically judge and change our inner experience—is particularly tricky. In fact, often being mindful involves practicing being nonjudgmental about our tendency to be judgmental!

We think that being mindful is a personal experience that can bring some flexibility to your life, and we will work together to find the best ways to apply this approach.

Here are a few points about mindfulness:

• *Mindfulness is a process.* We do not *achieve* a final and total state of mindfulness. It is a way of being in one moment that comes and goes. Mindfulness is losing our focus 100 times and returning to it 101 times.

• *Mindfulness is a habit.* Just like we have learned to go on automatic pilot by practicing it over and over, we can learn mindfulness through practice. The more we practice, the easier it can be to have moments of mindfulness.

(continued)

- *Mindfulness activities come in many different forms.* People engage in formal mindful practices like meditation, yoga, and tai chi. These practices can take hours or even days. People can also be mindful for a moment—attending to their breath at any point during the course of their day and noticing their experience. All forms of mindful practice can be beneficial. We will focus most on briefer, daily practice within treatment, but you may find that you also want to seek other, more formal modes of mindful practice outside of therapy or once therapy ends.

- *Mindfulness brings us more fully into our lives.* Sometimes, especially early in treatment, we will practice mindfulness in ways that seem very relaxing and removed from the stressors of our daily lives, but the ultimate goal is to use mindfulness to keep us more fully in our lives and to improve our overall life satisfaction. Mindfulness can allow us to pause and ready ourselves for some event (e.g., focusing on our breathing for a moment *before* we answer the phone) and bring us more fully into an event (e.g., being present and focused in the moment when we are interacting with someone rather than thinking about what they may be thinking or worrying about what might be coming next).

Awareness

We notice our experiences as they arise, including noticing what we notice. This awareness is:

- Expansive, rather than narrowed, so that we are taking in our full experience.
- In the present moment—this can include noticing when our minds go back to the past or forward to the future.
- An ongoing process—we lose awareness and regain it over and over.

Curiosity

We bring a perspective of curiosity and wonder to our experience so that we can notice it as it is.

- We can think of ourselves as scientists observing a phenomenon as one way to cultivate curiosity.
- Bringing "beginner's mind" helps us truly observe what is occurring in the moment with curiosity, rather than already assuming we know what is happening.

Acceptance

We gradually learn to put down the struggle to get rid of our experiences and instead to let them be as we notice them.

- Imagining "dropping the rope" can be an image to help with this.
- This isn't resignation—we are accepting what is already here in our present moment experience. We can still work to change things in the future.

Self-Compassion and Care

We develop an ability to bring kindness and care to our experiences, in place of judgment and self-criticism.

CHAPTER 7

Using ABBT Methods to Cultivate Self-Compassion

An overarching goal of our approach to treatment is to help clients cultivate a response of kindness, care, and compassion toward their experiences and themselves. Clinical theorists, researchers, and clinicians from a range of theoretical backgrounds have emphasized the central role that self-criticism and judgment plays in a wide range of clinical presentations and the ways that self-compassion can be a powerful mechanism of clinically meaningful change. We have already discussed how the therapeutic relationship, psychoeducation about the nature of emotional responding, and mindfulness practices can promote kindness and understanding toward one's own responses. In particular, the mindfulness strategies reviewed in Chapter 6 often naturally lead to self-compassion through the process of heightening nonjudgmental, decentered awareness of thoughts, feelings, sensations, and memories as they arise. However, clients often experience a number of barriers to cultivating compassion toward themselves. Therefore, in this chapter, we provide a more in-depth focus on strategies that can help to cultivate this important skill.[1]

What you will learn

- How to promote self-compassion using a range of ABBT strategies.
- Psychoeducation that addresses common misconceptions about self-compassion.
- Specific formal and informal practices that can cultivate self-compassion.
- How to address barriers to cultivating self-compassion.

---

[1]Many other clinicians and researchers provide in-depth guidance to therapists hoping to help their clients build self-compassion or directly guide clients in self-help books. For additional reading in this area, we recommend Germer (2009); Gilbert (2009); Kolts (2016); Neff & Germer (2018); and Tirch (2012).

DEVELOPING AWARENESS AND UNDERSTANDING OF REACTIONS AND REACTIONS TO REACTIONS

Psychologist Kristen Neff (2003) defines self-compassion as "being open to and moved by one's own suffering, experiencing feelings of caring and kindness toward oneself, taking an understanding, nonjudgmental attitude toward one's inadequacies and failures, and recognizing that one's experiences is part of the common human experience" (p. 224). Although this way of responding to ourselves can be learned and cultivated through multiple methods, it is challenging for those clients whose history has taught them the opposite response. People often have repeated experiences of being criticized and judged by family members, people in authority, communities, and society, and they internalize and fuse with the message that they are different from and less than others. Many aspects of ABBT inherently promote awareness of these learned patterns of responding and help clients to cultivate an understanding of both their original responses to challenging situations and the subsequent natural arising of judgment and critical reactions to these responses. This awareness and understanding helps to counteract this learned pattern of responding and sets the stage for new learning of a gentler, kinder response.

At this point, we have already described many elements of assessment and therapy in ABBTs that will cultivate this awareness and understanding:[2]

- The assessment process highlights the ways that a range of thoughts, feelings, sensations, and behaviors make sense, given what we know about humans and in the context of the client's life and learning history. This begins a process of understanding that counteracts judgments.
- The assessment process also begins to bring awareness to judgments and reactivity and the ways that these reactions perpetuate problematic cycles of responding.
- Within the therapeutic relationship, the therapist conveys understanding and care to the range of experiences and behaviors the client describes, further cultivating understanding of these responses. This therapeutic style also serves to highlight the contrast between the way the therapist responds, the client's own responses, and the responses they've experienced from others, further heightening awareness of these well-worn patterns and strengthening new patterns of responding. Just as clients have often internalized the responses they have received from others in their lives, they can begin to internalize these compassionate responses from the therapist.
- Self-monitoring, particularly of thoughts, increases awareness of the frequency with which critical, judgmental thoughts arise, as well as the impact of these thoughts.
- Psychoeducation about the nature of thoughts, emotions, and learned responses and actions further deepens the client's understanding of why their reactions and behaviors are natural and part of the human condition rather than signs that something is wrong with them.
- As described in depth in Chapter 6, mindfulness practices are aimed at cultivating awareness and compassion for whatever arises. When clients observe their

---

[2]Compassion-focused therapy (CFT) outlines a similar description of layers and processes that impact compassion, with more of an explicit focus on targeting compassion (e.g., Kolts, 2016).

BOX 7.1. TRY THIS:
Noticing Critical Thoughts As They Arise

Our ability to help our clients notice habits of self-critical thoughts and reactions and cultivate new responses of compassion and care is enhanced by our own experience of noticing and cultivating new responses. Over the next day, make a point of noticing as any critical thoughts arise for you and noting them in some form—carry a notebook, use a note function on your phone, or carry a piece of paper and write down the time, context, and thought. So, if I (LR) were doing this exercise, I first would have noted: *2pm, answering email, "Why can't I get myself started writing?" "I'm doing a terrible job working on this book!"* As you notice and jot down each thought, you might just take a moment to shift focus to your breath or sensations in your body and then return to what you're doing (or not doing as in my example!). If a day is too long, just try this for an hour, or even for 15 minutes. Any practice of noticing and noting these thoughts as they occur will help you to see how critical thoughts arise and unfold, and will also provide an opening for a different way of responding.

   You might notice that it feels unpleasant to recognize how often self-critical thoughts come up, and you might not want to keep doing the exercise—this is an important connection to our clients! On the other hand, you might also find that noticing a barrage of critical thoughts actually evokes empathy for yourself—it can be exhausting to wade through those thoughts and the feelings they elicit. Whatever you notice is useful, for you and for the clients you work with.

experiences, again and again, noticing how challenging it can be to be human, they often naturally develop self-compassion. The therapist's responses to each practice, aimed at highlighting this awareness and validating the naturalness of all responses, further deepens these skills.

PSYCHOEDUCATION ON SELF-COMPASSION: ADDRESSING COMMON OBSTACLES

Self-compassion and its potential positive impact on lives is commonly highlighted in the popular press and incorporated into many self-help and therapist-directed approaches to well-being and mental health. Nonetheless, self-compassion is often misunderstood in ways that create specific barriers to its cultivation. Addressing these potential sources of misunderstanding either implicitly or explicitly through psychoeducation and exploration of the client's experiences with compassion and criticism can facilitate clients' abilities to respond to themselves with care and kindness. Here we describe some of the psychoeducation we incorporate as needed in our work with clients.[3]

Self-Compassion Does Not Breed Complacency

We often receive messages that being "tough" on ourselves is the best way to make sure we accomplish things. We readily tell ourselves "Don't be a slacker" and make

---

[3]Neff and Germer (2018) have a section in their *Mindful Self-Compassion Workbook* describing what compassion is not.

comparisons to those we view as more motivated in an attempt to encourage our own productivity and success. Clients commonly share a concern that if they are kind and caring to themselves, they won't be able to get anything done. These perceptions can be supported by short-term experiential evidence—self-criticism does sometimes lead to increased productivity immediately as we are motivated and reduce the distress associated with it. However, this does not lead to sustained engagement or life satisfaction. For example, people often use self-criticism to strengthen their resolve to diet and exercise. Although this response style can elicit short-term increases in healthy behavior, if self-judgment and self-punishment continue or amplify after one eats a slice of cake or misses a workout, that can lead to discouragement and ultimately avoidance.

When clients raise concerns about complacency, or if we find this concern is getting in the way when we inquire about it, we often suggest that the client try out self-compassion for a couple of weeks and see what kind of impact it has on productivity over a period of time. We promise that we will drop the suggestion if, in fact, it leads to inaction and failure. So far, we have never found that to be the case. When we ask clients to pay attention to their lived experience (or when we pay attention to our own experiences), despite what they and we believe to be true, observation often teaches us that kindness and care (from both self and others) can help focus our actions on what matters personally and lead us to more sustained, rewarding behaviors. Sometimes a client might initially slow down their efforts, recognizing the toll that constant expectations and criticism has taken on their energy and vitality, and then they go on to engage in a more focused, invigorated way. In fact, self-criticism slows us down and interferes just as much as (or more than) it facilitates action, as you may have noticed in your own self-observation earlier in this chapter. Psychoeducation, supplemented with observation and behavioral experiments, can help clients to learn this for themselves.

Self-Compassion Is Not Overlooking Flaws

Self-compassion involves seeing ourselves fully and caring for ourselves in the midst of our humanness, inevitable mistakes, and shortcomings. It involves caring for oneself as a person, not in a way that is linked to performance or accomplishments. However, people often misrepresent or misunderstand compassion as engaging in false praise or overlooking flaws. This view is tied to mistaken beliefs that perfection or an absence of errors is what warrants care and kindness. When care and kindness are assumed to be something all humans deserve, rather than being viewed as something we earn, it actually creates a space in which we can more accurately recognize that humans are imperfect, with the potential to improve or grow and commit to trying harder or doing something different the next time we are in a similar situation. When mistakes and failures aren't seen as reflecting on our worth as a person, it is easier to notice, accept, and address them. Sometimes it is helpful to share the research summarized in Box 7.2 to invite clients to consider the potential benefits of self-compassion.

Self-Compassion Isn't Necessarily Selfish or Self-Indulgent

Often the "self" aspect of self-compassion evokes the impression that it is inherently selfish or self-indulgent to be caring or kind to oneself. A rigid, consistent focus on being kind to oneself to the exclusion of others could indeed be problematic, but in our

BOX 7.2. A CLOSER LOOK: Self-Compassion Enhances Self-Motivation, Self-Improvement, and Coping

Contrary to common misconceptions, self-compassion is associated with motivation toward and achievement of goals rather than inaction and complacency (cf. Barnard & Curry, 2011). For example, Breines and Chen (2012) conducted a series of experimental studies in which participants who were exposed to various manipulations that targeted self-compassion (e.g., a 3-minute self-compassion reflection: "Imagine that you are talking to yourself about this weakness from a compassionate and understanding perspective. What would you say?") were compared to participants exposed to various manipulations that targeted self-esteem (e.g., a 3-minute self-esteem reflection: "Imagine that you are talking to yourself about this weakness from a perspective of validating your positive (rather than negative) qualities.") and to participants exposed to a positive distraction condition or a no instruction control condition. In comparison to those in other conditions, participants who were assigned to the self-compassion conditions reported greater beliefs in their weaknesses being addressable/changeable; reported more motivation to make amends and address transgressions they felt bad about; spent more time studying after doing poorly on an exam; and engaged in more upward social comparisons with more motivation to change after reflecting on a personal weakness. A longitudinal study revealed that trait self-compassion predicted reduced avoidance-oriented coping and enhanced adaptive coping in response to a stressful life event (Chishima, Mizuno, Sugawara, & Migyagawa, 2018). These studies, consistent with many others, indicate that practicing self-compassion can help people to turn toward distressing material (personal weaknesses or transgressions, poor performance, a stressful life event) and make meaningful changes, making it a powerful skill to develop as part of therapy.

experience and observation of the practice of others, we continually see the ways that caring for oneself actually opens up generosity and care toward others. Seeing our own humanness and the ways we can make mistakes no matter how hard we are trying can often make it easier to recognize that same humanness in others. In addition, self-compassion helps to counter the resource drain of self-criticism, making more resources available to give to others. We often use the metaphor of putting on our own oxygen mask before we help the person sitting next to us on an airplane to illustrate how care for ourselves can help us to care more effectively for others. Further, consistent with our larger model of intervention, we emphasize that self-compassion, just like all the strategies aimed at changing the ways we relate to our internal experiences, is always in the service of being able to choose our actions and do what's important to us. So we aren't suggesting that self-compassion is a stopping point; rather, it is a step toward being able to be in our lives and with other people in the way we would like to be. Through cultivating self-compassion, we can lessen our emotional muddiness, clarify what's important to us, and then act accordingly.

That said, it is important to recognize that the concept of focusing on the self with compassion has an implicit (and maybe explicit) individualistic focus that may not resonate with all clients and should certainly be adapted and flexibly applied so that it matches the way that clients see themselves in relation to others. It may be more congruent to talk about compassion more broadly, rather than distinguishing self from other. Or it may be important with clients who are contending with systemic oppression to contextualize self-care within their experiences of marginalization and discrimination, perhaps referring to Audre Lorde's famous quote "Caring for myself is not self-indulgence. It is self-preservation and that is an act of political warfare." Still, for other clients, it may be more meaningful to speak of more communal care and compassion. Melissa Harris-Perry (2017), in describing the problematic individualistic focus of self-care, a concept closely connected to self-compassion, proposes instead communal care or "squadcare" in which it is acknowledged that one does not survive solely by caring for oneself and instead caring for one's "squad" or community is necessary.

Everyone Deserves Self-Compassion

Some clients tell us that they don't deserve compassion because of things they've done in the past, or things they haven't done, or messages they've received from important people in their lives. However, compassion toward ourselves doesn't mean endorsing everything we've done. Rather, it means accepting ourselves (and all humans) as inherently worthy and deserving of care and intentionally caring for ourselves. As we mentioned in the previous section, part of that care can absolutely include recognizing our mistakes and wanting to be different in the future, sometimes in very significant ways. We can share with clients the dialectics of acceptance and change (Linehan, 1993)—we can understand and care for ourselves exactly as we are, while also working to be different in certain ways. For example, someone who wishes that their body was leaner and stronger can accept their body for what it is, notice the ways in which their body in its current state functions to support life, and take actions to improve physical functioning. And someone who dislikes their habit of withdrawing when their partner shows love and affection can recognize and appreciate the ways that response was protective in the context of an abusive upbringing, while also considering new ways of responding in the current relationship.

Gilbert (2009) suggests that we help clients engage in compassionate self-correction in place of self-criticism. We can have compassion for the struggle that comes from our past learning at the same time that we work to make changes in the future. Clients often recognize the openness that comes from this kind of compassion, in contrast to the self-blame they have engaged in that creates muddy emotions and increases reactivity and actions that are counter to one's values. Self-monitoring and behavioral experiments can help to highlight this contrast and address this barrier to self-compassion.

Sometimes clients' beliefs that they do not deserve compassion go beyond wishing that they possessed a certain attribute or that they could remedy some past mistake. Clients with significant trauma histories, as well as those who have been exposed to repeated and prolonged invalidation and rejection, may be fused with a more generalized belief that they are fundamentally flawed and unworthy of self-compassion. Although therapists may feel pulled to convince clients that they do deserve compassion, in our experience this strategy can backfire in at least two distinct ways. Some clients might respond to therapist coaxing with a temporary shift in self-compassion during the session, but feel discouraged or even hopeless when critical and judgmental feelings arise at a later time. Another unintended consequence of therapists' assurances is that clients may feel pulled to argue even more persuasively against their worthiness. As discussed in Chapter 5, we are careful to offer psychoeducation as new information for clients to consider and rely on mindfulness and other practices (described later in this chapter) and client observations of their lived experience as major drivers of change.

BOX 7.3. TO SUMMARIZE
Correcting Common Misconceptions about Self-Compassion

- Self-compassion does not breed complacency.
- Self-compassion does not mean overlooking your flaws.
- Self-compassion isn't necessarily selfish or self-indulgent.
- Self-compassion is something everyone deserves.

PRACTICES THAT CULTIVATE SELF-COMPASSION

A wide range of practices can be used to help clients to specifically cultivate self-compassion. Again, we encourage readers to explore resources noted earlier that focus specifically on cultivating self-compassion for a broad array of methods to draw from (self-compassion websites and self-help books are also listed at *http://mindfulway-throughanxiety.com/resources*). We often find that an acceptance-based behavioral case conceptualization, a validating, compassionate therapeutic relationship, psychoeducation about how reactions and behaviors make sense, and self-monitoring and mindfulness practices inherently cultivate self-compassion and so, usually, few additional practices are needed. Nonetheless, we typically include the first two examples we provide here in our work with most clients, and we include the others when they seem indicated (and also have found them to be useful in our own practices).

How We Might Respond to Someone We Care About (or How Someone Who Cares about Us Might Respond to Us)

A common strategy for helping clients to cultivate self-compassion is to ask them how they might respond if a friend, loved one, or child was saying the things they say to themselves. Often people are much kinder to other people than to themselves, and so this simple inquiry can elicit a gentler response and can serve as an easy reminder to use as they notice self-critical thoughts arising in their daily lives. If this perspective is less accessible, therapists can ask clients to remember one specific time that someone they care about approached them with judgments about themselves and how they responded. When clients have caring people in their lives, therapists can also inquire as to how that caring person might respond if they shared these judgments with them.

AISHA: I just can't get anything done. I'm so lazy and unfocused.

THERAPIST: Those are really familiar thoughts, aren't they? I've noticed them in your self-monitoring forms, and sometimes they come up after a mindfulness practice.

AISHA: Yes, they're familiar because I can never focus and get things done. I'm just not motivated enough and I never try hard.

THERAPIST: I can hear how painful those thoughts are and how true they feel as you experience them. [First, the therapist validates the client's experience, slightly altering to thoughts *feeling* true, as a step toward decentering.] Would you be willing to spend some time exploring these kinds of thoughts and the way they affect you?

AISHA: Sure. They do feel very true and also very painful.

THERAPIST: I'd like to try a little thought experiment, just to see if it helps to get a slightly different perspective on these thoughts, a little bit of distance.

AISHA: Okay.

THERAPIST: What would you say if Tam [Aisha's son] came to you and said, "I'm lazy and unfocused. I can never get anything done."

AISHA: (*pauses, tears up a little.*) Wow. I'd feel so sad to hear him say that. I think I might start by hugging him. . . . And telling him that I believe in him and his ability to get things done. . . . I might remind him of things he's gotten done already. . . . Or I might say that it can be really hard to focus, when there are so many different things that can grab our attention and ask him if I could help him think of things that might help him to focus more.

THERAPIST: That's a lot of very compassionate responses that come very quickly when you imagine Tam saying these things.

AISHA: (*Smiles.*) It really is, isn't it? But I don't do that when I have the thoughts. I just take them as true and feel terrible about myself. Why can't I treat myself as kindly as I treat him?

THERAPIST: It's so much harder to bring that kind of compassion to ourselves than to someone else. As we've talked about, you've gotten these messages in the past and they've become such a well-worn habitual way of responding that it's hard to even notice them, never mind responding to them this way. And we certainly don't want you to now get caught up criticizing yourself for not being kinder! And it may be useful to try to remember how you would respond to Tam if he said the things you say to yourself and to see if you can start to introduce some of this kindness you so readily show to him into your own responses to yourself. Does that seem like something you might want to try?

AISHA: Yes. I think I can try that. And, you know what? I do get things done sometimes. Maybe I need to come up with a strategy that will help me focus on the tasks that I'm having trouble getting done, instead of just saying that this is another way I'm failing and being lazy.

THERAPIST: That sounds like a wonderful idea and like you're already starting to practice talking to yourself the way you might respond to Tam.

Of course, if clients don't have compassionate people in their lives, or they aren't able to generate compassion for others, these strategies won't be helpful and may instead generate even more pain and criticism. In those cases, other practices may be more useful.

Specific Mindfulness Exercises That Cultivate Self-Compassion

We have also collected a set of mindfulness exercises that we use with clients who are having a particularly difficult time cultivating compassion. Williams and colleagues

(2007) describe a practice, *Inviting a Difficulty In and Working It Through the Body*, aimed at softening toward one's own pain and distress, which we regularly use, with some adaptations (e.g., expanding the emphasis on bodily sensations to include all internal situations). We have clients begin by focusing on their breath and then expanding to their full body. Then we ask them to bring to mind a difficulty that is currently going on in their lives (see Appendix B for the text and listen to the recording on the Guilford website [see the box at the end of the table of contents]). Clients locate the sensations in their body associated with the distress and practice, allowing them and then softening in response to them. With some clients, we expand this awareness and softening to challenging thoughts and painful feelings as well. Practicing this regularly in a formal manner (e.g., with any discomfort a client notices upon waking or during their crowded subway commute) can help to strengthen the response so that clients can then also apply it in the midst of distressing life experiences, breathing and opening up to their experience, rather than trying to brace against, avoid, or judge it. Therapists and clients can also use phrases from this practice such as "Whatever it is, it's already here. Let me be open to it," as reminders to informally practice this expansiveness during sessions as well as daily life.

Another mindfulness practice that can be helpful is an adaptation (King, 2018) of the RAIN practice developed by the Vipassana meditation teacher Michele McDonald, for responding to distress. The acronym refers to four steps: Recognize, Allow, Investigate, and Nurture (initially Non-identification). In this practice, clients can begin by noticing (recognizing) what they are experiencing and simply naming their sensations, emotions, and other internal experiences. The next step involves allowing or being open to what is already happening (similar to Williams et al.'s [2007] practice). King (2018) suggests phrases like "This is hard. Let me be with it" or "Let's be here together, dear one!" to facilitate this practice. The third step is investigating how they are relating to what's happening—bringing curiosity to the distress they are experiencing. King suggests questions such as "What am I perceiving?"; "How am I relating to what's happening?"; "What assumptions am I making?"; "Do they support distress or freedom?"; "How is what's happening changing?" In the final step, clients nurture or care for the distress being experienced. King suggests asking "What's needed? What facilitates release from distress?" Clients may use a range of self-statements or images to facilitate this nurturing (including examples we provide in this chapter).

When clients struggle with their shifting thoughts about self-compassion by trying to hold on to thoughts that they are worthy and dispel their doubts or by blaming themselves for their frequently changing thoughts, we sometimes use the *pendulum metaphor* and the *accepting yourself on faith exercise* from ACT. The pendulum metaphor asks clients to imagine a swinging pendulum and consider that our minds work in a similar way. In one moment, we may have the thought that we deserve compassion and in another believe we are unworthy. If we try to "lift up" our thoughts and feelings too highly on one side (i.e., trying to convince ourselves we are absolutely worthy and trying to feel self-compassion and love), that action paradoxically powers the pendulum to swing up highly on the other side next (i.e., eliciting persuasive thoughts that we are unworthy and triggering self-criticism). We suggest to clients that this is just the way pendulums and our minds work.

As an alternative to what can be an endless search for confirmation that one is worthy of self-compassion, the *accepting yourself on faith exercise* from ACT asks clients to consider making the choice to accept themselves as worthy of self-compassion as a leap of faith, rather than needing to accrue sufficient evidence. In this exercise, we ask if clients are willing to try out living as if they are worthy and whole, just as they are, in this moment, even if their minds and emotions tell them otherwise.

A number of other self-compassion practices commonly used in mindfulness- and acceptance-based approaches have been drawn from traditional Buddhist practices. The Tibetan practice of *tonglen*, which involves breathing in (and opening ourselves up to) our own or others' pain and suffering and breathing out relief (Brach, 2003; Chodron, 2001), can be used to cultivate a nonavoidant, open response to any occurrence of pain or suffering. Continued practice with any suffering that arises can help clients develop a sense of their ability to hold pain and suffering, rather than needing to turn away from it. Loving-kindness meditation, or *metta* (e.g., Kabat-Zinn, 1994), can be used to cultivate a warm, caring response to oneself, and then in turn direct that loving kindness out toward other people. The intention of this repeated practice is to develop the habit strength of this kind of response, to counter the habit strength of judgmental responses. However, sometimes it is experienced as an instruction to feel other than one feels. Therapists should be sure to consider how clients experience the practice. When practices are congruent and presented flexibly, practicing compassion toward other people can be helpful in the context of interpersonal difficulties clients are having and can help clients to develop more skillful, effective ways of resolving conflicts they are having.

Applying Self-Compassion in Daily Life

Practices like those described above can help with developing and deepening the ability to respond with kindness and care to oneself. In addition to needing to develop this skill, clients often need ways to transport this newly developing response into their lives through reminders and strategies to recall the practice of compassion in a moment. In the previous therapy transcript, Aisha's therapist suggested that she think about how she might respond to her son when she noticed self-critical thoughts. Similarly, some of the phrases from mindfulness practices can serve as reminders (e.g., "It's already here, let me be open to it"). Neff (2015) suggests that people choose a term of endearment, like "Dear," "Sweetpea," or another personally meaningful term, and use that to refer to themselves when talking to themselves. Developing a habit of using this term can build a positive, warm association and a new response to counter the critical thoughts that arise. Bernhard (2013) suggests physical acts of care, like stroking one's hand, arm, or cheek with the other hand while acknowledging the feelings that are arising. Sometimes actions of care are easier to enact than feelings. Murphy (2016) shares his own practice of keeping on his phone the phrases he adapted from phrases Neff suggests: "This is a tough moment. Tough moments are inescapable. Tough moments call out for tender care. I'll give myself the kindness I deserve and need." Physical reminders can also be helpful—images or objects that are personally meaningful can serve as reminders to bring kindness and care to a given situation. Therapists can work with clients to identify the strategies that resonate most strongly with them and help them to add these reminders and daily practices to their lives.

BOX 7.4. TRY THIS:
Bringing Self-Compassion to Your Own Experience As a Therapist

Take a moment to remember a challenging moment you've had while conducting therapy recently. Think of a session that you didn't handle the way you wish you had—one about which you've had self-critical thoughts. Bring yourself back to the moments just after the session, noticing what you feel in your body as you remember the session, what you wish you'd said, what you wish you hadn't said, and the look on your client's face. Bring yourself back to that moment, and let that moment come into your body, exactly as it arises for you now. You may notice that you don't want to remember or that you try to push the feelings away. That's understandable. Just do your best to open up to the experience of the memory, again and again. And once you have the thoughts, feelings, and sensations, see if you can soften to the experience. Can you repeat "Whatever it is, it's already here. Let me be open to it"? Can you respond to yourself as you might respond to a friend or colleague who was telling you about a similar session? Or maybe just allow a sense of compassion to arise as you remember how hard this situation was for you. Can you see your own humanness?

Take some time to cultivate compassion in whatever way feels meaningful and useful. And when you're done, see what you've noticed. What was challenging about doing this? Were you able to have moments of compassion? What was that like for you? Did it lead the situation to change in any way? Do you feel more able to think about what you might do differently next time?

Actions Involving Caring for Oneself

We also view actions as an important way to cultivate care for oneself. In this context, we view behaviors that are often described as self-care as a way to manifest care toward oneself (or, more broadly, toward one's community), which will also naturally cultivate self-compassion. As we discuss self-compassion with clients and highlight the ways it can help to clarify our reactions and choose our responses so that we are living more consistently with our values, we suggest that clients take up daily or weekly practices that are aimed at caring for themselves in order to strengthen their "self-compassion muscle" and nourish themselves. We work to identify actions that can fit into their lives and be easy to make into habits. See Box 7.5 for a list of potential practices that clients might take up, or develop a list of your own that fits with the experiences of your clients. We ask clients to make a commitment to these practices, and then we ask them about the experience of integrating these practices into their lives, making sure to highlight and encourage the ways that they promote more self-compassion and help the clients move toward what matters to them, and, in addition, to address any obstacles that arise.

Addressing the Feeling That Practices Mean Feeling Other Than One Feels

As we noted briefly in the discussion of loving-kindness meditation, self-compassion practices can sometimes be experienced as instructions to feel other than one feels in a particular moment, which is inconsistent with psychoeducation that illustrates that we can't control our emotional responses on demand and that trying to control them can sometimes have paradoxical effects. Clients can easily become angry at and frustrated

---

BOX 7.5. Practices of Care for Self

- Take a walk.
- Listen to music you enjoy.
- Play with or pat a cat or dog.
- Read for pleasure/listen to an audiobook or podcast.
- Draw/paint.
- Take a warm bath or soak your feet and notice how it feels.
- Take care of your physical body by seeing the doctor for an annual check-up or going to the dentist to have your teeth cleaned.
- Light candles or incense and notice how they smell.
- Eat a food you enjoy and notice how it tastes.
- Take time to be with a friend(s) or family member(s).
- Cook something delicious (alone or with others).

- Work on a craft.
- Spend time in nature.
- Dance.
- Go fishing.
- Set a regular bedtime.
- Look at flowers, trees, or bodies of water.
- Watch something you enjoy or that energizes you.
- Attend a spiritual/religious/community gathering.
- Garden.
- Contribute to a community project that's important to you.
- Walk around the city and notice the sights, sounds, and smells.
- Any other activity that feels meaningful/ nourishing to you.

---

with themselves for not being able to feel more self-compassion, which can trigger a cycle of control efforts and self-critical thoughts.

For this reason, we present the practice of self-compassion as one possible way to respond differently to thoughts, emotions, sensations, and memories. We invite clients to consider trying to act with care toward themselves, as opposed to trying to engender caring feelings within themselves. We draw an analogy between practicing self-compassion and engaging in acts that soothe or nourish someone else (e.g., holding a crying infant, preparing a meal for a loved one, listening to our partner vent about a stressor, or running an errand for a parent), even if we are tired or angry and don't necessarily feel compassionate in the moment. Although people often believe they need to wait until they feel self-compassion to act compassionately, acting compassionately can at times lead to outside-in changes so that we actually feel more care after acting with care.

In his guide to compassion-focused therapy, Kolts (2016) highlights that a person who has learned to feel unsafe in relation to others may not be able to rapidly move from a history of learning that vulnerability is dangerous to cultivating self-compassion. Instead, he describes the way that people with these types of learning histories may engage in more of an unfolding process in which they first experience compassion from another (like the therapist) and deepen their understanding of themselves, and then may move on to directly cultivating compassion in time. In our experience, this process is also typically nonlinear and actually a life-long process in which old self-critical habits can continue to arise and ongoing practices of awareness and care, including compassion for moments in which compassion seems impossible to find, are an essential part of meaningful change. In addition, sometimes simply noticing that self-critical thoughts are just thoughts, rather than truths, can give clients the space they need to move toward what matters to them, and so the explicit focus on self-compassion may not be necessary. Relatedly, instead of trying to feel other than they feel, clients can gently invite themselves to cultivate caring responses, while still making room for the full range of their experiences. Larry Yang's (2017, p. 151) aspiration practice provides a model of this kind of expansive practice:

> May I be as loving in the moment as possible.
> If I cannot be loving in this moment,
>   may I be kind;
> If I cannot be kind,
>   may I be nonjudgmental;
> If I cannot be nonjudgmental,
>   may I not cause harm;
> If I cannot not cause harm,
>   may I cause the least harm possible. (p. 151)

BOX 7.6. WHEN TIME IS LIMITED:
Cultivating Self-Compassion

In brief therapy contexts, there may not be sufficient time to help clients effectively counter the extensive learning histories that have led to their patterns of self-criticism and their reluctance to be compassionate toward themselves. To plant the seeds for this process, you can:

• Introduce mindfulness practices, as described at the end of Chapter 6, that can begin to develop new habits, including recognizing self-critical thoughts as thoughts, and help establish patterns to maintain these practices.

• Provide psychoeducation to counter common misperceptions of self-compassion in order to address those barriers.

• Introduce the possibility of considering responding to oneself the same way you might respond to a friend.

• Suggest that clients engage in practices of care toward themselves and/or their communities.

CHAPTER 8

Articulating and Clarifying Personal Values

In an attempt to limit their exposure to painful and negatively evaluated internal events, clients frequently develop restricted behavioral repertoires. Some clients live relatively inactive lives, opting out of situations and activities that could elicit pain. Others spend the majority of their time and energy on chores and activities that "must" be done to prevent future feared outcomes or feelings of discomfort. Still others live their lives simply going through the motions, behaviorally participating in potentially valued activities without investing mindful intention or gaining any sense of fulfillment or satisfaction. Fortunately, once clients begin to cultivate acceptance and mindfulness, they often become more flexible and willing to expand their behavioral repertoire in ways that can enhance the quality and vitality of their lives. To support those efforts, an essential component of ABBT involves helping clients articulate and clarify their values. In this chapter, we provide a broad overview of the concept of valuing, a component of ACT that can be incredibly powerful in evoking meaningful behavioral change (Hayes, Strosahl, et al., 1999, 2012; Wilson & Murrell, 2004). We also describe the clinical strategies used to support clients in affirming their values.

What you will learn

- ೞ Clinical strategies aimed at helping clients to articulate and clarify their personal values.
- ೞ Common themes that may reflect stuck points in the values articulation process.
- ೞ Methods of working through stuck points and helping clients to clarify their values.

PSYCHOEDUCATION ON THE CONCEPT OF VALUES

Because "values" has multiple meanings within and outside of psychotherapy, including moral or religious connotations, we start values work with psychoeducation that involves sharing what we mean when we use this term in ABBT. Drawing from ACT, we define *values* as ways of being in our lives that are personally important or meaningful. For example, one might value being open and honest in relationships, seeking opportunities to learn and create at work, or being helpful in one's community. *Values-based actions* are specific activities that clients can engage in (or avoid) that are consistent with their personally held values, such as asking a friend to lunch, signing up to take a college class, or bringing food to a neighbor in crisis.

Values versus Goals

We also distinguish between values and goals (see Table 8.1). Although goals can sometimes be quite useful in directing behavior, they also have some characteristics that can limit their utility in promoting a healthy and fulfilling lifestyle. For instance, goals are future-focused and inherently favor where we *should be* over *where we are* currently. These properties can make goals quite motivating, but they can also engender feelings of discontent and promote nonacceptance of the present moment. In contrast, values are present-centered and encourage ongoing participation and engagement in meaningful activities. Whereas a goal is defined by an outcome that can potentially be achieved (e.g., losing 10 pounds, finding a dating partner), valuing is conceptualized as an ongoing process or direction (e.g., living a healthy lifestyle, being open in relationships) that has no endpoint.

We sometimes use one of the following two metaphors (if we are working with a client to whom it might be relevant) adapted from ACT to distinguish between goals and values (Hayes et al., 2012):

> "Suppose you really enjoy downhill skiing, and you plan a trip for weeks. Try to imagine for a moment . . . you start making coffee at home in the morning instead of stopping at your favorite coffee shop, you pack lunches to bring to work, volunteer for some overtime shifts, all so you can save up enough money to go on this skiing trip. . . . Finally, the day arrives. You wake up early and drive several hours to get up to the mountain. You purchase your lift ticket and wait in line, taking in the beauty of deep blue sky, the way the sun sparkles in the crisp white snow, and the clean scent of the evergreens. Finally, you arrive at the top of the hill and it's your turn to go. Just as you are about to push off, a worker asks, 'Where are you trying to get to?' When you reply, 'The bottom of the hill,' she ushers you back onto

TABLE 8.1. Values versus Goals

Goals	Values
• Future-focused.	• Present-focused.
• Can be met (or not met).	• Cannot be completed or fully achieved.
• Are often impacted by external, uncontrollable factors.	• Are dependent on our own actions.

Note. Adapted with permission from *Worry Less, Live More* by Susan M. Orsillo and Lizabeth Roemer. Copyright © 2016 The Guilford Press.

the chairlift and next thing you know you are on your way down. Consider for a moment what that experience would be like. . . . Although in theory the goal of skiing is to get to the bottom of the hill, what most people find meaningful about it is typically the process of swooshing down the powdered hill."

"Imagine that your goal is to find someone with whom you can have a committed relationship. You want to find someone who supports you, lifts you up, makes you laugh—someone you deeply love who deeply loves you back. Imagine that first moment the two of you meet. You are at a crowded social event and you catch each other's eyes and smile. Your heart quickens a bit—with excitement and happiness—as you notice the person walking toward you. Magically, your life fast-forwards through the process of falling in love and stops at the goal line—it's official, you found them! You got to skip the awkward moments, the first fight, but you also skipped the anticipation of the first kiss, the warm glow that arises when you feel connected to someone, and the experience of professing your love to each other. And now that you have met your goal, you've reached the endpoint. Consider for a moment what that experience would be like . . . how satisfying or fulfilling would it be to have achieved your goal, without getting to experience the relationship in an ongoing way before and after the point of commitment? Although in theory the goal of dating is to find a partner, what most people find meaningful about that is the moment-by-moment experience of being in a relationship."

Another characteristic we highlight in our psychoeducation is that our ability to meet a goal is often influenced by factors outside of our control. For example, with regard to the goal of losing 10 pounds, although diet and exercise absolutely influence weight, so do build, metabolic rate, and medication use. Similarly, if we are pursuing the goal of meeting a dating partner, we are more likely to be successful if we ask people out on dates, but we actually can't control whether or not they accept.

Because goals are future focused and not entirely under our control, they can sometimes feel out of reach. We might become frustrated, view our efforts as futile, and give up, concluding that we are flawed for not being able to achieve our goal. In contrast, because our ability to act consistently with values is under our own control, we can persist in our efforts regardless of external factors (although it may be hard or somewhat painful to do so). For example, we can choose to be open with our feelings regardless of how others respond.

Despite their different functions, goals and values are often interrelated: values can be thought of as the glue between goals. For example, one might pursue a college degree (goal) motivated by a deeply held value that seeking opportunities to learn is personally meaningful. Similarly, one might have the goal of going out on a date, which may be driven by a closely held value of nurturing intimate relationships.

In sum, goals can be helpful in propelling us forward, but focusing exclusively on goals has some downsides. Attending to a hoped-for future can distract us from, or devalue, our present experience. And if we don't have total control over the things we think we need to control in order to live a fulfilling and satisfied life, that increases our risk of feeling dissatisfied, frustrated, and hopeless.

Valuing as a Behavior

In ABBT, valuing is defined by actions and distinguished from emotions and thoughts. In other words, to order to enact a value of caring for one's children, one might get up in the middle of the night to comfort and feed a restless, hungry, unsettled infant. One might enact that value while having feelings of warmth and joy and thoughts such as, "I love this precious being." Alternatively, one might enact that same value in the same manner while having feelings of exhaustion and frustration, and thoughts such as, "This selfish creature won't sleep for more than 3 hours in a row." A core assumption of ABBT is that while we may not be able to control our physical sensations, thoughts, and emotions, we can exert some control over our behavior. Thus, although it may be easier to act in accordance with our values when we feel rested and loving, we can also take actions that are personally meaningful to us when those feeling states aren't present.

During psychoeducation, we try to choose examples of this phenomenon that our clients can relate to. For example, people who work out regularly can usually identify times that they opted to exercise even while encountering thoughts and feelings inconsistent with such an action (e.g., "I would rather be home watching television"; "I don't feel motivated"). Similarly, many clients attend important medical or dental appointments while also having thoughts like "I don't want to be here" and "This is really unpleasant." A more nuanced domain we explore that underscores the complicated association between behavior and internal states is that of relationships. Our feelings toward a friend, partner, or family member are likely to vacillate across time and context, yet, we often value remaining present and engaged so that these long-term relationships can weather fluctuations in our mood. Parents frequently value acting lovingly and consistently toward their children, even though the range of feelings they have in the presence of their children can extend from joyful and loving to frustrated and angry.

Values Are Choices

A final characteristic we share when providing psychoeducation about the nature of values is that we assume they reflect a deeply personal choice that cannot be logically evaluated or objectively judged. In other words, there are no absolute truths regarding "right" or "wrong" personal values as they are defined in ABBT. Instead, the way in which we determine the usefulness of holding a value is the extent to which living consistently with that value brings the holder a sense of meaning, fulfillment, and purpose over time.

Sometimes we use an experiential exercise drawn from ACT to help clients connect with this concept of choice. Starting with a relatively trivial preference (e.g., Coca-Cola vs. Pepsi or chocolate ice cream vs. vanilla), we ask our clients to choose their preferred flavor and then defend their choice. The first few queries (e.g., "Why chocolate?") are typically easy to answer (e.g., "Because I like the taste of chocolate better," "Because vanilla tastes too creamy for me"), but it quickly becomes difficult to generate logical answers to follow-up questions (e.g., "Why do you like the taste?"; "Why do you prefer a less creamy taste?"), and clients often get to the point of answering "just because" or "for no reason." Together, we consider the possibility that "just because, that is what I choose" can also be applied to the concept of personal values.

This feature of values is helpful to touch on during psychoeducation because many clients struggle with uncertainty and doubt during the values articulation process and may feel pressure to choose the "right" value. We will address some of the complexities related to choosing one's values, including importance of considering the roles of family and cultural identity, later in this chapter when we discuss working with stuck points in values writing.

PSYCHOEDUCATION ON THE BENEFITS OF DEFINING PERSONAL VALUES

Helping clients to recognize the costs associated with narrowing behavioral repertoires as a way of limiting contact with painful internal experiences and to articulate and affirm personal values can motivate meaningful life changes (Wilson & Murrell, 2004). When clients shift their focus toward what is most personally meaningful and discover they have some freedom to live their lives in a way that is consistent with these personal values, avoiding emotional discomfort becomes less important. An essential step in this process involves psychoeducation that provides a rationale for inviting the client to engage in values articulation.

Values as a Compass That Can Guide Behavior

We encourage clients to consider the different factors that influence our behavior. For example, many of the actions we take are driven by learned habits and enacted without intention. Someone might automatically turn on the television after work without considering the full range of possible leisure activities from which they could choose. Emotions can also strongly influence our behavioral responses. As we discuss throughout treatment, emotions function to alert us to changes in our environment and to prepare us to act. For example, when we're afraid, we experience a cascade of physiological responses that ready us to freeze, fight, or flee our way to safety. When we feel sad, our attention is drawn inward, and we are predisposed to withdraw and self-reflect (Huron, 2018).

Although emotions *prepare* us to take particular actions, they do not automatically *cause* us to enact particular behaviors. Instead, a *pause* exists between our experience of emotion and our behavior, which gives us the option to respond in emotion-incongruent ways. One reason we might choose an action that is different from the one our emotions *recommend* is that the recommended behavior may be inconsistent with our values or what matters most to us personally. We use the examples in Client Handout 8.1, *Intentional Responses That Differ from Emotion-Driven Reactions*, to illustrate this point.

Fully engaging in our lives requires a willingness to experience a range of emotions. In order to experience love and connection, we need to open ourselves up to potential loss and rejection. Taking risks and trying new experiences requires a willingness to feel fear and uncertainty. We can observe a friend's behavior across different contexts to see if they act in trustworthy ways, but the way we truly come to trust a friend is by exposing our vulnerabilities and discovering how our friend responds. In other words, there is no way to achieve fullness and vitality in our lives without accepting the fact that we will feel fear, sadness, disappointment, and anger. Thus, although it is adaptive for us to notice our emotional responses and consider their messages, we may not always choose to act on their advice.

Values as an Opportunity to Enhance Quality of Life

Every day we make countless choices about how to spend our time. Upon awakening, we might check our phone, stretch our bodies, let out the dog, or kiss our partner. We might prepare breakfast for ourselves or others or race out the door without eating. Even if the bulk of our day seems predetermined by our responsibilities at work, class schedules, or caretaking demands, we actually have innumerable choices to make regarding the way we move through these experiences. We might listen intentionally and share our ideas openly at work, or we may daydream through meetings and keep our ideas to ourselves. We might be gruff with a coworker or take a minute to notice that they seem upset and choose a word of kindness instead. We might involve our children in our morning chores or let them watch television while we wash the dishes and put away the laundry. We can make these choices out of habit or impulse, a sense of obligation, or an attempt to avoid pain or stress. Or we can make those choices in ways that are consistent with our personal values.

Making large, life-altering choices is certainly one way to improve quality of life. The choices to initiate a new relationship, switch jobs, start an exercise routine, or join a mosque can make a measurable difference. Yet, as clients become more aware of their personal values and mindful of their moment-to-moment experiences, they will notice limitless opportunities to make small but intentional values-consistent choices that can enhance well-being. Daily activities that are previously seen as chores, such as cooking breakfast, can be appreciated as opportunities to engage in self-care or to demonstrate care for others. Small opportunities to engage in values-consistent behaviors can be woven into daily life, like enacting the value of engaging in healthy behaviors by climbing the stairs instead of taking the elevator or enacting the value of opening up to others by offering to play a board game with one's partner after dinner instead of watching television in separate rooms.

Values as a Guide for Finding Meaning in Challenging Contexts

Many of our clients exist in situations or contexts that bring considerable pain. They grapple with poverty, discrimination, injustice, chronic and acute illness, disability, work and school challenges, and interpersonal stressors that are beyond their control. Fortunately, one subtle, but powerful, benefit of articulating and affirming personal values is that doing so can help clients to find ways of being true to themselves in these challenging contexts. We might share an example like this one with clients to illustrate this possibility (adapting the story so that the example is relevant to the client's lived experience):

> "Pablo's closest childhood friend Leon was recently diagnosed with small cell lung cancer, and the prognosis isn't good. Leon smoked cigarettes for over 20 years, but he quit when his wife became pregnant. At that time, Leon told Pablo he wanted to be the best father and husband he could be to his family. Pablo feels extremely angry that such a good man who made such hard sacrifices could still develop

cancer. He worries that Leon's family will be financially and emotionally devastated by this experience. And as Leon grows sicker and weaker, Pablo is filled with sorrow that his best friend is dying.

"It can be hard to imagine how awareness of one's values could help in this situation or to see where values-driven actions could be taken. So many aspects of this extremely painful situation are completely out of Pablo's control. But let's consider some of Pablo's options.

"Pablo's deepest wishes are that he could cure Leon's cancer and prevent Leon's family from suffering emotionally and financially. Because those actions are outside of Pablo's control, he may feel helpless and, in an attempt to avoid painful thoughts and feelings related to Leon and his family, unintentionally act in ways that are inconsistent with his core values. For example, Pablo may stop visiting Leon or spend his visits searching the Internet to find cancer survival rate statistics. Struggling with the pain that comes from wishing he could help Leon's family financially and recognizing his own financial struggles, Pablo may stop visiting Leon's family as well. Pablo may spend time getting drunk or high in an attempt to suppress his feelings of sorrow, and he may stop attending church out of anger that God could allow this to happen.

"On the other hand, even though Pablo can't undo Leon's diagnosis or avoid feeling pain, there are values-consistent actions he can choose that might bring some meaning to an otherwise tragic situation. For example, he can make regular visits to Leon and Leon's family and be present and engaged during those visits, reminiscing about happier times and sitting with the pain of all that has been, and will be, lost. Because doing so is personally important to him, Pablo can continue attending church and meet with a spiritual leader to discuss confusion and anger. Pablo might offer to start a social media campaign to raise money to help Leon's family pay their bills, or he might volunteer to help with some home repair work. Although these actions won't erase Pablo's pain or change the outcome of Leon's cancer, they can allow Pablo to be the person he wishes to be in this painful context."

EMOTIONAL PROCESSING/WRITING EXERCISES

We also use a series of writing exercises to help clients articulate and clarify their values, modeled on the emotional processing task developed by James Pennebaker (1997; Pennebaker & Smyth, 2016) and adapted by Kelly Wilson (personal communication, 2000). The first set of exercises invites clients to reflect on how their current struggles are interfering with what matters most to them personally in three life domains: relationships, work/education/household management, and self-nourishment and community activities. The second asks them to articulate and affirm their personal values in these same three domains.

These exercises also draw from the principles underlying motivational interviewing, an approach that aims to strengthen the client's own personal motivation and commitment by helping them explore and resolve their natural ambivalence about making behavioral changes (Miller & Rollnick, 1991, 2012). The underlying assumption of motivational interviewing and these writing exercises is that ambivalence about change is

BOX 8.1. A CLOSER LOOK:
Research Evidence for Values Affirmation

Research on acceptance-based behavioral therapies provide support for the idea that increasing engagement in valued action predicts improved psychological functioning (e.g., Hayes, Orsillo, & Roemer, 2010; Michelson, Lee, Orsillo, & Roemer, 2011). In addition, numerous studies in social psychology demonstrate the widespread benefits of values affirmation. Studies using a wide variety of methods to encourage participants to connect with their personal values have shown that values affirmation reduces defensiveness (e.g., McQueen & Klein, 2006; Sherman & Cohen, 2006), increases openness to new information, strengthens intentions to change, and positively impacts subsequent behavior (e.g., Epton, Harris, Kane, van Koningsbruggen, & Sheeran, 2015). When student veterans affirmed their personal values, they reported increased intentions to seek counseling both immediately following the intervention and at a one-week follow-up (Seidman et al., 2018). Affirming values has been shown to decrease the gaps in academic achievement across gender (e.g., Miyake et al., 2010) and racial (Cohen, Garcia, Apfel, & Master, 2006; Cohen, Garcia, Purdie-Vaughns, Apfel, & Brzustoski, 2009) identities that are fueled by stereotype threat (i.e., beliefs that one will be judged on the basis of a negative stereotype about the intellectual ability of one's identity; Steele & Aronson, 1995). Finally, values affirmation instructions reduce cortisol responses to stress (Creswell et al., 2005).

natural. Both experiential and behavioral avoidance negatively impact quality of life, but they also reduce distress in the short term. Willingly and mindfully engaging in valued activities improves quality of life, but doing so also increases our contact with a range of painful internal experiences. Values writing exercises help clients to more fully encounter the costs of their avoidance and the discrepancy between their current experience and the ways in which they would like to be living their lives. Doing so may help them to resolve their ambivalence and move forward with change. A growing body of research has demonstrated the widespread benefits of values affirmation (see Box 8.1).

Exploring the Costs of Distraction, Avoidance, and Inaction

Although it can be challenging for clients to connect with the real pain of noticing the costs of avoidance and inaction in valued domains, this exercise can lay the foundation for deeply meaningful life change, particularly if it is done within a relational context of validation, acceptance, and hope.

We encourage clients to set aside 20 minutes a day, for 4 days, to engage in an emotional processing/writing activity. On each of the first 3 days, clients write about how their struggles are interfering with their satisfaction in one life domain. On the fourth day, clients are asked to reflect on anything important they may have noticed when completing the assignments. We include specific prompting questions for each life domain to help clients more fully engage in this process. Client Form 8.1, *Values Writing Exercise I,* from our client workbook, *Worry Less, Live More* (WLLM), is written for someone struggling with worry and anxiety, but this assignment can be personally tailored to whatever concerns are most central to the client.

BOX 8.2. TRY THIS:
Disconnection from Values

We encourage therapists to complete an adapted version of the first writing exercise themselves before recommending it to clients in order to experientially connect with the clear (and
often muddy) pain it can elicit. Doing so reminds us how easily we can all unintentionally stray
from our values, particularly when learned habits and reactivity override purposeful, mindful
action.

Think about what is important to you in your relationships, work/education/household
management, and self-nourishment and community activities. How might your general busyness, stress, or struggles with worry and anxiety be interfering in these three life domains? Try
to set aside 20 minutes to write about what comes to mind for you. In your writing, try to really
let go and explore your very deepest emotions and thoughts about the topic.

Not surprisingly, clients have varied reactions to this initial writing. Both discussing the challenges *that can arise* when first introducing the exercise and sufficiently
processing those *that do arise* after the client completes the exercise are essential. Clients may feel motivated and empowered by the process. They may be surprised by the
subtle shifts they have made to accommodate their clinical challenges and the widespread costs of those shifts. Many clients find that the exercise elicits strong feelings of
sadness as they notice how consumed they have become with internal struggles and
how distant they feel from the things that really matter to them. All of these responses
are validated and explored in session. Clients are encouraged to use their mindfulness
practices to make room for the full range of their responses.

This first values writing exercise can uncover several different patterns of behavior. Some clients describe significant avoidance and narrowed behavioral repertoires.
For example, Rodney had been struggling with posttraumatic stress disorder (PTSD)
for over a decade before he initiated ABBT. In his values writing, he described the ways
his attempts to suppress painful memories and images, including the use of substances,
pulled him away from valued life activities. Rodney was extremely close to his family,
but his parent reluctantly told him that he could no longer live at home if he continued
to get high around his younger siblings. Rodney felt unable to give up that habit, so he
moved out and fell out of contact with his family. Rodney tried to protect his partner by
limiting contact with her when he was struggling with symptoms. This distance, and
Rodney's refusal to seek couples counseling, ultimately led to their breakup. Rodney
also wrote about how he valued fostering his creativity through music, but recently he
felt too empty and sad to pick up his guitar. Rodney concluded that his struggle with
his symptoms left him little time or energy to engage in values-based actions.

Other clients discover that while they have been behaviorally active in valued
domains, they have not been actively engaged and present. For instance, Tony had a
strong relationship with his family of origin and his partner to whom he had been committed for over 10 years. Tony was a talented electrician who owned his own business
through which he had grown a loyal customer base. He was also an involved father who
coached his daughter's baseball team, and he volunteered in his son's preschool classroom. In short, Tony was active in many valued life domains. However, during the first

writing assignment, Tony poignantly described feeling like a spectator in his own life. When he was at work, he frequently worried about his mother's health, his partner's level of commitment to their relationship, and his children's happiness and well-being. At home he found himself ruminating about events from his day at work and worrying about the challenges the next day's schedule would bring. Tony shared the perspective that despite the fact that he was regularly "going through the motions," his struggle with worry left him feeling completely disengaged from his values.

Finally, many clients learn that they have lost their sense of choice and purpose in valued life domains. Their daily activities are focused on tasks that "have to" or that "should" get done. Our client Lei, a graduate student in history, reported a disconnect from the values that had initially pointed her toward graduate school, an interest in challenging herself intellectually and a desire to engage in work aimed at improving the lives of others. She had become increasingly focused on the goal of obtaining her PhD, and she began to view her daily activities (e.g., reading, writing, and conducting research) as tasks she needed to complete so that she could stop worrying about them and avoid the potential feelings of self-loathing that would arise if she fell behind. Lei felt as if program requirements were controlling her life, and she no longer experienced the inherent value of her work.

Another common response is for clients to fail to complete the exercise. Exploring this understandable response in session can help us better understand our clients, deepen the therapeutic relationship, and generate personalized recommendations for how clients might overcome obstacles to change. Sometimes these discussions uncover the fact that we did not provide a sufficient rationale for why we think the exercise may be helpful or did not provide clear enough instructions about how to complete it. Recognizing our mistakes provides us with an opportunity to try again. Other times, we may underestimate how fearful clients are to engage in this exercise. Offering recommendations about how clients may use the skills they are developing to work with the painful thoughts and feelings that arise during values writing can be helpful. Alternatively, we sometimes have clients work through the exercise in session where we can offer scaffolding and support. Some clients face very real limits on their time. The multiple demands they're juggling make it challenging for them to devote sufficient time outside of session exercises. To address this obstacle, we brainstorm creative ways of finding time, which may include completing an abbreviated version of the exercise in session. Finally, many clients are hesitant to express their most strongly held personal values in writing. Although we believe there are benefits to emotionally processing values-related material through writing, we are open to having clients recording their spoken thoughts instead of simply talking to us about their values in session. Recording spoken thoughts is also a good option for clients with limited writing abilities and for those who are less comfortable writing because English is not their first language or because of negative experiences they have had in educational contexts.

Articulating and Clarifying Personal Values

Once clients have had the opportunity to become more aware of the ways in which their struggle with internal content has pulled them away from valued pursuits, we encourage them to articulate a set of personally relevant values that can serve as a compass to guide their behavior. The first step in the articulation process is to invite clients to write

BOX 8.3. TRY THIS:
What Matters Most?

Take a few moments to write about what is important to you in your relationships with others, work/education/household management, and self-nourishment and community activities. For the purpose of this therapist exercise, you just need to jot down a few of your thoughts—the first ones that come to mind. We will ask you to refer back to your notes later in this chapter.

about what matters most to them in each of three important domains of valued living (see Client Form 8.2, *Values Writing Exercise II*).

IN-SESSION VALUES EXPLORATION AND CLARIFICATION

For most clients, this exercise is only a starting point for the exploration of values. Significant session time is devoted to learning about the clients' experience with this exercise and reviewing the material they generate. We start by reinforcing clients for their willingness to engage in values articulation and validating any painful emotions or thoughts that arose. We also review our clients' values writing for themes that can signal a potential obstacle or stuck point that could interfere with the next phase of values work.

Setting the Stage for Values Clarification

The process of reviewing values writing for possible stuck points should be a collaborative one, approached with considerable clinical sensitivity. We certainly don't want to invalidate our clients' lived experiences that factors outside of their control have significantly impacted their well-being. We also don't want to imply that we as therapists know more about what is personally meaningful to our clients than they do themselves. On the other hand, we do want to help clients generate values that can be used in therapy and after termination to guide engagement in personal meaningful activities.

To that end, in setting the stage for values clarification, we acknowledge the broad array of factors that impact our quality of life, including our *current context, preferences, and values*. External stressors in our current context such as financial burdens, caretaking responsibilities, and incidents of bias can elicit an ongoing stream of challenging thoughts and feelings that can be quite painful. The people in our lives play an important role; some providing love and support and others criticism and neglect. Depending on our context, we may be given opportunities or we may be excluded from them. And while we may have some influence over the context in which we reside, we rarely have total control over these factors despite their influence on our quality of life.

Preferences also have considerable influence on our life satisfaction. We all hold preferences about the type of people with whom we would like to interact and the situations we hope to encounter. We may prefer a partner who is adventurous and outgoing, or one who is dependable and reserved. At work, we might prefer a supervisor who provides a lot of oversight or one who grants us considerable independence. We often choose to take actions informed by our preferences. For example, someone might join a group that plans weekly excursions with the hope that they find a dating partner who shares their taste for travel. An employee might directly ask a supervisor to provide more hands-on training and attention. But even though our preferences are an important part of who we are, and we can express and act on them, we can't always ensure that our preferences will be met when they involve people and situations out of our control.

Values, as they are narrowly defined in ABBT, are the ways we choose to be in the world. Although values are only one part of what defines our experiences, they are the part over which we have control. For that reason, they have the potential to serve as a compass that can guide our clients' behavioral choices and empower them to act in life-fulfilling ways even in challenging contexts. That is not to say that our context and preferences don't matter or that clients shouldn't consider contextual factors or preferences when making choices. We are simply asking clients if they are willing to expand their focus and articulate and clarify personal values as another important piece of their experience. If clients are willing, we work with them to go over their writing, identify potential stuck points that might reflect goals and preferences, and clarify their values.

Identifying Common Stuck Points

Beginning ABBT therapists are often surprised when clients write about wanting to change their internal experiences or achieve goals, given that these topics are covered earlier in treatment. But psychoeducation simply lays the groundwork for change, it is not sufficient in and of itself. Given the central role that goals play in our lives, it makes sense that many clients include at least some "goal language" when writing about what matters most to them personally. Clients also frequently write about the ubiquitous desire we have as humans to change our internal experiences, change other people's emotions and behaviors, and control situations and circumstances beyond our control. For example, a client might write:

> "I would like to be a happy, self-confident person. I think if I were more positive and fun I would have a stronger relationship with my partner and I would have more friends. Right now, I avoid talking to the other students in my classes because I don't feel good about myself. I value developing more relationships and strengthening the ones I have. Once I can shake this depression I will feel more confident about putting myself out there."

When people are asked to reflect on the things that matter to them, it is no surprise that our most strongly held values often involve others. Although relationships often bring great satisfaction and comfort, they can also elicit pain and distress. A natural response is for us to wish that others would change. For instance, a client might write:

> "I wish that my partner would really listen to me and be willing to do some of the things I am interested in. We spend so much time going to the movies, which she loves, but she isn't willing to go to concerts or listen to music, which is something I really value. I also wish my friends would be a little bit less selfish. Whenever they have a problem, they call, but no one is there for me when I need a true friend."

Another common theme is the desire to be perfect or rise about our "humanness" in different domains of one's life. For example, a client may write:

> "I would like to be a loving, caring person who is always there for my partner. I also want to be a patient, fun-loving parent who is always attuned to the needs of my children. I want to be a loyal friend. It is really important to me that I am the kind of person that all my friends can depend on—whenever they need me."

Finally, some clients include specific behavioral changes they wish to make (e.g., "I want to attend temple every week") in their values writing, rather than describing more overarching life directions (e.g., "I value being a spiritual person"). A summary of these common stuck points and examples of the types of statements that reflect them are displayed in Table 8.2.

We find it helpful to name these themes and use them to guide the values clarification work. We often invite our clients to read Chapters 10 and 11 in *WLLM* (Orsillo & Roemer, 2016) so that they can work through their own writing outside of session as well to identify the presence of these potential "traps." However, these categories overlap, and thus many values statements can fall into more than one category. We don't approach the task of values clarification with the goal of labeling each stuck point exactly right; we simply use this list as a way of increasing our awareness of these common themes.

TABLE 8.2. Common Stuck Points in Values Writing

Common stuck points	Sample statements
Emphasizing goals	• "I want to lose weight." • "I want to get my college degree." • "I want to get promoted at work."
Focusing on specific behaviors	• "I want to spend time with my friends every weekend." • "I want to read to my children." • "I want to go for walks in nature."
Striving to control the uncontrollable	
Internal states	• "I want to be happy and feel confident." • "I don't want to be disappointed in my family when they let me down." • "I want to fall in love."
Other people	• "I want my partner to be more responsive." • "I want my sister to appreciate the things I do for her."
Situations and circumstances	• "I want my children to have a safe and secure future." • "I don't want to be limited by my chronic illness." • "I want my children to be accepted into the school in our neighborhood."
Aiming for perfection	• "I always want to be there for my neighbors." • "I want to excel in school."

BOX 8.4. TRY THIS:
Clarifying Values

If you completed the "Try This" in Box 8.3, take a look back over your answers. Notice if you wrote about values, as we define them in ABBT, or if you were pulled to express goals and preferences. Take note of whether you can see some of the stuck points discussed in this chapter in your own writing. If you can, take a moment to recognize how common it is for us to focus on things that may be somewhat out of our control when thinking about what matters most to us personally.

WORKING WITH STUCK POINTS IN VALUES WRITING

Goals

As noted earlier, our purpose in identifying stuck points in our clients' writing is to broaden their awareness of these patterns and to help them identify opportunities to engage in present-focused actions that are personally meaningful. If we notice a goal in a client's values writing (e.g., to lose weight; to graduate college), we acknowledge the importance of the goal *and* we try to explore the underlying value (e.g., to live a healthy lifestyle; to learn). If clients find themselves struggling to differentiate values and goals, we might recommend that they complete Client Form 8.3, *Values versus Goals*, on their own, or we may walk through it together in session. This form asks a number of prompting questions that clarify the difference between these two closely related concepts. See Figure 8.1 for an example of how a client might complete this form.

Internal Experiences

Given the inherent pleasure and pain associated with certain internal states, and the messages we receive about which thoughts, emotions, and physical sensations are acceptable and desirable, it's not surprising that many clients write about valuing internal experiences such as happiness or confidence. We always validate the very natural wish that we could think and feel in ways that bring constant peace and happiness. And we ask the client to consider the potential downsides to holding values connected to internal states, given that they are not entirely in our control. Most clients can acknowledge that if we value experiences we can't control, we can get pulled into an endless loop of trying; these futile efforts can leave us feeling chronically helpless and dissatisfied.

We recommend two strategies to clients who find themselves valuing internal states. First, we invite them to practice self-compassion and remind themselves that it is natural both to have a wide range of thoughts and emotions and to want to try to avoid pain. Second, we ask them to consider how things would be different if they had the ability to control their internal experiences, to see if underlying values emerge. For example, Derek wrote about wanting to feel more confident and less shy. When his therapist probed, Derek shared that if he had more confidence he would open up more to his neighbors and make efforts to get to know them. When asked, Derek confirmed that opening up to others was one of his core values.

Potential Value	Could you take an action today that would be consistent with this value?	Can you ever complete or fully achieve this value? Will you ever be done?	Do you have complete control over the execution of this value?	Value?
	For a value, the answer would be "yes."	*For a value, the answer would be "no."*	*For a value, the answer would be "yes."*	*Yes or No?*
I want to be promoted to manager.	Yes—I could tell my boss.	Yes—there is a clear endpoint.	No—the ultimate decision is my boss's.	No.
I want to fall in love.	Yes—I could look at a dating site.	No.	No—I can't make myself feel an emotion.	No.
I want to be dependable and responsible.	Yes—I could spend time working on a project for work.	No.	Yes—I can choose whether or not to act this way.	Yes.
I want to maintain a healthy diet.	Yes—I could choose what to eat.	No.	Yes—I can choose what I eat.	Yes.
I want to be an A student.	Yes—I could study.	Yes.	No—I may have natural limits in my ability to understand; I may have an unfair teacher.	No.

FIGURE 8.1. Example of Client Form 8.3, *Values versus Goals.*

Other People

Social connectedness is core to our human nature. Thus, when clients write about what they value, they often express the desire for the important people in their lives to respond in particular ways. We always validate this wish. And we support our clients taking actions aimed at getting what they want and deserve in their relationships. However, we also ask our clients if they are willing to expand their focus and consider what matters to them personally about how *they* act in their interactions with others. Once again, we try to increase our clients' awareness of the frustration and helpfulness that can arise when we define values that are out of our personal control. We also share with clients our experience that, ironically, sometimes when we are trying unsuccessfully to control other people, we end up acting in ways that are completely inconsistent with our personal values.

For example, Grace valued being responsible and dependable in carrying out her assignments as a volunteer. And she understandably expected the same of her peers and became frustrated when they took multiple breaks to get coffee and interact with their phones. Grace tried to inspire her peers by leading by example, and when that failed she gave clear feedback directly to her peers and then to their supervisor. Despite these admirable efforts, nothing changed. Demoralized by her inability to change her peers' behavior, Grace started canceling her own shifts and taking more breaks herself.

When the therapist asked Grace to explain her motivation, Grace first offered that she made the choices she made to "get back at her peers." Then she justified her behavior by noting that it was only fair. The therapist validated Grace's wish for things to be fair and shared her understanding of how tempting it can be to act out of revenge. The therapist also asked Grace if these actions were effective, at which point Grace became teary. Grace described feeling guilty and unfulfilled by her current behavior, but also feeling stuck. Grace expressed the concern that letting her peers "get away" with being "lazy" would feel like "giving in" and letting them off the hook, and she feared that made her seem weak. The therapist validated the humanness of Grace's responses and shared her belief that Grace had the wisdom to choose the right response for herself. The therapist suggested that Grace practice defusing from thoughts that were telling her the "right" and "wrong" ways to respond, observing her lived experience using her newly developed mindfulness skills. Grace was able to notice that although she believed that changing the behavior of her peers or "getting back" at them were the "right" options, her efforts had not left her feeling whole or fulfilled. She was also willing to try out practicing acceptance over her limited control of others and focusing on and enacting her own personal values at the site, which she found more fulfilling. She also considered the possibility of leaving the site and instead finding a volunteer opportunity where other volunteers were more engaged. However, she identified that the work at this site remained meaningful and important to her, and so she chose to continue there.

The Desire to Be Perfect or Super-Human

Sometimes, when a client writes about values using extreme language (e.g., "I want to excel at my job"), it simply reflects the aspirational nature of the exercise. During the in-session discussion, the client might clarify that by "excelling" they meant they value putting in effort and being responsible at work. Other times, values written with extreme language accurately reflect a deeply held desire to rise above one's humanness and achieve unreachable goals (e.g., "I *always* want to be emotionally present with my children" or "I want to be a *model* Christian"). Although defining lofty values may provide initial motivation, they can ultimately lead to feelings of hopelessness and burnout, as well as extensive self-criticism when perfection cannot be achieved or maintained.

To avoid this stuck point, we encourage clients to consider tweaking their values in ways that reflect more sustainable action. One method of tweaking is to simply remove extreme language ("I value being emotionally present with my children"; "I value living consistently with my Christian faith"). However, it's also important for clients to go beyond the grammatical edit and use acceptance and compassion to practice accepting the limits of being human.

Some clients strive to be perfect because they believe they will be accepted and loved by others only if they achieve perfection. We sometimes invite our clients to bring mindful awareness to their experience with this belief, encouraging them to examine whether their attempts to be perfect bring them closer to others. For example, Mia wanted to be more open and connected to the people she met at her new job. She considered inviting them over to her apartment, but she was embarrassed by its small size and gently used furnishings. Mia was hoping to be able to move to a new place once she had been working for a while or at least save up enough money to buy some nicer things. In the meantime, given the less than perfect state of her home, Mia limited her socializing to sitting with her coworkers during breaks and lunch. Unfortunately, Mia noticed the conversation seemed to become stilted when she joined them. Desperate to make a good impression, Mia talked about her recent successes at work and the praise she received from their supervisor. She also tried to portray herself as a good parent to her coworkers who had children. Mia imagined one day becoming good friends with some coworkers and inviting them to visit with their children. In an attempt to earn their trust and to be perceived as a good parent, Mia used her time during breaks to talk about the ways she limited her children's use of electronics and fed them healthy snacks.

Through treatment, Mia began to notice that these attempts to become the perfect worker and mother living in the perfect apartment were not bringing her a sense of fulfillment. Warily, she accepted her therapist's suggestion that she try a different approach to see what could be learned. Mia invited some coworkers over to her home and was surprised when they commented on how cozy it seemed. As the night went on, Mia intentionally shared some of her struggles at work and as a parent. To Mia's surprise, the next day at lunch, one of her coworkers, Luisa, waved Mia over to her table. Mia felt warmth and affection from Luisa, who confided, "I never realized we had so much in common. You always seemed to have it all together, and honestly, I was intimidated by you before I got to know you better. It was really validating to hear that you are confused by the new process we are supposed to use to enter the monthly reports. Maybe we can figure it out together."

Often the belief that we must be perfect develops through a history of receiving conditional attention and love for certain behaviors or achievements. Helping clients to recognize the origins of their desire to be perfect, validating the need we all have for love and acceptance, and being present with clients as they sit with the pain of not being able to control how others feel toward us and treat us can help clients consider articulating values that reflect their desire to be open and present with others.

Specific Behaviors

Sometimes clients define their values using specific behaviors (e.g., "I want to attend events at my daughter's school"). Generating specific actions clients can take that are consistent with their values is definitely a focus of ABBT, but we also want clients to be able to articulate the general principle guiding these actions. Grounding values in specific behaviors can limit our flexibility. For example, if Dimitri values attending events at his daughter's school, but an event conflicts with another commitment he has made (e.g., taking his mother to a doctor's appointment), he is likely to feel stuck and unable to enact his value. Instead, if he values demonstrating his love and care toward his daughter, he can choose from a wide array of actions to enact this value (e.g., spend time in the evening listening to his daughter describe the event, donate snacks to the school to be shared at the event, or text his daughter a picture of Dimitri and his mother wishing her good luck at her event).

Narrowly defining values as specific behaviors that seem inaccessible to us can lead to feelings of hopelessness. Amelia was the single parent to a toddler and a law student who sought therapy for help with stress. Previously, Amelia used to relax and engage in self-care by taking long hikes in the woods or renting a kayak and paddling around a lake near her house. In her current context, Amelia could not find the time to engage in those activities. She felt she desperately needed the enjoyment and self-care those activities used to bring her, but it felt impossible for her to carve out the necessary time. Amelia's mother recommended that Amelia practice mindful breathing during her commute, but Amelia felt that such a small change would be completely insufficient. Amelia's therapist validated Amelia's sadness over having less time to go hiking and kayaking and Amelia's skepticism about the potential benefits a few minutes of mindful breathing could bring given Amelia's considerable stress. The therapist also suggested that affirming a general value of self-care, rather than grounding self-care in hiking or breathing during a commute, might create flexibility and allow for more opportunities. Together, Amelia and her therapist generated a large list of self-care behaviors that could fit in her current life. For example, they discussed planning and packing meals and snacks that could sustain Amelia during long days at school, creating a more comfortable study space (adding a pillow to a hard, uncomfortable chair, burning a fragrant candle, replacing a harsh light bulb with one that cast an easier glow), and choosing parenting activities that also reflected Amelia's interests and hobbies (e.g., taking her daughter for a bicycle ride, walking her daughter home from day care on sunny days, attending a child-friendly event at the art museum). Although Amelia was initially skeptical that these activities could be sufficiently self-nourishing, over time she found broadening her view of self-care and integrating multiple valued actions into her daily life gave her a stronger sense of self-fulfillment (although she still went hiking and kayaking whenever she could!).

WORKING WITH STUCK POINTS RELATED TO VALUES ARTICULATION

Indecision

In addition to the stuck points that are sometimes apparent in values writing, sometimes obstacles arise that are related to the overall process of defining and articulating values. It's not uncommon for clients to feel nervous and indecisive about the process of affirming what matters most to them. Clients may be unsure about what they value, feel motionless and stuck, or believe they need to change internally (e.g., feel less depressed, improve their self-esteem) before they can fully lean into valued action.

We validate these responses while also gently encouraging clients to consider the alternative. Whether or not we articulate values, something is guiding the large and small choices we make on an ongoing basis. In other words, "values" are already guiding our behavior, even if those "values" are to minimize risk and avoid pain. By inviting clients to articulate and clarify their values, we are asking them to bring attention to a process that is already ongoing and to consider being more intentional in their choices.

When clients are indecisive, they often believe that continuing to ponder their possible values is the best method of attaining clarity. Unfortunately, the distinction between reflecting on one's values and entering into an endless worry loop about choosing the "right" values can be hard to make. We suggest that our clients practice living consistently with values, even if they are not "certain" about their choice in order to see what can be learned from their experience. Mindfulness practice can also help clients who struggle with significant self-awareness, or who are chronically disconnected from their sense of self, to choose valued directions reflexively rather than reactively (Shapiro, Carlson, Astin, & Freedman, 2006).

Given that values are seen as a compass that guides our behavior, one assumption is that we remain committed to personal values even when we experience thoughts, emotions, or sensations that suggest an alternative action. And to some degree that is true. For example, if caring for one's baby is a personally held value, one's intention would be to do so both when the baby was serene and cuddly and when she was irritable and colicky. On the other hand, what we hold as values might change as a function of growth and experience. For example, as a teenager and young adult, Olivia defined autonomy as one of her core values. As she grew older, she found that value less compelling, and she became more focused on actions consistent with her value of connecting with others.

Avoidance and Hopelessness

Some clients, often those who are the most distressed, avoid completing values writing because they are entangled with thoughts that behavioral change is impossible. A rush to challenge this assumption can leave clients feeling invalidated, as if the therapist does not understand the extent of the client's struggle. Instead, we recommend that therapists both make room for this hopelessness in session and use ABBT skills to work with it. Hopelessness about the possibility of change typically reflects both clear and muddy emotions. For example, clients may feel sadness over the recognition that they become so disconnected from their personal values. They may also engage in self-criticism, recall previous experiences of loss and disappointment, and worry that things will never change in the future—all understandable responses that muddy their current emotional state. Validating our clients' sadness and the challenging ways our minds work, modeling compassion, and encouraging them to practice acceptance and mindfulness can be effective ways to move forward. These moments can also be an opportunity for clients to practice acting in ways that are inconsistent with their thoughts and emotions. In other words, clients can be encouraged to consider taking a leap of faith and attempting to engage in behaviors that seem impossible or pointless.

Influences That Shape Our Values

The question of what motivates us to hold particular life directions as values has been the focus of considerable theory and research (see Box 8.5 for a closer look at the research on this topic). Hayes and colleagues (Hayes, Strosahl, et al., 1999; Hayes, 2016) draw from relational frame therapy (RFT; Hayes, Barnes-Holmes, & Roche, 2001) to highlight the potential influence of external factors on clients' articulation of their values in the context of ACT. Specifically, they recommend considering how *pliance* could potentially impact clients' articulation of their values. Pliance is defined as rule-governed behavior that is under the control of a socially mediated history of reinforcement for following the rule. For example, a client might endorse pursuing life-long learning as a value because doing so is reinforced by an increase in parental love/affection and a reduction in parental criticism and ridicule. Similarly, clients might write about holding social justice and volunteerism as values because in the past they were given approval and acceptance for talking about valuing these constructs.

Although it can be useful to consider the potential influence of external factors on a client's values articulation, this exploration should be guided by an understanding of, and appreciation for, the role of cultural identity in values development. Values are a culturally bound construct. In other words, the extent to which we see values as personally relevant, individualistic strivings, as opposed to ways of being and acting that reflect others' expectations, is at least partly influenced by our cultural identity, particularly as it relates to our construal of the self as independent or interdependent (Markus & Kitayama, 1991). Research has shown that people from an individualistic culture (United Kingdom) most strongly endorse values that represent personal ideals, whereas those from a collectivist culture (India) endorse values representing personal ideals and the expectations of others similarly (Cheung, Maio, Rees, Kamble, & Mane, 2016). Values that reflect one's cultural identity or that are consistent with one's family or larger community can be powerfully motivating and life enhancing when clients also personally identify with the values or have integrated them as their own. For example, Desmond's personal value of being responsible and committed at work reflects his family's emphasis on the importance of reliability. Living consistently with this value brings Desmond a deep sense of fulfillment because it is personally meaningful for him, as is honoring the values of his family.

On the other hand, Brad wrote extensively about valuing creativity and how it was motivating him to pursue his master's in fine arts in the values articulation exercise. But when discussing this exercise with his therapist, Brad expressed some doubt as to whether it was an authentically held value. Brad explained that his parents were both highly creative people who were clearly disappointed with Brad's initial inclination to study economics in college. Brad described feeling proud when his parents complimented his artistic pursuits and enjoyed their shared interest in visiting museums and

BOX 8.5. A CLOSER LOOK:
Intrinsic versus Extrinsic Motivation to Pursue Values

Our motivations can be broadly characterized as intrinsic or extrinsic; intrinsic motivation is assumed to reflect authentic, integrated core values, whereas extrinsic motivation assumes that values are controlled by external factors (e.g., Deci & Ryan, 1985; Sheldon & Elliot, 1999). Research generally suggests that holding values for internal, authentic, self-concordant reasons leads to more frequent goal attainment and enhanced well-being than holding values that are externally controlled (e.g., Bailey & Phillips, 2016; Ferssizidis et al., 2010; Sheldon & Kasser 2001).

However, important subtleties are missed by this broad distinction. Ryan and Deci (2000) defined four subtypes of extrinsic motivation processes that vary in both the degree to which they are accepted and integrated into one's own sense of values and the impact they have on values-consistent behavior and psychological well-being. According to these authors, values that are held or enacted because of *external regulation* (social pressure to satisfy an external demand) or *introjected regulation* (internal pressure to behave in a way that will reduce guilt or anxiety or enhance feelings of self-worth) are less likely to contribute to a sustained sense of self-fulfillment and meaning. In contrast, when extrinsic factors motivate values that are congruent with someone's sense of self, in the case of *identified regulation*, or that become an integral part of who they are through *integrated regulation*, they may enhance satisfaction and quality of life (Ryan & Deci, 2001).

galleries. But he also described feeling lost in his graduate program and approaching his coursework with a sense of dread and obligation.

The therapist validated Brad's desire for love, affection, and admiration from his parents and helped Brad to identify his limited control over their behavior and the costs associated with consistently trying to elicit those expressions from his parents. The therapist also helped Brad to identify personal values that could guide Brad's behavior in his relationship with his parents and in his education/career. Through this process, Brad was able to share his doubts about graduate school with his parents and ask for their support. Although Brad continued to feel some guilt about leaving his graduate program and his parents occasionally made condescending remarks about his career choice, Brad was able to derive a sense of inner strength and stability by living consistently with what mattered most to him personally both in his career choice and in his orientation toward his parents.

INCREASING AWARENESS OF ACTION AND INACTION IN VALUED DOMAINS

As the final step in the process of identifying values, we ask clients specifically to define one or two values in each of the three domains and then to identify opportunities to take values-consistent actions that naturally arise in their daily lives. For example, clients might identify the following values:

- Interpersonal relationships
  - "I want to share my thoughts and feelings openly with my partner."
  - "I want to make time to nurture my relationships with friends."
- Work/school/community
  - "I want to be responsible in my actions at work."
  - "I want to set challenges for myself so that I continue to learn and grow."
- Self-nurturance and community involvement
  - "I want to promote my physical health."
  - "I want to pursue social justice for my community."

Once clients articulate these values, we ask them to use the mindful observation skills they have been cultivating to complete Client Form 8.4, *Monitoring Opportunities for Valued Action*. Using this form, clients monitor the times they engaged in values-consistent actions, the degree to which they were mindfully engaged during the valued activity, missed opportunities to engage in valued behavior, and obstacles that made engagement in valued behavior difficult.

An example of the kind of information that can be derived from clients filling out this form is what we learned about Zac, a client who came to treatment for help with generalized anxiety and substance abuse. Zac identified values related to being more open and accessible in his relationships. The first time he completed Client Form 8.4, Zac noted a day during which he spent some time with his children, consistent with his values, but he rated his mindfulness during that activity as low because he was distracted by ruminations about an argument he had with his brother earlier in the day. Zac also recorded a missed opportunity later in the week; he canceled lunch plans with his brother. Although Zac used work as an excuse, he noted on the form that his primary motivation for canceling was to avoid the discomfort that was lingering from their earlier argument. Later that week, Zac took a valued action and called his brother on the phone to discuss their conflict. He rated this as a valued-consistent activity and noted that he was mindfully present during the conversation. Zac also noted that he took a values-consistent action in choosing to mindfully play catch with his son one evening after work.

As noted on this form, it's essential that clients practice self-kindness and compassion when completing this activity. All of us have moments when we intentionally or unintentionally pass up opportunities to take actions that would be consistent with our values. Thus, the goal of this exercise isn't to demonstrate perfect compliance with one's values. Instead, its primary aim is to help clients and therapists become more aware of how values-consistent actions could be interwoven into a client's existing activities. The knowledge gained through this activity can be used to inform choices about the types of behavioral practices clients can pursue later in therapy, as we discuss in the next chapter.

BOX 8.6. **WHEN TIME IS LIMITED:**
Articulating Values

When we have less individual time with clients in session, we rely more heavily on outside of session handouts and exercises to:

- Provide psychoeducational resources about the nature of values (using Chapter 9 from the *WLLM*).
- Build motivation by asking clients to complete Client Form 8.1 and begin to notice the ways in which their struggles with internal states and attempts to engage in avoidance are eroding their quality of life.
- Articulate their values using Client Form 8.2.

We reserve in-session time for helping clients to identify stuck points and working with them to clarify and articulate values that have the potential to serve as a compass to guide behavior and enhance quality of life.

Struggles with worry and anxiety often interfere with people's relationships, work/education/ household management, and self-nurturance and community involvement. Worrying can distract us and make it hard for us to be present with the people and activities that we care about. And sometimes, in an attempt to try to minimize our stress, we may avoid certain situations or activities—even if those situations and activities are important to us.

Sometimes the effects of worry, anxiety, and avoidance on our lives are very obvious; other times the effects are harder to see. Anxiety and worry can lead us to develop habits and responses that are so automatic we don't even think about them as choices. It just seems like "this is just how things have to be."

This assignment offers an opportunity for you to take some time for yourself to really focus on how your life may be affected by worry and anxiety. Set aside 20 minutes on four different days during which you can privately and comfortably do this writing assignment. In your writing, we want you to really let go and explore your deepest emotions and thoughts about the topics listed below. Use a notebook or your computer to record your answers to each of the questions below.

As you write, try to allow yourself to experience your thoughts and feelings as completely as you are able. This work is based on the evidence that pushing these disturbing thoughts away can actually make them worse, so try to really let yourself go. If you can't think of what to write next, repeat the same thing over and over until something new comes to you. Be sure to write for the entire 20 minutes. Don't be concerned with spelling, punctuation, or grammar; just write whatever comes to mind.

Day 1

Write about how you think your anxiety and worry might be interfering with your relationships (family, friends, partner, etc.).

- What are some ways that your struggles with anxiety, worry, or avoidance has affected your current relationships?
- Does your anxiety and worry hold you back in relationships? What do you need from others in your life? What do you want to give to others? What gets in the way of asking for what you need and giving what you want to give?
- Do you make choices in your relationships that are driven by avoidance? Does fear get in the way of developing new relationships?
- Are you present and engaged when you are with others? Do you find yourself frequently distracted by worry?

(continued)

Note. Adapted with permission from *Worry Less, Live More* by Susan M. Orsillo and Lizabeth Roemer. Copyright © 2016 The Guilford Press.

Day 2

Write about how you think your anxiety and worry might be interfering with your work, education, or training or your family/household management.

- What are some ways that your struggles with anxiety, worry, or avoidance has affected your job/ studies/household management?
- How does your anxiety and worry hold you back in your work/schooling? Have you passed up new opportunities?
- Are there changes that you would like to make in this area of your life?
- Do you make choices in your work/studies/household management that are driven by avoidance?
- Are you present and engaged when working, studying, or managing your household?

Day 3

Write about how you think your anxiety and worry interfere with your ability to take care of yourself, have fun, and/or get involved with your community.

- What are some activities in these areas that you would like to spend more time doing?
- How does your anxiety/worry hold you back?
- Do you make choices about your leisure or community-based activities that are driven by avoidance?
- Are you present and engaged when participating in leisure or community-based activities?

Day 4

This is your last day of writing, so take some time to reflect on what came up for you over the last few days as you allowed yourself to focus on the issues raised in the first three parts of the writing assignment. Have you noticed any important areas that need more attention? Feel free to write about whatever comes up for you about these three areas of living.

Clarifying what matters most to you is an important part of the process of defining your own personal values. First, create a space for yourself to focus intentionally on what matters most to you. One way to do this is to practice mindfulness. You might start by focusing on your breath for a few moments and then expanding your awareness to notice and acknowledge the worries, stressors and demands of your life that may be pulling at your attention and gently bringing your attention toward this exercise.

Next, spend 20 minutes writing about what matters to you in each of the three areas of your life described below. Use a notebook or your computer to record your answers to each of the questions below. It can be tempting to just think about what matters to you without writing about it or to spend less time on the exercise, especially if you are busy with other tasks. Sometimes it's painful to reflect on what matters most to you because it can seem out of reach or it can remind you of how much of your time is spent on "shoulds" rather than "wants." Yet, investing time in this exercise and opening yourself up to pain in the service of making some meaningful life changes can be an important step in the process of change.

Day 1

Choose two or three relationships that are important to you. You can pick either actual relationships (my relationship with my brother) or relationships you would like to have (I'd like to be part of a couple; I'd like to make more friends). Briefly write about **how you'd like to be** in those relationships. Think about how you'd like to communicate with others (e.g., how open vs. private you'd like to be, how direct vs. indirect you'd like to be in asking for what you need and in giving feedback to others). Consider all of the ways people can be in their relationships—caring, supportive, genuine, open, honest, attentive, respectful, accepting, dutiful—and identify what matters most to you.

Day 2

Briefly write about the sort of work, training, education, or household management you would like to be engaged in and why that appeals to you. Next write about the kind of worker and/or student and/or household manager you'd like to be with respect to your work habits and your relationships with your boss/coworkers, or co-students. What's important to you about how you approach your work? Do you value learning, teaching, being reliable, being creative, taking on challenges, figuring out solutions to problems, taking on responsibility, or being industrious? What matters most to you? How would you like to communicate to others about your work? How would you like to respond to feedback? Are there any additional challenges you would like to take on?

(continued)

Note. Adapted with permission from *Worry Less, Live More* by Susan M. Orsillo and Lizabeth Roemer. Copyright © 2016 The Guilford Press.

Day 3

Briefly write about the ways in which you'd like to spend any additional time, whether or not you actually have additional time in your life right now. Do you enjoy creative pursuits, participating in physical activities, connecting with nature, developing yourself spiritually, engaging in self-care, taking actions in line with your political and social views, or engaging with or contributing to your community?

Potential value	Could you take an action today that would be consistent with this value?	Can you ever complete or fully achieve this value? Will you ever be done?	Do you have complete control over the execution of this value?	Value?
	For a value, the answer would be "yes."	*For a value, the answer would be "no."*	*For a value, the answer would be "yes."*	*Yes or no?*

Note. Adapted with permission from *Worry Less, Live More* by Susan M. Orsillo and Lizabeth Roemer. Copyright © 2016 The Guilford Press.

CLIENT FORM 8.4. Monitoring Opportunities for Valued Action

At the end of each day, reflect on your values. Think about *actions you took that were consistent* with one of your values and *opportunities to take values-consistent actions that you missed.* (1) Briefly describe the action. (2) Mark *T* for taken or *M* for missed. (3) On a scale of 0–100, rate how mindful you were during the action or the missed opportunity, and for missed opportunities, note any obstacles you noticed that stopped you from acting.

Practice self-kindness and compassion when completing this activity. It's natural to miss some opportunities to engage in valued activities. And we all have moments during which our desire to avoid discomfort holds us back. This practice is simply aimed at helping you to become more aware of moments in your daily life where you can make some choices to act in values-consistent ways.

Date	Action	Taken (*T*) or Missed (*M*)	Mindfulness (0–100)	Obstacles

Note. Adapted with permission from *Worry Less, Live More* by Susan M. Orsillo and Lizabeth Roemer. Copyright © 2016 The Guilford Press.

Intentional Responses That Differ
from Emotion-Driven Reactions

Situation	Emotional Response	Action Tendency	Behavior We Might Choose
Child misbehaves	Anger	Attack; assert dominance	Model understanding and teach appropriate behavior
Asked to attend a social event by someone you just met	Fear	Avoid; escape	Accept the invitation because doing so is a potential opportunity to build new relationships
Relationship breakup	Sadness	Withdraw; isolate; self-reflect	Open up and reach out to family and friends for support, continue to engage in hobbies and activities that are personally important

PART III 🐞 🐙 🐙 🐙 🐙 🐞 🐞 🐙 🐙 🐙
Putting It All Together:
Promoting Mindful, Valued Action

In Part II, we provided in-depth discussions of the central clinical methods used in ABBT. This final Part is focused on how we bring these different clinical strategies together in an integrated way, address internal and external challenges that arise as we encourage clients to engage more deeply in their lives, revise our approach based on ongoing assessment, and end therapy. Because ABBT is a flexible, conceptualization-driven approach to intervention, there is no set protocol for this integration. Instead, clinicians should make decisions based on their case conceptualization, the client's context, and the context of treatment. As we have throughout the book, we provide a description of why we make clinical choices and a lot of examples so that readers can flexibly apply this approach with their own clients in their settings.

To help therapists build idiographic treatment plans targeting the three goals of ABBT, here we provide a brief overview of the strategies we presented in the previous section that can serve as a summary and reference for your ongoing work. The following strategies can be used to help clients address the first two goals of ABBT: (1) change the nature of their relationship to their internal experiences and (2) reduce rigid experiential avoidance:

Within the **therapeutic relationship**, you can:

- Treat reactions, behaviors, challenges as natural responses that "make sense" and that we all (including therapists) experience.
- Provide validation and model acceptance and willingness.
- Name responses precisely (thoughts, feelings, urges, actions).
- Provide opportunities in therapy that promote new learning.

You can provide **psychoeducation** on topics that include:

- Principles of learning.
- The nature and function of emotions, the differences between clear and muddy emotions, and habits that can muddy emotions.
- The nature of mental content and processes, including similarities and differences between the concepts of worry, problem solving, reflection, and rumination.
- Limits to control and consequences of rigid, habitual attachment to, and use of strategies aimed at controlling internal states, others' thoughts, emotions, and actions, and external circumstances
- Describe and address any misinformation about mindfulness and self-compassion.

You can recommend and work through **self-monitoring practices.**
You can teach and encourage practice of formal and informal **mindfulness.**
You can share methods of cultivating **self-compassion.**
Finally, the following strategies can be used to address the third goal of increasing intentional, mindful engagement in personally meaningful actions:
You can provide **psychoeducation** on topics that include:

- Defining values as used in ABBT (valuing as behavior, values as a choice).
- Distinguishing between values and goals.
- Providing a rationale for defining values (compass that guides behavior, method of improving quality of life, guide to finding meaning in challenging contexts).

You can assign **writing exercises** that help clients explore the costs of distraction, avoidance, and inaction, and also articulate and clarify their personal values. You can follow this with **in-session exploration** of values and identifying and working through values articulation stuck points (e.g., unachievable values, those that are dependent on the actions of others, indecision, avoidance, hopelessness, and confusion about external influences).

You can assign **self-monitoring practices** and **mindfulness exercises** that increase awareness of action and inaction in valued domains.

As we described previously, ABBT consists of two phases. The first is a skills-building phase, while the second is focused on applying skills in daily life. So the first phase involves developing the skills described above, and the second phase applies those skills, while also returning to skills building as new challenges or setbacks arise. In Chapter 9, we describe how to integrate these skills in the skills-building phase and also how the second phase of treatment unfolds. In Chapter 10, we describe strategies and considerations in addressing external stressors and barriers throughout treatment, but particularly in the second phase of treatment (i.e., in relation to attempts to engage in mindful, valued actions). Finally, in Chapter 11, we describe the ongoing assessment of progress, how to address stuck points that emerge, relapse prevention, and how to end therapy. We provide numerous examples so that you will have a wide range of options to choose from in meeting the needs of your clients.

Integrating the Three Goals of ABBT into Each Session

Although ABBT is designed to be flexibly adapted so that it can meet the individual needs of particular clients and fit within the constraints of different treatment settings, two overarching principles guide its application. First, ABBT therapists strive to target all three of the psychological processes thought to contribute to clinical problems (e.g., problematic relationship with internal experiences, rigid experiential avoidance, limited engagement in personally meaningful actions) in each session. Also, ABBT is typically delivered in two phases, each with a distinct structure. In the *first phase,* therapists prioritize (1) establishing a validating, genuine, ABBT-consistent therapeutic relationship, (2) delivering psychoeducation material related to the overarching model and most relevant to the client and their presenting concerns, and (3) developing and practicing mindfulness and related skills. In the *second phase,* therapists shift their focus toward helping clients to apply ABBT principles in their daily lives and promoting skills generalization. In this chapter, we will describe how each of the distinct ABBT goals and strategies can be woven together to create treatment plans that meet the individualized needs of clients in the particular contexts in which they receive treatment during both phases of treatment.

What you will learn

- ⧉ How to structure sessions during the first phase of ABBT and use complementing clinical strategies to promote learning.

- ⧉ How to shift into the second phase of ABBT and encourage clients' commitments to valued actions.

- ⧉ Methods of promoting values-based action that have the potential to improve clients' quality of life.

- ⧉ Ways to help clients apply ABBT when they are struggling with difficult emotions and in their daily lives.

- ⧉ How ABBT strategies can help clients choose actions in challenging moments.

BRINGING THE COMPONENTS OF ABBT TOGETHER IN EARLY SESSIONS: TEACHING THE ABBT MODEL AND PROMOTING SKILL DEVELOPMENT

As described in Part I of this book, careful assessment and case conceptualization guide the development of client-specific ABBT treatment plans that are feasible in a particular clinical setting. Figure 9.1 delineates how therapists should choose which comprehensive set of clinical strategies described in Part II to include in a treatment plan. It also shows how to integrate strategies so that each session targets the three overarching goals of ABBT: cultivate an expanded awareness and a compassionate decentered stance toward internal experiences; increase acceptance of/willingness to have internal experiences; and encourage mindful engagement in personally meaningful behavior.

We recommend that therapists first consider how each of the three psychological processes thought to contribute to the development and maintenance of clinical problems from an ABBT perspective relates to clients' presenting problems and goals. For example, Nadia presented to an outpatient ABBT practitioner with a principal diagnosis of generalized anxiety disorder (GAD) with comorbid social anxiety disorder and major depression. During the assessment, Nadia provided several examples of the ways in which (1) she was often narrowly focused on threat cues; (2) she was fearful of and distressed by her emotions and associated physiological sensations and frequently tried to suppress them; and (3) worry consumed her attention. Nadia also described widespread avoidance of social situations and little engagement in valued activities. Thus, her therapist determined that the treatment plan should include a balance of strategies aimed at addressing all three components of the ABBT model (i.e., all three goals). In contrast, Raven was referred to an ABBT therapist in the context of integrated primary care after she talked with her pediatrician about her desire to gain clarity on parenting values. After a brief assessment meeting, the ABBT therapist developed a treatment plan that primarily included values articulation and clarification strategies (a component of goal three) that were responsive to Raven's specific needs.

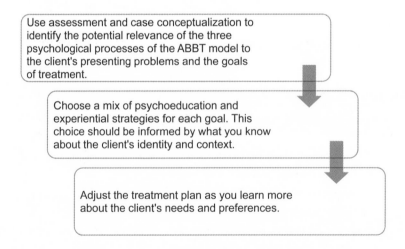

Use assessment and case conceptualization to identify the potential relevance of the three psychological processes of the ABBT model to the client's presenting problems and the goals of treatment.

Choose a mix of psychoeducation and experiential strategies for each goal. This choice should be informed by what you know about the client's identity and context.

Adjust the treatment plan as you learn more about the client's needs and preferences.

FIGURE 9.1. Process to follow when selecting clinical strategies to integrate into early sessions.

Once ABBT therapists determine the relevance of each of the three overarching treatment goals to their client, they choose a mix of psychoeducation and experiential strategies that can be integrated into each session. The choice of specific strategies and the number of sessions devoted to the first phase of treatment should be informed by the therapist's knowledge and understanding of a client's presenting concerns, treatment history, cultural identity, and current context. For example, Hector's therapist reflected on a few key points from the assessment when choosing how to integrate and balance multiple strategies in each session. First, Hector clearly had a solid understanding of the role of learning in the development and maintenance of anxiety. Hector was employed as a mental health counselor and had previously participated in cognitive-behavioral therapy for an anxiety disorder he struggled with as a teen. Given Hector's preexisting knowledge, the therapist planned to provide him with psychoeducational material that he could read outside of session and focus in-session psychoeducation on topics unique to ABBT, as well as any topics about which he had questions. Despite (or perhaps because of) Hector's deep knowledge of the factors that cause and maintain anxiety, the therapist noticed that Hector seemed to talk about his anxiety in a somewhat detached, intellectualized manner. Thus, the therapist noted that he should use metaphors, stories, and experiential practices to promote new learning of ABBT concepts in session whenever possible. Hector and his therapist discussed their similarities and differences across several visible identity characteristics and how those could impact their therapy relationship. Hector shared his concern that the therapist might assume Hector was less intelligent and an inferior counselor because of his personal struggles, given that they had similar professional and educational backgrounds, but Hector played the "client" role in their interactions. The therapist disclosed his view that all humans, including therapists, struggle with challenging thoughts and emotions, and he expressed respect for Hector's willingness to explore this struggle in therapy. The therapist also made a personal note to prioritize use of the therapy relationship as a method of validating Hector's struggles with anxiety. The therapist also committed to noticing and taking any opportunities he could to appropriately disclose his own habits of trying to control his public speaking anxiety and slipping from problem solving to worry.

> For a summary of strategies used to achieve each of the three ABBT goals, see the introduction to Part III.

Minnie, an older adult with mild cognitive deficits, who had never received previous therapy, needed a somewhat different balance of ABBT strategies to meet her treatment goals. Understandably given her background and history, Minnie showed little knowledge of psychological constructs and appeared to have a limited understanding of her own behavior. Minnie also seemed particularly confused and uncomfortable when her therapist tried a brief mindfulness practice in their first meeting. In response, Minnie's therapist decided to shift the balance of the treatment plan so that the first few ABBT sessions focused almost primarily on psychoeducation. The therapist personalized the handouts to better fit Minnie's learning style (i.e., making sure that each handout had no more than three main points supported by client-relevant examples and using a larger font size; see Box 9.1). Minnie's therapist also predicted that self-monitoring practice was going to be a crucial piece of Millie's learning, given Millie's limited psychological insight, but she also recognized that Minnie would need considerable scaffolding to be able to use the forms outside of session. The therapist developed

BOX 9.1. A CLOSER LOOK:
Adapted Client Handout 5.1, *Fear Is Learned* with Examples

- **Fear is helpful in dangerous situations. It can help us stay safe!**
  - Ethel loves to drive her car.
  - But she can't see very well at night.
  - One night, Ethel gets into a car accident!
  - The next week, after dinner, Ethel notices she is out of milk.
  - It's already dark and Ethel is afraid of getting in a car accident.
  - Ethel waits until the next morning to go to the store.
  - Ethel's fear kept her safe!
- **Because staying safe is important, "helpful" fears can grow and spread.**
  - Ethel enjoys visiting her grandchildren.
  - The best time to see them is after dinner.
  - Ethel's daughter, Franny, offers to pick Ethel up and bring her over for a visit.
  - Franny is a safe driver who can see perfectly well at night.
  - Ethel is still afraid of getting in a car accident.
- **If our fear spreads too far, we can miss out on the fun things in life.**
  - Just to be on the safe side, Ethel stops going out at night altogether.
  - It gets really hard for Ethel to find a time to visit her grandchildren.
  - Ethel is sad and lonely.

a treatment plan in which a significant portion of the early sessions was devoted to working through monitoring forms in session. Despite the fact that it seemed like psychoeducation and self-monitoring might require considerable in-session attention, the therapist also understood the importance of integrating experiential methods of learning into the treatment plan. The therapist found some mindfulness practices that had been adapted for use with older adults, including aromatherapy and hand massage (McBee, 2008) that she felt would be helpful in promoting Minnie's experiential learning.

In sum, there is no one, "right" way to choose and integrate multiple strategies in the early sessions of ABBT. The combination of strategies should be intentionally informed by the treatment plan and adjusted as the therapist's understanding of the client deepens. In Appendix C, we provide a model of one way that topics, exercise, and practices could be integrated into weekly therapy sessions for clients seeking outpatient individual therapy for GAD and related concerns. If you choose to use this model, we encourage you to adapt it for your own use. As noted earlier, during the first phase of treatment we follow a particular structure. Sessions typically start with a mindfulness practice, followed by a review of any outside session practices and the presentation of a new ABBT topic supported by psychoeducation, metaphors, stories, or experiential exercises. Clients usually complete some sort of mindfulness practice and self-monitoring between sessions to deepen

> For more details on how sessions are structured in the early phase of therapy, see Table II.1 in the introduction to Part II.

learning. We give them handouts to read or direct them to outside readings such as the *WLLM* (Orsillo & Roemer, 2016), and we ask them to complete several values writing exercises across this phase of treatment.

SHIFTING INTO THE SECOND PHASE OF THERAPY: ENCOURAGING CLIENTS' COMMITMENTS TO VALUED ACTIONS

Many clients seen in ABBT initiate therapy because they want to make significant changes in their lives, but they feel stuck. From an ABBT perspective, "stuckness" arises when the barriers to change are perceived as too punishing (e.g., painful thoughts and emotions are viewed as intolerable and dangerous) and the potential rewards too minimal. The inherently rewarding characteristics of previously valued activities may be underestimated by clients with broad and generalized avoidance. Moreover, any sense of fulfillment that might come from pursuing values in those who are less avoidant is often overshadowed by worry and rumination. When the obstacles to valued action often seem insurmountable and the potential for reward seems remote, it makes sense that clients would be ambivalent and sometimes even hopeless about the prospect of change.

The early stages of ABBT are designed to help clients shift this balance by providing skills and practices that help to (1) minimize the punishing qualities of uncomfortable internal experiences and (2) increase the salience of valued activities. The therapeutic relationship, psychoeducation, and mindfulness practices used in the first phase of ABBT are all aimed at breaking down barriers to change. The assessment, psychoeducation, and emotional processing practices that help clients to see the costs of avoidance and encourage values articulation and clarification are designed to increase clients' contact with the potentially rewarding aspects of engaging in personally meaningful activities. Once this balance begins to shift, clients may be ready to make a commitment to act consistently with their values. To start this work, we sometimes suggest another writing/emotional processing practice aimed at preparing clients to make meaningful, enduring behavioral changes and identifying any final barriers to action.

Client Form 9.1, *Values Writing Exercise III*, asks clients to set aside 20 minutes a day on three different days to write as openly and honestly as they can about the thoughts and emotions that come up for them as they consider making significant changes in the way they live their lives, the importance of the values they've chosen, and the biggest obstacle that stands between them and the changes they want to make. Although many clients have fears about their ability to commit to making a change, they may be hesitant to disclose them. We encourage clients to express their concerns, we validate their reactions, and we encourage and support them in using the skills they have learned thus far in ABBT to work with internal barriers to change.

Introducing the Concept of Commitment

Commitment can be a loaded term, particularly for clients who have struggled with making changes in the past. Thus, we start this phase of therapy by clarifying how commitment is defined in the context of ABBT. Specifically, we describe commitment as a process, characterized by an intention to behave consistently with one's values. We are clear that part of being human means that, even with this commitment, we will often miss opportunities to engage in valued action and respond to challenges in ways that are not values consistent for several reasons. Sometimes opportunities to act consistently in one valued domain may conflict with actions to be taken in another (e.g., passing up a chance to go to a concert in order to visit a friend who is ill), old habits

 Helping clients balance actions in different values domains is discussed in Chapter 10.

and strong emotions can influence our behavior in less mindful moments, and particularly intense or chronic life stressors can sometimes distract our focus from valued activities.

It is actually in these challenging moments, when we experience a lapse from behavioral change, that a commitment to values can be the most beneficial. When we are able to notice, acknowledge, accept, and learn from our lapses, while also renewing our intention to live in accordance with our values, we can more easily reintegrate valued actions into our daily lives. In contrast, if we view a missed opportunity to take a valued action as a broken commitment or a sign of failure, fusion with guilt, self-criticism, and the dread associated with setting unreasonable expectations can elicit avoidance, making it difficult to recommit to our values (see Box 9.2 if you are interested in learning more about research related to the concept of "lapse").

The struggle some clients have with the notion of commitment is illustrated in a conversation between Daqwan, a client who was struggling with erectile disorder and related relationship problems, and his therapist.

BOX 9.2. A CLOSER LOOK:
Commitment and the Abstinence Violation Effect

Alan Marlatt's theory and research on the factors that contribute to relapse in those struggling with a substance use disorder can be helpful to draw from when considering the concept of commitment. Marlatt and Gordon (1980, 1985) argued that a person's emotional and cognitive/attributional response to an initial slip or lapse (e.g., sipping champagne during the toast at a wedding) would be predictive of whether or not they would relapse (e.g., resume regular use/misuse of alcohol). Specifically, they proposed that people who attributed a lapse to internal, stable, and global factors (e.g., "I drank because of a character flaw—I have no willpower and I am a failure—and I will never be able to change") would be at higher risk for relapse than those who attributed the lapse to external, unstable, specific, and controllable factors ("I was in a unique high-risk situation and forgot to use my coping strategies, but moving forward I can practice saying no and draw on my social support"). The effect of this cognitive/attributional and emotional response to a lapse or relapse or return to a problematic pattern of behavior, coined the *abstinence violation effect* (AVE), has been demonstrated on a wide range of behaviors, including smoking (e.g., Curry, Marlatt, & Gordon, 1987), binge eating (e.g., Grilo & Shiffman, 1994), and repeated episodes of domestic violence (King & Polaschek 2003). Although the AVE theory has been critiqued, expanded, and reformulated (Ward, Hudson, & Marshall, 1994; Witkiewitz, & Marlatt, 2004), teaching people effective ways to respond to lapses (i.e., relapse prevention) is considered among the most important and influential clinical innovations in the treatment of substance use disorder. Moreover, mindfulness practice appears to be a skill that can be helpful in coping with the challenging thoughts, emotions, and sensations associated with behavioral lapse (e.g., Bowen et al., 2009).

DAQWAN: The idea of making a commitment to living consistently with my values is bringing up a lot of challenges for me.

THERAPIST: Tell me a little more about what you are noticing.

DAQWAN: Well, I started thinking about how Yvonne and I tried to commit to making regular "date nights" to improve our relationship last summer. We went through this period when we had a standing babysitter every Saturday night, and we would go into the city to listen to music or have dinner. We started feeling really close, and I had some hope that our sex life would improve. Except there were also some real rough points. A few times I had to cancel on Yvonne last minute to pick up an extra shift at work. It's not like I wanted to—it's just that the bills were piling up, plus there had been a few layoffs at work—so when they asked me to work extra, I didn't feel like I could say no. Yvonne said she understood, but I hated how guilty I felt canceling. Plus, I started thinking things like"Why can't I get a better paying job so I can provide for my family without working all the time?" and "I should just stand up for myself and say no to the extra shifts."

Then, one night I had too much to drink on our date, and I wanted us to try to have sex. We had been working with our therapist on taking it slowly—spending time just kissing and touching each other—but I felt good and relaxed and I just wanted to have sex like a "normal" person. We started getting intimate, but then I couldn't get hard. It was so embarrassing. I felt like a complete loser, even though Yvonne kept telling me she didn't care. I ending up sleeping on the couch and Yvonne and I barely spoke for the next few days.

THERAPIST: What happened after that?

DAQWAN: We never really talked about it. We just got swept back up into our work and the kids, and things mostly went back to normal, except we pretty much stopped going on dates and trying to be intimate. At the time, I wrote it off to us both being really busy and under a lot of stress. But after our last session when we talked about making a commitment to work on my values, I started thinking about it more and now I think it was avoidance. I'm not gonna lie—I thought about trying again—talking to Yvonne about getting a babysitter, asking her if she wanted to get physical. But every time I did, thoughts would come up, like "I am not a real man" and "I'm such a loser," and I couldn't stand how guilty and ashamed I felt. And honestly it just didn't seem worth it to go through all that again. I am starting to feel that way now, thinking about a commitment.

THERAPIST: It makes a lot of sense to me that those memories, and thoughts, and feelings would come up for you now. And that certainly sounds painful. I can see why you would be hesitant to make another commitment. But it sounds like last summer, for you, making a commitment meant never canceling a date and making sure every date was "successful." Does that sound right?

DAQWAN: Yeah, I guess. . . . I think I know where you are going with this.

THERAPIST: What do you mean?

DAQWAN: As I hear you say that, I'm starting to think about how what we've been talking about in here might apply to commitments.

THERAPIST: What are you thinking?

DAQWAN: Well, one big thing is that my value is to open up and connect with Yvonne. And to show physical affection. But I don't have control over what she thinks or feels or acts. Plus, I can choose to show affection, but I can't control whether or not I get an erection. I hadn't really made a connection between what we have been talking about in here to last summer until now.

THERAPIST: That's great. Any other thoughts about that?

DAQWAN: Just how I guess I could use my skills when those really upsetting thoughts and feelings come up, so that I could still act with my values.

THERAPIST: I definitely know that all this is easier said than done.

DAQWAN: That's true. But thinking about it this way at least gives me a little hope. I am not dreading the idea of making a commitment as much as I was before.

THERAPIST: This is all really important. I am so glad you noticed your reactions and brought them up in here. It sounds like when you made a commitment before and then missed an opportunity to act in a way that is consistent with your values, you'd notice some really painful feelings, thoughts that you were a failure, and a behavioral urge to move away from your commitment. Is that right?

DAQWAN: Yeah. But I am open to trying again . . . and using mindfulness to help when I get stuck in my head.

THERAPIST: That's great. What about also thinking about commitment as an intention rather than as a contract that one misstep can break? That you are committing to *holding* that value of opening up and showing affection, even knowing that there are times you might not enact it, because you're human and we humans are imperfect. And committing to renewing your focus on your value whenever you notice you've drifted away from it.

DAQWAN: Sort of like returning to my breath every time I notice my attention moves away?

THERAPIST: Exactly!

DAQWAN: That seems more doable. I feel more hopeful—like I can actually follow through on my word if there is room for me to make a mistake.

A metaphor we learned from a Zen teacher can also be helpful in conveying the concept of commitment as an intention. If we are asked to shoot a target with an arrow, we can control many aspects of the situation. For example, we can learn about the physics behind archery and incorporate that knowledge into our practice. We can choose the level of attention and care we bring to taking aim, be intentional about how far we draw back the bow, and decide when to release the arrow. But myriad factors outside of our control also influence an arrow's path and landing point. For example, the weight and balance of arrows impact the trajectory of their curve, and we may be handed an arrow different from the one we used in practice. A sudden and unexpected gust of wind that comes after the arrow is released can alter the arrow's course. Our intentions as we prepare to shoot the arrow are appropriately focused on hitting the target, yet once we release the arrow we accept that it will land where it lands. Similarly, we can do our best to choose actions we think will contribute to optimal outcomes, yet we need to accept that the outcome may be out of our control. All we can do is aim our arrow.

Introducing the Concept of Willingness

Committing to valued actions requires a willingness to accept the range of internal experiences that inevitably arise when one fully engages in meaningful life activities. The "passengers on the bus" metaphor from ACT can be a useful illustration of how a client can demonstrate a willingness to pursue a valued direction, even while still noticing unwanted or uncomfortable thoughts, emotions, sensations, or images. In this metaphor, the client is asked to imagine being the driver of a bus filled with passengers who represent the internal experiences with which the client is struggling. The client is asked to imagine driving the bus following their own valued directions and chosen path and then to consider how in the past they have taken both large and more subtle detours off-course in an attempt to appease the unruly and unwanted passengers.

A client may have once driven her bus toward intimacy, but in an attempt to avoid the unpleasant passenger of vulnerability deviated from that route. Another client may have stopped his bus journey toward taking creative pursuits to head to the back of the bus to try to convince difficult passengers of the worthiness of this life choice. In both examples, the clients stopped pursuing valued actions in an attempt to control or change internal experiences. As we discuss in more detail below, taking a willing stance means driving the bus on one's own chosen path even while the passengers threaten, criticize, and complain.

Qualities of Willingness

Hayes and colleagues (Hayes et al., 2012; Hayes, Strosahl, et al., 1999) describe several qualities of willingness that can be useful to share with clients. First, *being willing* to experience painful internal responses is not the same as *wanting* to experience them. We aren't asking clients to contact their pain because it is an inherently noble thing to do. In fact, we share the wish many of our clients have—in our own lives and for our family members, friends, and clients, we wish there were a way to live a fulfilling, rich, connected life without experiencing pain, vulnerability, and loss. Unfortunately, the reality of being human is that to live an engaged and active life we need to be willing to have the full range of responses that accompany it.

We often use the *swamp metaphor,* adapted from ACT (Hayes et al., 2012; Hayes, Strosahl, et al., 1999; Wilson, 1999, 2016) to illustrate our view of willingness.[1] On our journey guided by personal values, we may encounter a disgusting, murky swamp on our path. To further distinguish willingness from wanting, we note that we wouldn't

---

[1]In this section, we describe several metaphors that can be useful in helping clients to experientially connect with sometimes abstract concepts. We rarely present all of these metaphors to a client in one session. They are typically spread out across sessions, or we simply choose those metaphors that seem most necessary to highlight a point. Intentionally trying to share too many metaphors in too short a time can undermine the effectiveness of the strategy.

necessarily dive into the swamp or roll around in it, just for the sake of getting dirty. Instead, we would consider whether it was necessary to wade through the swamp to continue our journey, as well as the costs of stopping or changing paths. If we concluded that, in order to follow our valued directions, we would need to wade through the swamp, willingness involves accepting that reality and moving forward.

We also point out that some strategies, like wearing rubber boots or using a plank, might reduce the mess one encounters when crossing a swamp, similar to the ways that using ABBT skills can potentially help ease the pain associated with engagement in valued actions. On the other hand, we acknowledge that sometimes swamps surprise us, no matter how much we've practiced encountering them. For example, we might underestimate the size of the swamp and run out of plank to walk on or the seams of our boots might rip. Or we might trip and fall. If we choose to cross the swamp and continue our journey, we need to be willing to accept the possibility we could get dirty and smelly despite our preparations.

Similar to earlier discussions we've had about the ways in which emotions and behaviors can be distinct (see Chapters 5 and 8), we highlight the fact that willingness is an *action* and not a *feeling*. We assure clients that it is natural to feel fear and doubt about trying new things, and we dispel any misunderstanding clients may have about needing to feel confident and calm before taking valued actions.

Another important characteristic of willingness is its all-or-nothing quality. The client's first attempts at being willing to take valued actions often involve conditions. For example, Leo was willing to bring concerns to his shift supervisor as long as Leo didn't feel himself start to blush during the conversation. Delaney was willing to commit to a trip to the bookstore over the weekend as long she didn't feel "depressed." Chloe was willing to be open with her partner Alex, as long as Alex didn't show any signs of frustration.

Although these conditions certainly seem reasonable, if rigidly adhered to, they are all limiting. All of these conditions suggest that the clients are willing to live consistently with their values as long as some experience outside of their control (i.e., physiological sensations, emotions, other people's behavior) does not occur. Making values-based actions contingent on experiences out of our control limits our choices and leads to feelings of helplessness and despair. Moreover, clients who leave a situation when a feared event begins don't get the opportunity to create new learning. In other words, Leo can't learn that he can be effective in raising concerns even when he blushes. Delaney can't learn that she can engage in values-consistent actions even when feelings of sadness, fatigue, and challenging thoughts are present. And Chloe can't learn that, although she was unsafe when her parents became angry, she is safe with her partner, even when he feels angry.

We sometimes use a modified metaphor from ACT to illustrate these points:[2]

"Imagine that you are new to your neighborhood and you decide to host a party. You put up a poster in the lobby of your building, inviting all of your neighbors. The party is going strong, and you are truly enjoying connecting with your neighbors

---

[2]Readers interested in additional metaphors that might fit with ABBT may want to review Jill Stoddard and Niloofar Afari's (2014) *Big Book of ACT Metaphors: A Practitioner's Guide to Experiential Exercises and Metaphors in Acceptance and Commitment Therapy.*

until Joe shows up. Even though your poster said everyone was welcome, you actually didn't include Joe in that category. Joe isn't threatening at all, but he is loud, opinionated, and sometimes crude.

"If you're not actually willing to have everyone who lives in the building at the party, your experience of the party is going to have to change. You can ask Joe to leave, but knowing how he is, he might try to sneak right back in when you aren't paying attention. So, you will probably need to spend the rest of the night with one eye on the door to make he doesn't return. If you are willing to have Joe at the party as long as he doesn't talk about politics or bother too many people, you are going to have to spend the rest of the evening trying to manage him. Unfortunately, both of these options, being unwilling and having conditional willingness, severely limit your ability to participate fully in the party. Instead of mingling with the guests, enjoying some tasty snacks, and maybe even dancing with your next-door neighbor, you're stuck managing Joe.

"Another option would be for you to practice willingness—for you to allow Joe to be at your party and to be who he is while you engage with the party. You can hold a negative opinion of Joe and even wish he did not show up while accepting the fact that he is there and intentionally bringing your attention to your party."

Finally, it's useful to explain the ways in which willingness can be challenging to distinguish from tolerance. Someone who boards an airplane despite having a fear of flying may exhibit similar behaviors whether she is willing to encounter her internal experience or is simply tolerating it. However, in spirit, willingness and tolerance are polar opposites. Tolerance implies that we are grimly enduring what we have to just to get through an experience. It suggests we're resigned to the fact that we simply have to do certain things even if we'll be miserable doing them. Although a tolerant stance may help clients to take actions they may have previously avoided, it is unlikely to bring a sense of meaning and fulfillment to clients' lives. In order for clients to reap the benefits of engaging in values-based actions, they may need to notice when they are tolerating and practice bringing a willing stance to their experience.

APPLYING THE COMPONENTS OF ABBT IN LATER SESSIONS

The second phase of ABBT is structured a bit differently from the first. Although each session starts with a mindfulness practice, we don't follow a particular progression. Sometimes the therapist will recommend a particular practice. For example, if a client is struggling with worries that keep hooking her attention, the therapist might suggest a mindfulness of thoughts exercise. Or if a client is engaged in considerable self-criticism, a practice aimed at promoting self-compassion might be useful. As we move toward the end of therapy, we usually encourage clients to choose the practice that starts the session.

We may also introduce some "advanced" psychoeducational topics if we haven't covered them earlier and if they're relevant to a client's experience. For example, if a client is struggling to differentiate between experiential avoidance and

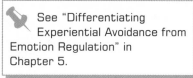

See "Differentiating Experiential Avoidance from Emotion Regulation" in Chapter 5.

emotion regulation, or facing considerable external barriers to valued action, we would spend time in session on those topics. Struggles related to attempting to control other

> See Chapter 10 for a discussion of how to identify, validate, and help clients work with external barriers.

people's thoughts, emotions, and actions is another psychoeducational topic that may be too advanced to cover during phase one but might require attention in the second phase of treatment. We also commonly revisit "foundational" psychoeducation from the first phase of therapy if it becomes clear that a client needs a refresher.

Another characteristic that differentiates the second phase of ABBT from the first is that we often encourage clients to apply mindfulness or to deploy some other ABBT skill in the midst of session in response to a difficult moment. This approach helps underscore the ways in which skills can be integrated into the client's ongoing experience outside of therapy. Also, when clients use their ABBT skills in session, the therapist can observe the client's level of effectiveness and provide scaffolding and feedback that will hopefully facilitate the generalization of skills.

In addition to these clinical strategies, most of the session time in the second phase of ABBT is devoted to one or more of the following topics, depending on the client's current functioning and treatment goals: (1) planning and implementing values-based actions into daily life, (2) working with painful emotions as they arise in daily life, and (3) identifying actions to take in challenging situations. Each of these goals is described in more detail below. The number of sessions devoted to each of them can be tailored to meet the goals of the client. Appendix C includes one example of how we might address each component in this second phase of treatment in a session-by-session format.

Helping Clients to Plan and Implement Values-Based Actions in their Daily Lives

Many clients have severely restricted lives when they first seek therapy, and their goals involve improving life satisfaction in one or more valued domains. Much of the work in the second phase of treatment for clients with this type of presentation is focused on brainstorming ways in which they can incorporate values-based activities into their daily lives, monitoring these actions using Client Form 8.4, and then reviewing how it went the following week to address barriers that arose. As discussed in Box 9.3, this aspect of treatment overlaps with behavioral action and exposure-based approaches. Drawing on our training as behaviorists, we encourage clients to operationally define specific actions they can take that are consistent with their values. Further, we help them to schedule activities in a way that increases the likelihood of their occurrence, as can be seen in this brief exchange between Lorie and her therapist.

LORIE: I would like to take some actions this week consistent with my value of contributing to my community.

THERAPIST: Great. Have you given some thought to your options?

LORIE: I have a friend who volunteers at the Zuni Wellness Center, and I thought I might want to volunteer there.

THERAPIST: That sounds like a great idea. So, what would be the first step you would need to take?

LORIE: I am not exactly sure. I could email them. Or maybe it's better if I stop by.

THERAPIST: Is there some day this week when it would be convenient for you to stop by?

LORIE: I haven't really thought about it. I guess I don't know what hours they are open. But I am only working until noon on Wednesday, so that could work.

THERAPIST: Should we look up their hours now while we are together to see if that is an option?

The therapist would also explore any potential barriers Lorie might encounter (e.g., limited access to reliable transportation, center is not in need of volunteers at this time) and brainstorm several other possible actions Lorie could take. Internal barriers to values-based action, including difficulties with challenging emotions that can arise when we attempt to engage in values-based actions, also deserve considerable attention during this phase of therapy.

Chapter 10 provides on overview of the range of external barriers clients might face and guidance on how to support clients in acknowledging, accepting, and working with them.

BOX 9.3. A CLOSER LOOK:
Values-Based Action, Exposure, and Behavioral Activation

In ABBT, values-based action involves helping clients to engage in actions that they intentionally choose regardless of the internal experiences that arise before, during, and after these actions. This aspect of treatment is grounded in behavioral principles that underlie evidence-based strategies such as behavioral activation (Addis & Martell, 2004; Martell, Dimidjian, & Herman-Dunn, 2010) and exposure (e.g., Craske & Barlow, 2014; Craske et al., 2014). These three treatment approaches share some common features.

Behavioral activation (BA), an evidence-based treatment for major depressive disorder that has also been applied to other clinical presentations, encourages clients to monitor their activity, observe the impact of their specific actions on mood, and then increase the frequency of those actions shown through monitoring to enhance mood (i.e., activity scheduling), while they also practice intentionally bringing attention to their experience (particularly whenever they notice their attention is pulled toward ruminative thoughts). Although earlier versions of BA emphasized the importance of focusing on activities that bring a sense of pleasure or mastery (e.g., Martell, Addis, & Jacobson, 2001), more recent versions recommend encouraging clients to take actions consistent with their personal values (Kanter, Santiago-Rivera, Rusch, Busch, & West, 2010; Lejuez et al., 2011; Martell et al., 2010). BA's recent focus on values assessment, engagement in valued-based actions, and the importance of remaining mindful while engaged in values-based actions are all consistent with both the spirit and the strategies used in ABBT.

(continued)

Exposure-based approaches, which are effective for a range of anxiety disorders, also have some overlap with ABBT in that both treatments encourage clients to approach previously avoided situations and activities in an effort to increase behavioral flexibility and broaden behavioral repertoires. Historical models of exposure therapy (e.g., Foa & Kozak, 1986) emphasized within-session fear reduction, or a decrease in fear during exposure exercises, as a key indicator of treatment success. Thus, earlier forms of exposure therapy that emphasized fear reduction as a goal may seem inconsistent with an ABBT approach. However, advances in our understanding of learning have led to an evolution in both the theory used to account for the effectiveness of the exposure therapy and the recommended treatment strategies in ways that align exposure more closely with ABBT. Currently, clinical researchers recommend that exposure therapy treatment plans be designed to *maximize new learning* rather than to explicitly reduce in-session fear (Craske et al., 2014). The approach is more consistent with an ABBT values-based action approach in that the goal is not to alter internal experience but rather to learn to relate differently to it. An ABBT approach also shifts the selection process and rationale for exposure a bit in that situations are selected because they are related to what matters to the client, not solely because they elicit anxiety. This may help the client to be more motivated to engage in the feared activities, facilitating compliance and engagement in this aspect of treatment.

The recommendation toward maximizing new learning in exposure therapy is informed by inhibitory learning theory (ILT). According to ILT, the original association between a neutral and threatening stimulus that is formed during fear acquisition is not erased or unlearned during exposure therapy when the neutral stimulus is presented without the threatening stimulus. Instead, the stimulus takes on an ambiguous quality; that is, it has both fear-activating (threat) and fear-inhibiting (no threat) qualities that depend on context (e.g., Bouton, 1988; Bouton & King, 1983; Rescorla, 1996). Thus, in order to target clinical levels of fear and life-interfering avoidance in sustainable ways, "modern" exposure therapy is aimed at optimizing inhibitory learning (Craske et al., 2014).

Several of the clinical strategies that have been recommended to optimize new learning in exposure therapy are consistent with clinical strategies frequently used in ABBT. For example, exposures that maximally violate outcome expectancies are presumed to be most effective in promoting new learning (e.g., Craske et al., 2014; Rescorla & Wagner, 1972). In other words, exposure assignments that help clients to have a very different experience than they expect to have when approaching a feared and previously avoided situation or activity are presumed to be most helpful in producing positive treatment outcomes. In ABBT, when clients are encouraged to engage in values-based actions that have traditionally elicited fear, and their attention is broadened such that they also attend to those aspects of their behavior that are meaningful to them, they often describe their experience as unexpected and different. Thus, values-based actions may be a way to help clients violate their expectancy about the experience and consequences of approach, values-consistent actions.

Another recent recommendation for improving exposure outcomes that is consistent with ABBT involves adding affect labeling or describing one's emotional experience during exposure to a feared stimulus. Specifically, research suggests that affect labeling during exposure may reduce arousal and facilitate the behavioral approach (Kircanski, Lieberman, & Craske, 2012). Affect labeling during exposure is consistent with the emphasis ABBT places on encouraging clients to practice present-moment focused awareness while engaged in values-based actions.

Given these clear overlaps in rationale and function across these approaches, ABBT therapists can easily incorporate BA and exposure-based techniques, while remaining consistent with the ABBT model.

Attending to Emotions That Arise during Committed, Values-Based Actions

Sometimes the challenging thoughts and emotions that arise when we engage in valued action are clear emotions giving us important information. As we discussed in Chapter 8, clients can sometimes get stuck when they are trying to articulate their values because it is impossible to truly know in advance what it will be like to live consistently with a particular value. Also, given our social and cultural contexts, we might feel pressure to endorse a value that we later conclude does not represent who we want to be. Living consistently with a set of values and mindfully attending to our experiences can lead to an authentic and life-enhancing shift in values. For example, although Opal initially prioritized acting consistently with her value of independence, as she began practicing mindfulness more regularly and turning toward her experiences, she noticed feelings of loneliness and a desire to be more connected to others coming up when she was enacting her value of independence. Her willingness to turn toward painful, but clear, experiences led her to realize that her "value" of independence was motivated by a habit of avoiding the discomfort that comes from opening up to others.

On the other hand, waxing and waning feelings about committing to a particular valued direction and ambivalence and doubt about one's values are also a natural part of the commitment process. For example, committing to showing affection toward one's partner may feel effortless during an enjoyable walk on the beach on a quiet Sunday afternoon when feelings of warmth, joy, and love are easily accessible. Acting consistently with that value may be much more challenging in a moment when one is grappling with feelings of annoyance and frustration listening to their partner complain about a family member after having a long, exhausting, and stressful day at work. Similarly, living consistently with one's value to teach others can be exhilarating and rewarding when a student reaches out to describe the positive impact of a particular lecture, while it can be discouraging and draining when the student is asking for an undeserved grade change. Part of living consistently with our values is intentionally

> We examine working with internal barriers in more depth later in this chapter.

noticing the ways the activity allows us to engage in behavior we find meaningful, even in situations we can't fully control and those that may prompt a range of painful thoughts and emotions.

On the surface, it can be quite difficult to know if a particular shift in values represents growth or avoidance, particularly for therapists! In ABBT, we describe both possibilities and encourage our clients to mindfully engage in valued activities and use the wisdom that will come from their direct experience to determine the activities most likely to add meaning to their lives. Sharing an adapted version of the *gardening metaphor* from ACT shown in Box 9.4 can be one way to help clients understand the shifting emotions that can accompany commitment.

> The "paddling out" metaphor in Chapter 10 also illustrates some complexities of values-based action.

BOX 9.4. A CLOSER LOOK:
The *Gardening Metaphor*

It's often exciting to plan and start a new garden—the idea can be full of possibilities. But that excitement might wane a bit when it seems like it's taking forever for things to grow. It's disappointing when some seedlings just don't take, regardless of the care you provide. Frustration may set in when it seems like weeds are overtaking the plants. Yet, the first bloom of a flower that brightens up the yard or the first meal that is made with a homegrown vegetable can bring great satisfaction and pride. Living consistently with values can be similar to gardening in that doing so can prompt different emotions at different moments in the process.

As you grow your garden, you may have doubts about whether you chose the best spot, especially if you notice that another area seems sunnier or has fewer rocks. The tricky thing about gardens is that most spots have imperfections. If you dig up your plants and move them too soon or too often, it's hard for the plants to truly grow and mature (and for you to accurately evaluate the quality of the plot). On the other hand, if you bring your best gardening efforts to the plot year after year and find the yield unfulfilling, it might be time to choose another option. We can learn a lot about gardens and values by committing to fully engage with them and attending to our experience as we do.

Working with Painful Emotions as They Arise in Daily Life

Another focus in the second phase of therapy is helping clients to use the skills they've learned in ABBT to work with painful emotions as they arise in daily life. Clients who have been highly avoidant regularly encounter challenging internal experiences as they integrate valued actions into their experience. However, clients who have been engaging in values-based actions all along may also continue to struggle when challenging thoughts, painful emotions, or uncomfortable sensations arise.

When clients find themselves struggling with particularly intense emotions or painful thoughts and feeling stuck or when they find themselves unwilling to engage in valued activities because internal experiences seem like obstacles, we encourage them to work through Client Form 9.2, *Clarifying Emotions in the Moment*. This form is an advanced version of Client Form 5.3, *Clarifying Emotions Reflection*, introduced in Chapter 5, and provides concise guidance through a synthesis of the strategies described in Part II. Clients are first prompted to bring their attention to a few breaths and then to bring that same observing, present-moment, compassionate awareness to their experience as they answer a number of questions. Clients describe the current situation, identify any emotions that may be present, rate their intensity, consider whether any of their emotions might be clear responses to a current situation, and, if so, explore the message the emotion may be trying to send. After noticing their clear emotions, clients are prompted to practice a brief mindfulness exercise, bringing attention to their clear emotions and any related physical sensations, while simply allowing those responses to be present, noticing that emotional responses to situations are a part of being human, and cultivating self-compassion as they notice how challenging situations that elicit clear emotions can be.

The next section of this form asks clients to reflect on whether they might be responding in any of the habitual ways that can contribute to muddy emotions, and for each habit they identify, a practice is recommended. For example, if a client notices that their emotional response is muddied because their mind has been pulled to the past or future, they are asked to acknowledge that shift and to practice guiding their attention back to the present moment. If clients are having critical, judgmental responses or if they are trying to alter or suppress their experience, they're reminded that humans are hard-wired to have a full range of emotions and asked to practice self-compassion, noticing how natural it is to wish for feelings of calmness and happiness, while also acknowledging and allowing their emotions to be as they are. Finally, if clients observe that they are tangled up in their thoughts, they are reminded about why we are so easily pulled toward emotions and emotion-laden communications and how we can make an intentional choice about whether to purposely engage with our inner experience or shift our focus toward valued actions.

The final question on Client Form 9.2, *Clarifying Emotions in the Moment,* asks clients to consider whether there is some action to be taken in the situation that brought up challenging emotions. If clients need more help and support sorting through behavioral choices, therapists may want to recommend that they also complete Client Form 9.3, *Values-Consistent Actions Reflection,* described in more detail below.

Clients are encouraged to note any questions that come up, or struggles they encounter, applying ABBT skills in their daily lives. Reviewing and brainstorming ways to address these challenges in session is a primary focus of the second phase of treatment. Therapists validate successful application of skills and dedicate in-session time to troubleshooting difficulties. During these discussions, therapists are encouraged to bring in previously reviewed concepts (e.g., the function of emotions, the problem of control) and recommend previously used self-monitoring and mindfulness practices to their clients, as relevant. Given the long learning history most clients have in judging and trying to change or control their internal experiences, and the fact that their current context may be reinforcing old habits, it may be necessary to reintroduce and review material multiple times to promote and support new learning. We also recommend that **therapists** review the stuck points that were described as potentially arising during the first phase of treatment and the options for addressing them, discussed in Chapters 5–8.

> Client Form 11.2, *Treatment Progress Exploration,* in Chapter 11 can also be helpful when progress is stalled.

Regardless of whether or not a client completes Form 9.2, *Clarifying Emotions in the Moment,* therapists should guide in-session discussion of the obstacles their clients encounter trying to apply skills outside of session by asking them to describe their moment-by-moment experience (e.g., "I noticed that my attention was drawn away from my breath and toward worry thoughts") rather than simply providing a general evaluation (e.g., "I tried mindfulness of breath, but it didn't work"). One of the most useful questions therapists can ask when clients describe difficulty applying skills is, "What did you do next?" It's not uncommon for clients to try a mindfulness practice outside of session, get distracted or entangled with their thoughts, and give up. Those types of responses are totally expected, but clients can sometimes get derailed from practicing if they view them as a sign of failure and react with self-criticism. We frequently remind clients that the moment they notice distraction, self-criticism, or entanglement is the moment they have become mindful and that noticing creates an opening for them to try a different response. Although it can be frustrating, the most hopeful characteristic of mindfulness practice is that it is a process. So, no matter what happens in one moment, the next moment brings an opportunity to try something new. And even a new response of compassion instead of criticism can alter the problematic cycle.

IDENTIFYING ACTIONS TO TAKE IN DIFFICULT SITUATIONS

As noted earlier, one way to encourage clients to live consistently with their values is to help them identify new activities that they can build into their daily life (e.g., helping a client who values self-nurturance find some quiet time in the midst of a busy schedule). Another is to help clients become more intentional in the small and large choices they are already making, particularly in difficult situations, to see if there is an opportunity to respond with values-consistent actions (see Box 9.5 for a summary of the ways session time is used in the second phase of ABBT). In Chapter 8, we suggested that people often respond in habitual or emotion-consistent ways, especially in challenging moments. Once clients clarify and articulate their values and become more tuned into their emotional experience, responding in values-consistent ways becomes an option to consider.

At times, distinguishing between one's choices in a challenging situation may seem reasonably straightforward (even if taking the action is not). For example, Rosie put significant effort into the group project she was working on for her political science course. The project was worth a large portion of her grade, and Rosie hoped to do particularly well on it because she planned to ask her professor for a letter of recommendation for graduate school. Rosie was in the midst of an incredibly busy semester. She was working a part-time job, taking five classes, and sharing caretaking responsibilities for her younger brother with her mother. Despite these demands, Rosie made sure her contribution to the project was finished in advance of the due date. Unfortunately, just a few days before the due date, one of the group members, Brett, sent Rosie his contribution to the project and his work was incomplete and of very poor quality. Even worse, Brett boasted to Rosie that after graduation he had a job lined up at his father's company, so he didn't care at all about his final grade in the class. Rosie was understandably angry. She had several options as to how she could respond. She could call Brett out for his selfishness and let him know that his actions jeopardized her grade and plans for the future; this would be a response consistent with her anger. Alternatively, Rosie could redo Brett's part of the project. She frequently took on more than her fair share even when she didn't have the capacity, so opting to do so now would be consistent with her habitual response. From Rosie's perspective, an action that would be consistent with her values would be for her to contact the professor, explain the situation, and get the professor's advice as to how to proceed. Although Rosie was nervous about enacting her values-based response, she was able to sort through and differentiate between her potential options.

However, there are also times when sorting different options out can be quite complicated. Sometimes the same behavior falls into two of the categories. For example, Jenny was home alone in her apartment, and she noted that she was feeling sad and that her attention was repeatedly drawn to memories of her recently deceased grandmother. An emotion-consistent response would be for Jenny to withdraw even more and remain

BOX 9.5. TO SUMMARIZE:
Focus of Session Time in the Second Phase of ABBT

1. Planning and implementing values-based actions into daily life.
2. Working with painful emotions as they arise in daily life.
3. Identifying actions to take in challenging situations.

alone. Jenny's habitual response when she felt sad was to engage in avoidance efforts. A values-based action for Jenny would be to reach out to friends and invite them over to watch a movie. Jenny opted to call her friends. She noticed that doing so was consistent with her relationship values, yet she also wondered if it reflected her strongly ingrained habit of avoidance. Jenny definitely had the thought that she might feel less sad spending time with friends and that she would be relieved to feel less sad.

When clients find themselves in a situation like Jenny's, experiencing difficulty in determining whether their actions are motivated by avoidance or values, we recommend that they reflect on how attached they are to potential outcomes and the potential costs and benefits of different actions. If Jenny spends time with friends because it is a values-based action, she can find some meaning in her choice even if she remains sad. On the other hand, if she seeks out her friends as a method of changing her mood, she is likely to be frustrated and possibly even compelled to try other avoidance strategies if she doesn't achieve her intended outcome. Jenny ultimately decided that reaching out to friends was a valued action, and she made sure to practice mindfulness toward her sadness as it waxed and waned across the evening. Completing Client Form 9.3, *Values-Consistent Actions Reflection,* is one method clients can use to work through some of these challenges.

Vijay also chose a values-consistent action when faced with several options, but after reflecting on his experience, he concluded that it was also strongly motivated by avoidance. Vijay values being a loyal friend and also participating in recreational sports. Over the winter, he moved to a new city and contacted a few different sports-oriented groups with the hope that he could line up an activity for spring. Despite that valued action, Vijay's struggle with social anxiety made it difficult for him to commit to a particular group. As spring grew nearer, Vijay finally arranged to join a tennis league. The weekend before the season opened was a rough one for Vijay. He was consumed with worry about the social demands he would face as a member of the team, and his stomach felt like it was tied in knots. That Sunday evening, Vijay got a call from his friend Dev. A member of Dev's soccer league team had to suddenly quit because of an injury, and Dev wondered if Vijay was interested in serving as his replacement. Vijay readily agreed and felt a wave of relief as he sent off an email canceling his tennis league membership.

Vijay was grateful for the opportunity to play on Dev's team because it would allow him to enact his friendship and recreational values. But he also recognized that choosing the soccer league over the tennis league was strongly motivated by fear, and he knew that, although avoidance brought relief in the short term, if he was unwilling to act with fear, his life would be restricted. Thus, Vijay decided to contact the head of the tennis league and volunteer to fill in when regular members were on vacation. Also, instead of just sending an email, Vijay opted to call, even though he knew that doing so would elicit some feelings of anxiety, because sincerely apologizing for the last-minute cancellation was a values-based action.

We all have moments when an opportunity to act in a values-consistent way presents itself and we let it pass. Sometimes choosing a habitual or emotion-driven response instead negatively impacts our lives. Yet, at other times, the cost of passing up an opportunity to act consistent with our values may not be as great and may even be restorative. For example, Jocelyn was committed to fighting for social justice. She devoted countless hours working to create more inclusive policies in her workplace, she engaged in volunteer work and attended protests and marches in her community, and she participated in social media groups aimed at educating followers about instances and consequences of oppression. Jocelyn found that being on social media presented her with limitless opportunities to engage with posters making racist and misogynist comments, to correct misconceptions about privilege, and to advocate against oppression. She found it challenging to let any opportunities pass, given the importance of her value. However, Jocelyn also noticed that she was feeling exhausted and burnt out, and she recognized that in order to sustain her social justice efforts in the long term, she would need to let some opportunities go. As Jocelyn practiced more self-compassion and awareness, she began to notice that the cost of passing up some potential valued actions (e.g., joining in with several other posters to call out a racist post made on the page of a distant acquaintance) was lower than the cost of passing up others (e.g., missing a crucial policy meeting at work). She used that awareness to guide her choices and increase her self-nurturance.

Client Form 9.3, *Values-Consistent Actions Reflection*, can help clients to fully consider their choices in difficult situations. Clients can be more intentional in their responses to difficult situations in many ways: reflecting on whether any choices are aimed at trying to control things that are potentially out of their control (e.g., internal experiences, other people's behavior); noticing whether choices might have the potential to provide a short-term sense of relief (e.g., help them calm down, avoid conflict, feel less guilt or pain); considering whether they are attached to the outcomes of their efforts or focused on the process; working through the costs, if any, of those choices; and considering whether their actions are leading them toward something meaningful. Regardless of the choices made in each given moment, clients can continue to bring awareness and compassion to their experience and use these skills to continue to refine their choices about values-based living.

BOX 9.6. WHEN TIME IS LIMITED:
Integrating the Three Goals of ABBT into Each Session

In contexts where time is limited, it's even more critical that the treatment plan be individualized to the specific needs of clients and that the mix of psychoeducation, experiential practices, and values work be balanced to fit learning style. Some specific recommendations include:

- If appropriate, consider providing psychoeducation material (handouts, chapters) for clients to read outside of sessions and/or deliver this material through psychoeducational groups and limit in-session individual therapy to discussion of highly relevant themes and concepts the client finds unclear.
- If feasible, mindfulness and other experiential practices can also be offered through group therapy, again with the idea that individual contact time can be reserved for working through client-specific obstacles. Clients can also use online recordings (like those available on the Guilford website [see the box at the end of the table of contents]) or individualized recordings created by the therapist so that they can engage in guided mindfulness practice outside of session.

In our experience, individualized coaching is one of the most helpful elements of ABBT. Thus, we highly recommend encouraging clients to use Client Form 9.2, *Clarifying Emotions in the Moment*, and Client Form 9.3, *Values-Consistent Actions Reflection*, frequently in the second phase of therapy, so that session time can be focused on skill scaffolding, brainstorming methods of working through obstacles, and refreshing client knowledge of previously covered topics relevant to their stuck points.

CLIENT FORM 9.1. Values Writing Exercise III

First, create a space for yourself to intentionally focus on willingness and the changes you may be preparing to make in your life. You may want to practice a mindfulness exercise to help you be attentive and aware. Next, spend 20 minutes a day for 3 days writing in response to each of the following prompts. Use a notebook or your computer to record your answers to the questions below. As with all the writing exercises, painful thoughts and emotions may come up. Acknowledging and allowing them is an opportunity for you to practice cultivating willingness.

Day 1

What comes up for you as you think about making some significant changes in the way you live your life?

Day 2

What's the importance of the values you have chosen? What do they mean to you?

Day 3

What do you think is the biggest obstacle that stands between you and the changes that you want to make?

Note. Adapted with permission from *Worry Less, Live More* by Susan M. Orsillo and Lizabeth Roemer. Copyright © 2016 The Guilford Press.

CLIENT FORM 9.2. Clarifying Emotions in the Moment

Use this form when you are struggling with complicated, intense emotions. Make note of questions that come up or struggles that you have applying the suggested skills, so that you can discuss them in your next therapy session.

Start by bringing your attention to your breathing for a few breaths. Try bringing that same mindful (*i.e., observing, present-moment, compassionate*) stance to your experience as you answer the questions below.

A. Describe the current situation. _____

B. Expanding your awareness and mindfully observing, try noticing all the emotions that are arising.
   - Rate their current intensity from 0 to 100.
   - Check the "Clear Emotion" box if you think some parts of your emotional response are directly related to the current situation. For each clear emotion, describe the message your emotion may be trying to send you about the current situation.

Emotion: _____ Intensity: ____ ☐ Clear Emotion: Message: _____

Emotion: _____ Intensity: ____ ☐ Clear Emotion: Message: _____

Emotion: _____ Intensity: ____ ☐ Clear Emotion: Message: _____

Emotion: _____ Intensity: ____ ☐ Clear Emotion: Message: _____

C. Practice bringing your attention to your clear emotions and any related physical sensations; allowing those responses to be just as they are while you take a few mindful breaths; noticing that part of being human means that certain situations (e.g., facing risks, losing something we care about) bring on certain emotions (e.g., fear, sadness); noticing that feeling emotions can be difficult. . . . ; and bringing compassion to yourself as you notice that.

D. Check any of the boxes below that describe habits in the first column below that could be muddying your emotional response. For each box that is checked, practice the new habits described in the second column.

Habits That Muddy Emotions	New Habits to Try
☐ I am thinking about the past	It's natural for our minds to drift to the past or the future, and when this happens our current emotional response is affected. Bring your attention to your breathing for a few breaths and then expand your awareness to take in your current thoughts, emotions, and sensations. Notice each time your attention is pulled to the past or the future, and with kindness and compassion, gently guide your attention back to the present moment.
☐ I am imagining the future	

(continued)

Habits That Muddy Emotions	New Habits to Try
☐ I am having critical/ judgmental thoughts about my current emotions	Even though humans are hard-wired to have a full range of emotions, we often learn to judge certain emotions as "good" or "bad," and we try to hold on to "good" emotions and push away "bad" ones. Practice acknowledging and allowing your emotions to be as they are for just a few moments, without judging or fighting them. Try practicing self-compassion, noticing how natural it is to wish for feelings of calmness and happiness; also noticing how judging and trying to change emotions often brings more distress.
☐ I am trying to avoid, suppress, or change my current emotional experience	
☐ I am tangled up in my emotional experiences/ thoughts.	Strong emotions pull our attention because their job is to communicate a message. Yet, sometimes we get stuck in our emotions, particularly if we don't want to have them or the experience that triggered them. Try one of the following: • If the emotion is "suggesting" a behavioral response that is in line with your values, shift your attention toward your actions. • If you are entangled in thoughts, try working through Client Form 5.4, *Worry or Problem Solving* • If the emotion is alerting you to a painful challenge in your life that you don't have the ability to change or control, practice noticing and accepting the limits of control; acknowledging the pain and challenge of being human. Bring compassion to yourself for trying to make the situation better, while also observing how control efforts can amplify distress, leave you feeling helpless, and take you away from other important experiences in your life. Practice letting go of that struggle for just a moment. Consider taking a valued action in this present moment—whether or not the action is related to the situation triggering the painful emotions.

E. Finally, consider what options you have for taking actions.

CLIENT FORM 9.3. Values-Consistent Actions Reflection

Are there choices I could make here that would give me a short-term sense of relief? For example (check off those that apply):

☐ Help me calm down

☐ Please other people

☐ Help me avoid conflict

☐ Make me feel less guilty

☐ Distract me from pain

☐ Other: _____

If so, are there any costs to those choices? What are they? _____

_____

_____

_____

_____

Is my focus turning toward something that is meaningful or turning away from pain? _____

_____

_____

_____

_____

- How attached am I to the possibility I may feel less pain if I make this choice? _____

  _____

- Are there any costs to that choice? If so, what are they? _____

  _____

Are there choices that I could make here that are likely to influence other people who are involved? What are they? _____

_____

_____

- If so, how tied am I to that outcome? Am I accepting the limits of control? _____

  _____

- Are there any costs to those choices? What are they? _____

  _____

(continued)

Note. Adapted with permission from *Worry Less, Live More* by Susan M. Orsillo and Lizabeth Roemer. Copyright © 2016 The Guilford Press.

Values-Consistent Actions Reflection *(page 2 of 2)*

Are there choices I could make here that could possibly make it less likely something bad will happen? What are they? _____

_____

_____

- If so, how tied am I to that outcome? Am I accepting the limits of control? _____

_____

- Are there any costs to those choices? What are they? _____

_____

Are there choices I could make here that are consistent with what matters most to me? What are they? _____

_____

- Is my unwillingness to have certain thoughts or feelings holding me back? In what way? _____

_____

CHAPTER 10

Working with Contextual Inequities and External Barriers to Values-Based Actions

In Chapters 8 and 9, we reviewed two major components of helping clients to engage in values-based action: clarifying values and using strategies to accept and decenter from the internal experiences that arise as barriers to values-based engagement. In our previous therapist guide, we focused almost exclusively on these strategies while including a brief mention of addressing external barriers through taking actions to address these barriers (e.g., joining a basketball league to address the obstacle of not knowing a lot of people in a new town). However, over the years, clients and therapists have helped us appreciate the multitude of external barriers that clients often face, and we have identified a broader range of strategies to address these barriers. As we have noted throughout the book, a vital first step in addressing any barriers that arise is validating the reality of the external barriers a client is facing.

What you will learn

- Strategies to help clients address constraints on their time.
- How to help clients balance actions across domains.
- Ways to identify and address barriers that arise in relationships.
- How to skillfully and empathically respond to physical, societal, and systemic barriers and use values-based actions to help clients empower themselves.

PROBLEM SOLVING

Often when clients identify a values-based action they would like to take, external barriers interfere with their ability to engage in a meaningful action. For instance, clients may want to be open and intimate with others, but they may have limited social contact.

In these cases, the therapist can help the client notice opportunities in their daily life they may be overlooking (e.g., practicing openness with the neighbor they see at the mailbox, the receptionist at the doctor's office, or people at work). Therapists can also help clients generate possible actions that will increase their social contact (e.g., joining a group of people with shared interests, volunteering someplace they may meet people, becoming involved with activities at their place of worship, joining a neighborhood action group). Once potential actions have been identified, then they can use their mindfulness and acceptance-based skills and Client Form 9.2, *Clarifying Emotions in the Moment*, to address the internal barriers (like social fears and anxiety) that may arise as they think about taking any of these actions. Role-plays and skills-building may help clients to engage in new contexts that they have previously avoided, as they address external barriers to taking meaningful actions they've identified.

ADDRESSING THE BARRIER OF LIMITED TIME

A common barrier that arises for clients (and therapists, graduate students, and humans in general) is not having enough time to do all the things that we value. For instance, Sean identifies that he values connecting with his friends and spending time alone on projects, and he also would like to develop an intimate relationship and hasn't met anyone who interests him lately. He works 60 hours a week and has trouble figuring out which of these things to devote time to when he isn't working, so he always ends up feeling like he isn't doing what's important to him. Ayanna values spending time with her extended family, alone with her partner, and with friends and neighbors, and often feels like she isn't doing enough of any of these things outside of work hours. Chuck values teaching new employees the ropes at work, but he also values new challenges—a new position would bring him new challenges but reduce the time he can spend with new employees. Lina values spending time with her family and helping around the house, and she also values learning and challenging herself—the time she spends on her homework from her university classes interferes with her ability to help her family in the ways she used to. Each of these clients can identify what they value and still faces challenges in deciding what to do when.

Examining How Time Is Spent

Our first step as therapists is always to validate the reality a client is sharing with us. In this case, we often share our own challenges with time constraints and recognize that we each have many values but not enough time to engage in actions consistent with all of them. Also, sometimes engaging in actions consistent with one value can interfere with engaging in actions consistent with another. As we discuss in more depth later in this chapter, accepting this reality and learning to choose within these constraints, while also having compassion for what isn't possible, is one important aspect of responding to the limits of time.

A second step that can often be useful is taking some time to attend to exactly how time is being spent in order to see if the client (or we) can bring more intentionality to their choices and potentially find more time for some actions, or maybe identify actions they can take concurrent with other activities. (As we've discussed in previous chapters, we also use this strategy when clients are having trouble finding time to engage in skills practices between sessions.) This strategy needs to be used sensitively—clients who have to work multiple jobs to support themselves or their family or who are going to school full-time while also working to support themselves or caring for family members may not, in fact, have flexibility in their time, and we certainly don't want to suggest that their perception is inaccurate. At the same time, bringing attention and intention to the ways we spend our time can often bring to light some potential places for either significant or even slight changes that can enhance values-based actions. Client Form 10.1, *How Do You Spend Your Time?*, provides guidance for one method of engaging in this exploration.

Just as the process of clarifying values can be emotionally challenging, as clients (and we) recognize the ways we haven't been living consistent with our values, the process of examining how we use our time can be similarly challenging emotionally. It is human and natural to develop habits that drain rather than replenish our energy, and it is easy to get caught up in doing things we think we "should" do, rather than finding the meaning in the actions we take. Bringing compassion to this process is essential; it's easy for this kind of self-examination to elicit muddy emotional responses of self-blame and regret that can make it even harder to engage in values-based actions.

An example of pie charts from Client Form 10.1 is presented in Figure 10.1. Preston would like to have a relatively balanced life—spending about 45% of his time with family and friends and about 15% engaged in some kind of physical activity, and very little time on chores or in front of a screen. However, in fact, he spends 40% of his time on chores or in front of a screen and spends almost no time engaged in physical activity and relatively little time with family or friends. His therapist helps him explore the time he spends on chores and in front of a screen to better understand how his actual time has come to differ so much from how he would like to be spending his time. He describes coming home from work and intending to work out, but instead deciding to watch a little TV or check his email first, then continuing to engage with different content on the computer or TV for the rest of the evening, and finally going to bed feeling discouraged. He and his therapist generate several potential strategies to help Preston align his actual time investment with his values. For example, he could join a gym or take up running so that he can get in the habit of engaging in physical activity before he gets home; he could wake up earlier and work out then; and/or he could start engaging in physical activity with his friends (e.g., hiking or playing basketball), so that he can increase engagement in both of these valued domains at once. His chores present a different challenge. He realizes that there are a lot more things needed around the house

---

 BOX 10.1. TRY THIS:
How Do You Spend Your Time?

In order to explore how awareness of how we spend our time can be helpful in enhancing values-based actions, take some time to complete Client Form 10.1 and reflect on the way you're using your time and whether there are any adjustments you'd like to make based on what you've identified as being important to you. Be sure to also acknowledge the real constraints on your time and to have compassion for how you may get caught up in habitual ways of using your time that aren't as meaningful as you'd like them to be.

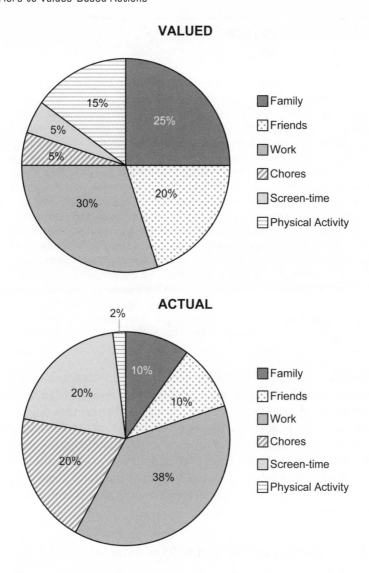

FIGURE 10.1. Example pie chart of valued versus actual actions.

than he was imagining when he filled out his "valued" pie chart. In discussing his different chores, Preston and his therapist are able to identify a few adjustments that may increase his satisfaction. His children are old enough to help with some of his weekly chores, so he could involve them in these tasks and increase his family time while also making the chores feel like less of a burden. He also realizes that sometimes he appreciates time alone, something he hadn't put in his valued pie chart. So he decides that some tasks, like washing the dishes, could be an opportunity for him to have some quiet time on his own, and so these tasks could be paired with a valued action. Finally, in discussing the chores, he recognizes that some of them (like cooking dinner) include caring for his family, so he is able to see the value that connects to the chore, which alters his experience of that chore. (Sometimes we use the *paddling out* metaphor described in Box 10.2 to help clients connect tedious tasks to their purpose and meaning.)

BOX 10.2. A CLOSER LOOK:
The *Paddling Out* Metaphor

A metaphor that we sometimes use to capture the experience of doing something that seems boring or undesirable in service of something else that is meaningful and valued comes from Jamail Yogis's *Saltwater Buddha*. He describes a realization he had while surfing: When you spend the day surfing, the goal is to spend time standing on your board, riding a wave. However, a large part of your day will be spent "paddling out" so that you are in a good position when the next wave comes in. Although no one goes surfing because they want to spend time paddling out, this paddling out is an essential part of the process of surfing. An example of this in my (LR) life is reviewing about 100 graduate applications each year. It is a tedious process and one that is not intrinsically rewarding in the moment. In fact, the process can feel counter to my values because I read about so many wonderful applicants, and yet I can only interview a subset of them and I much prefer encouraging to rejecting people. However, mentoring graduate students is one of the most rewarding things I do and is very consistent with my values. And so I "paddle out" through the applications so that I'll be able to "surf" and help usher fantastic new people into the field. And bringing attention to the connection between reading applications and mentoring graduate students helps me to find meaning in the task. Sharing this metaphor and our own personal examples can help clients when they have to do some "paddling out," like studying for an exam that will help them pursue a meaningful career or going on a lot of first dates so that they can eventually make a romantic connection with someone.

An alternative method of exploring use of time is having a client monitor and record activities through the day to get a real-life accounting of what they are spending their time on. This exercise often leads to changes as the process of just noticing how time is being spent can lead to a realization that one wants to do something different in the moment. Clients also may recognize some of the challenges they face in making choices about how to spend their time and bring those to session when the therapist can help them sort through different aspects of their lives and come up with potential solutions to try out in the coming weeks (see Box 10.3 for a summary of strategies for adjusting how time is spent).

Finding Balance and Accepting the Limits of Time

Although examining how time is spent often leads to more flexibility and some new approaches that can be taken, many of us continue to face the challenge of how to fit in everything that is important to us and how to negotiate conflicts that may arise between different things we value. Validating this reality can help to address the guilt and self-blame that often arise from the reality of the limits of time. Similar to the ways we address values that involve being perfect or super-human (Chapter 8), we explore the impossibility of doing everything we care about all the time, or even as much as we would like to, and we encourage clients to recognize the real constraints of time. Exercises like those described in the previous section can help clients to see these limitations more clearly.

Broadening Our Definitions of Balance

In addition to accepting limitations of time, self-compassion and satisfaction can be increased when we (and clients) are able to broaden or adjust our sense of what balance

BOX 10.3. TO SUMMARIZE:
Adjusting How Time Is Spent

After clients identify how they would like to spend time and assess how they are spending time, they can work with the therapist to:

- Identify activities that occur out of habit and aren't nourishing/meaningful and consider reducing time spent this way.
- Identify activities that are necessary but could be done in a different manner to make them more rewarding.
  - Consider bringing mindfulness to these activities.
  - Consider connecting to the underlying value of the activities.
  - Consider pairing the activities with another valued domain (e.g., other people, reflection).
- Identify activities that occur due to a desire to control something or reduce distress and use mindfulness and acceptance skills in place of those activities.
- Recognize and accept the limits of time, using some of the principles from the next section.

or valued living will actually look like. This broadening might involve (1) looking at a longer time period for balance (rather than trying to achieve balance in the course of a day or even a week), (2) addressing some values in other domains of life, or (3) recognizing that smaller, briefer actions can still be values-consistent and satisfying. For instance:

- Winnie valued being a team player at work and spending quality time with her family. When work was busy, she really wanted to put in extra hours to support the efforts of her team and the success of their joint project, yet she missed spending evenings with her extended family.
  - Winnie decided that she would regularly take a day or two off after completing a particularly intensive project at work so that she could spend evenings working on the project during the busy time and then spend a long weekend with family to take actions consistent with that value.
- Erin valued providing for their family and they also valued working to be of benefit to others. They were offered a well-paying job with excellent benefits that didn't provide any opportunities to help others.
  - Erin decided to take the position so they could support their family, and to begin volunteering on weekends to engage in actions consistent with her value of helping others.
- Nadia valued spending time with family and friends, and also valued learning new things and challenging herself. She was very excited about the doctoral program she had just started, and yet was saddened when she realized she would have to work on weekends to keep up with the workload. Previously, she had spent all day Saturday with friends and all day Sunday with family, and she wanted to continue to act consistent with those values.
  - Nadia realized that she was rigidly defining the values-based action of spending time with friends and family, in that she felt like it required a whole day

to act consistent with that value. Although she continued to prefer spending a full day on these actions, she decided that she would instead make sure that she could set aside a meal or a few hours each weekend for each of these values-based actions.

One obstacle that can arise as clients explore broadening or adjusting their definition of balance is the thought that not taking a particular action means that they no longer hold the underlying value. Often this thought also arises when clients face conflicts between two different values-based actions. We remind clients (and ourselves) that valued living is a process and isn't defined by a single concrete action. We can continue to value something even when we choose not to engage in a consistent action in a given moment, week, or month. A small example of this is when I (LR) had to choose between (1) fulfilling a professional (and personal) commitment to present at a conference and to support my students' presentations, or (2) attending a family wedding. Although I ended up going to the conference, this decision didn't mean that I didn't value the family member. I did my best to communicate that valuing and also to choose a gift that I knew would be meaningful to the family member as a way of continuing to express this value, even though I didn't engage in the obvious action that would convey this value. Of course, even if we and our clients are able to recognize that not engaging in an action doesn't mean we don't value it, other people in our lives may sometimes react differently. We can help clients to communicate clearly when these reactions arise and also to accept that our choices won't always please other people.

BARRIERS THAT ARISE IN RELATIONSHIPS

Given the centrality of social connectedness in our lives, it's no surprise that relationships are one context in which external barriers often arise. As we described in Chapter 8, any valued action that involves another person is inherently limited by the constraints of our lack of control over that other person. In Chapter 9, we describe the ways that we can think of valued actions as "aiming our arrow," so that we are attempting to act consistent with our values (e.g., by opening up emotionally to another person, by sharing with that person something we wish they would address in their behavior, or by trying to strike up a new relationship with someone), while recognizing that we can't control how the other person responds to these attempts. Accepting the reality of our limited control in this domain is essential, but it is also extremely painful and challenging given the relational nature of our lives. Therefore, we often find it useful to more deeply explore some of the complexities raised by values-based action in this domain.

Recognizing What Can (and Can't) Be Controlled and How to Navigate Preferences and Disappointments

Simply acknowledging that we can't control the behavior of other people doesn't change the reality that we often want people to whom we are relating to be different in both small and large ways. Wanting people to be other than they are can increase our own reactivity and muddiness (as can realizing that we can't necessarily change them and therefore getting angry at ourselves for still expecting them to be different). This muddiness can, in turn, lead us to behave in ways that we don't like or value, leading to further reactivity and muddiness. Therapists can work with clients to interrupt this cycle in several places and help them make intentional decisions about how (and whether) to continue to interact with people. These decisions will depend on things like the nature of the relationship, the potential for change by the other person, the relative positionality and power of each individual, and the importance of the behavior that clients want the other person to change. Emotional clarity achieved through mindfulness- and acceptance-based practices can facilitate this complex process of discernment. Riva's discussion with her therapist provides an example of navigating this interpersonal challenge.

> RIVA: I spent time with my family this weekend, like we talked about last week. But it was awful.

> THERAPIST: Well, I'm glad you were able to take an action that was important to you, but sorry to hear that you found it so challenging. What came up when you were with your family?

> RIVA: Well, I know I'm supposed to focus on being the person I want to be in the situation, and I walked in with an intention to be warm and loving to people and to really be present with them and bring myself back each time I thought about something that was frustrating me at work, just like we said. And then, as soon as I walked in the door, my Aunt Mary came over, hugged me, and said "Have you gained weight? You could be so beautiful if you only lost a few pounds."

> THERAPIST: Ouch. That is a painful way to be welcomed to a family event. What kinds of things came up for you when she said that? [The therapist is validating the painful experience and is also helping Riva attend to the reactions she had in the moment.]

> RIVA: It was like she hit me in the stomach.

> THERAPIST: Of course, that's so understandable. So you felt that pain in your body. Any thoughts or feelings you noticed?

> RIVA: First, anger, then sadness. And thoughts that she's a terrible person, and that I'm fat and unlovable. And then pretty quickly thoughts that I'm an ungrateful person, and she's old and doesn't know better, and I shouldn't let her get to me. And then, after I said something snarky to her, I felt even worse and thought that I wasn't being the person I want to be.

> THERAPIST: That is such a challenging and very human cycle of responding. And I can really hear how that led to the thought that it was awful. I want to come back to exploring how these reactions unfolded, but I'm wondering what happened next.

> RIVA: Well, I walked away feeling terrible, and then my Aunt Viv came up and about 5 minutes into our conversation she asked if I was dating anyone, and I thought I was going to scream, and instead just said that I wasn't at the moment and walked away from her as well.

THERAPIST: Well, nice job not screaming. I'd imagine, given what we've talked about, that that question seemed pretty connected to the comment on your weight.

RIVA: Yes, definitely. It fed right into that whole cycle of my family wanting me to be partnered and wanting me to look a certain way so that I can be partnered. And no matter how many times I tell them how those comments make me feel, those two aunts never stop. My mom has gotten a lot better about it after our conversation. And I actually went over to my mom at the party and told her what happened, and she gave me a hug and said I was beautiful just as I am.

THERAPIST: Oh! Well, that moment doesn't sound awful. You continued opening up to your mom even after two very difficult interactions with family members. And it sounds like you felt heard by your mom and that you've noticed she's made a change?

RIVA: (*smiling*) Yes, that was really nice. And, good point, the whole thing wasn't awful. I spent some nice time with my nieces, and I made a point of telling them how beautiful and strong they are too.

THERAPIST: Well, that definitely sounds like being the person you want to be.

RIVA: Yes, it was. I just was so mad at myself for being rude to my aunts. I couldn't even look at them for the rest of the day, and part of why I'd wanted to go is because I don't see them often and I want to be closer to them. So that's what made the whole thing feel awful. I just feel like I went in there thinking they were different people, and then I reacted so badly when they were exactly the way they always are. And that just feels so stupid—we always talk in here about how we can't make people be different, we can only aim our arrow. And I know my arrow isn't going to hit them, no matter how hard I aim it. So why do I let them get to me? And, also, who am I to judge how they are? I know that my grandmother said the same things to them, and it's not their fault that they haven't been able to change that. It feels disrespectful and unkind that I don't accept them as they are.

THERAPIST: Wow—so much going on in this situation, and it's all so understand- able and so human. And before we look at it a little more closely, I just want to point out that you're really noticing so many things—your thoughts, feelings, sensations, the actions you feel compelled to take, and the actions you would like to take. I can really see you using all of your skills. And, as we've talked about, other people, particularly family, are one of the most challenging con- texts for our valued actions. So it makes a lot of sense that you found this so hard. I guess the first thing I noticed is that a lot of self-criticism arose for you.

RIVA: Yeah, I noticed that while I was telling you. I don't think I noticed in the moment. But I was being really harsh with myself. I just really want to be more kind, and I hate it when I'm not.

THERAPIST: Yes, I know you value that. And I also heard that you engaged in a lot of kindness that day, although not all the kindness you wanted to. You were kind to your nieces. And not screaming at Aunt Viv was a kindness.

RIVA: Yeah, I guess that's true. I could have been more unkind than I was. But that's still not how I want to be.

THERAPIST: I know. And we can talk about what options were available to you in that moment and other choices you can make next time. But I do want to first make sure that we acknowledge that feeling sad and angry in response to those comments was a valid, understandable response. If someone we love criticizes us, sadness and anger are clear emotional responses—and it's helpful to recognize that and make room for them—even if we expect the criticism or understand why they act the way they act. And, remember, even if we'd rather not let others sense our emotional responses, that's not always possible. One of the main functions of our emotions is communicating important information to others, through our words, behavior, or facial expressions—information like—that comment hurt.

RIVA: But thinking my aunt is terrible and getting pissed at myself were muddy reactions.

THERAPIST: Agreed. And having those reactions arise is hard and also somewhat expected. We don't choose to respond in muddy ways, we learn to. And we can't simply unlearn our learning. All we can do is practice noticing and bringing compassion to ourselves for being human—in difficult moments or later when we have more space—and see what can be learned from our experience. Sometimes being less unkind is the best we can do in a moment. Or even being unkind and then later apologizing.

RIVA: I did manage to hug them both good-bye and say I loved them.

THERAPIST: That's wonderful. I wonder if it would be helpful for us to consider what all the options for responding could be in that situation like that. I think we both wish that your aunts wouldn't say those things and that their words didn't have to cause you pain or trigger muddied thoughts and emotions. Yet those are responses that we need to practice making room for and bringing compassion to. Given that you can expect to continue to have very real, very human responses to your family, what are some possible ways of responding to them that are values consistent?

Riva and her therapist went on to bring awareness to the sadness and pain that these exchanges elicited for Riva, doing a brief version of the *inviting a difficulty in . . .* mindfulness practice (Appendix B). They then discussed what choices Riva would like to make in future interactions with her aunts. Riva clarified that she valued closeness with her aunts, even though she was aware that they were not going to change this particular style of relating to her. Although she had made the choice of explicitly telling her mom a comment made her feel sad or angry, Riva opted not to have that same conversation with her aunts. However, she did decide to accept the fact that they might (or might not) notice her emotional response in her facial expression or subsequent behavior. Riva decided that she would try to engage in shared activities with her aunts that might engage their focus elsewhere (like watching their favorite shows together or knitting) and would bring compassion to herself when these comments were made. She would also make sure that she took time after these interactions to engage in more self-affirming actions and also use Larry Yang's aspiration practice (p. 178) before and after these visits to help her stay connected to her value of being as kind as possible (including to herself).

A basic, painful challenge that emerges in relationships is unreciprocated feelings and desires. A client who values being more vulnerable with others may also wish to develop a closer, more intimate relationship with a specific person. Discovering that the person does not want the same things can naturally lead to the clear emotion of sadness and an action tendency to withdraw and to give up trying actions that are consistent with this value. Therapists can help clients to make room for their emotional responses, cultivate self-compassion, and grieve these losses. Then they can turn to identify other contexts or people in which to continue to engage in these valued actions. Making the choice to enact values in other relationships doesn't diminish the clear pain associated with the loss of a specific, desired relationship; it's just a reminder that we have the ability to continue engaging in relationship values-based actions even when some relationships disappoint us or don't work out. These actions may not be as inherently satisfying initially and may be accompanied by ongoing feelings of sadness and loss. Yet, they can still elicit a sense of connection and relating that is intrinsically rewarding and a sense of agency that is empowering. Mindfulness practices can help clients to expand their awareness and notice all aspects of these emotional responses.

 Revisit Chapter 7 for more details on how to do this.

Another complexity in relational values-based actions is that we all have preferences for a range of qualities in others—our partners, friends, coworkers, neighbors, and family members—and may have to navigate the reality that people don't meet some of these preferences or have characteristics or behavioral patterns that we dislike. Again, our disappointment in not finding all of our preferred qualities in the people in our lives needs first to be acknowledged and validated. Then we can explore our choices. Considering the relative importance of the qualities that are present and missing in a specific person can inform whether or not one chooses to continue to foster or end the relationship. For example, after Ann recognized that integrity and mutual respect were qualities she prioritized highly in her relationship with coworkers, she shifted her attention and resources away from relationships with some colleagues and increased her efforts to cultivate new relationships with others. Clients might also recognize that preferred qualities can be spread across relationships. Marta appreciates her considerate and generous partner, Lynda, although she wishes Lynda were more adventurous. Fortunately, Marta's friend Roberto shares her taste for adventure, and so Marta feels sustained by both relationships. Finally, clients might find it helpful to clearly communicate their preferences to, and ask for changes from, others, while recognizing that others might not be willing or able to make those changes. Exploring options allows clients the opportunity to choose whether they want to stay in particular relationships and accept others as they are, end the relationship, or alter it in some way. Of course, these choices and the freedom clients have in negotiating them will vary depending on the nature of the relationship and the nature of the qualities desired and undesired.

Choices about Emotional Expression and Communication

One challenge that often arises relationally is how and whether to communicate to people in our lives. As we noted in Chapter 5, emotional expression varies culturally, and research suggests that emotional suppression may not have negative effects for people from cultures in which more indirect forms of emotional communication are valued.

Therefore, when working with clients about whether and how to communicate with people in their lives, therapists need to keep this cultural variability in mind (see Hall, Hong, Zane, & Meyer, 2011, for an in-depth discussion).

While clarifying and engaging in values-based actions in the domain of relationships, clients often identify that they are having reactions to other people and struggle with how to effectively work with these reactions in the context of these relationships. Integrating skills building into ABBT can be one way to help clients learn how to more effectively communicate with people in their lives, which can be consistent with values of honesty, emotional connectedness, and attempts to create reciprocity in relationships. Skills in communicating emotionally can also help clients to counteract the tendency to either automatically express or habitually suppress reactions in ways that are contributing to relationship conflict.

We also explore with clients moments in which they might intentionally choose to wait before expressing their responses. When emotional reactions are muddy, clients may want to take some time to use the skills they've developed to clarify their responses before communicating with someone else. This could involve explicitly asking for a break or creating an opportunity to take one (e.g., saying something like "I have to answer this call from my daughter's teacher; can we continue this conversation later?") before taking up the topic again. Similarly, some contexts may not be as conducive to effective communication as others, and so a client may decide to wait for a different opportunity to share their responses. For instance, a group context may not always be the most effective place to resolve an interpersonal conflict. Sometimes a client may weigh the relative importance of two relationship-related, values-based actions in a moment (e.g., intending to remind one's son that he is expected to complete his assigned chores after noticing dishes in the sink and wanting to express empathy upon learning that he just received an email that he was not hired for a job he really wanted) and choose to pass up one of the opportunities (e.g., let the conversation about dishes go this time). In all of these situations, as with the previous discussion of balancing values, we encourage clients to remain attentive to whether any of these responses are becoming habitual and potentially avoidant of the distress that might arise from clear communication, thus leading to longer-term distress through not sharing with another person.

We also need to acknowledge that there are contexts in which a client may purposefully choose to never intentionally disclose their emotional responses to some people. When they have less power than the other person and could be harmed as a result of sharing (e.g., an adult living with a difficult parent while they try to save money to move into their own apartment, or a worker whose boss makes the work environment very challenging for those who complain), clients may choose to keep their responses to themselves in that context and focus on other values-based actions available to them. For example, clients may choose instead to enact self-care and seek social support from others. Unfortunately, clients facing interpersonal challenges that are related to systemic inequity and injustice may frequently face these choices, given that injustices are so prevalent and so often denied and ignored. It's essential that therapists recognize that intentionally choosing not to respond in a potentially dangerous or damaging context is very different from automatically avoiding that situation. When working with clients who face these difficult choices, we do our best to convey validation, acceptance, and compassion for both the understandable reactions they are having and the choices they are making to not express these reactions. We also encourage them to find other methods and contexts that provide them with this same validation and self-compassion, rather than denying or criticizing their reactions or choices.

ADDRESSING PHYSICAL, SOCIETAL, AND SYSTEMIC BARRIERS AND INEQUITIES

As we work with clients to help them make meaningful changes in their lives, we need to recognize the contexts in which they live, including the messages they receive and the systemic inequities they encounter, which produce genuine barriers and limit access to opportunities. Unfortunately, we as individuals, and even the therapeutic context, are part of systems in which people receive different opportunities and costs based on aspects of their identity. We need to be particularly attentive to these factors so that we don't perpetuate these inequities, and we can actively work to challenge and dismantle harmful systems. For instance, if a therapist dismisses fears that a Black client expresses about the possibility that they will be less likely to be hired for a job due to race-based discrimination, that therapist is perpetuating a system that denies the reality of hiring discrimination (Quillian, Pager, Hexel, & Midtbøen, 2017), adding invalidation and erasure to the stress of the existing inequity.

Actively countering these tendencies involves an ongoing process of self-exploration and investigation to better see the inequities and injustices that therapists may be socialized to overlook, whether or not they involve aspects of one's identity. As two White, heterosexual, cisgender women who are not currently living with a disability or facing significant economic barriers, we are aware that we have been socialized to overlook many areas, and we are constantly working to turn toward and see the injustices and inequities that we may be missing.[1] It's also important to recognize that even when we hold identities that are associated with marginalization, we may have been socialized to overlook these inequities as well.

As we have noted throughout this book, an essential first step in addressing systemic external barriers to values-based action is to validate the reality of these constraints. Given how pervasive invalidation of these realities of injustice and inequity is, a therapist genuinely acknowledging these societal constraints will often be therapeutic in and of itself. Concurrently, therapists can emphasize how understandable a range of emotional responses, such as anger, fear, sadness, and disappointment, is to these realities. Clients often receive harmful messages that suggest they shouldn't get so upset about these chronic realities (i.e., "Can't you just let it go and get over it" or "What did you expect? This is how it always is") or share their responses because it makes others feel uncomfortable or guilty. Creating a context in which clients can feel what they're feeling may help to counter the additional reactivity, entanglement, and fusion that naturally arises from invalidating messages. Helping clients to develop self-compassion for their natural reactions to systematic barriers often requires that we first provide clients time to grieve the reality of these injustices and their impact on clients' lives.

---

[1]We acknowledge that our writing in this area is necessarily constrained by the limits of our perspectives and encourage therapists to also seek training from, and consult with, therapists with other identities for exposure to a range of perspectives and lenses.

BOX 10.4. TRY THIS:
Exploring Areas of Privilege

Privilege refers to "having preferred status in a social system of hierarchy that benefits some, but not others, in ways that are not connected to effort or ability" (Okun & Suyemoto, 2013, p. 22). Part of being a culturally responsive therapist includes an ongoing practice of noticing any areas of privilege that may lead us to fail to recognize the marginalization and barriers that clients we work with are facing (Hays, 2016). Revisit the aspects of identity reviewed in Chapter 2 (the ADDRESSING framework, pp. 37–40) and think about which aspects of identity are areas in which you hold some privilege—where you receive some benefits that people with different identities do not. Remember that receiving these benefits doesn't mean you're doing something wrong. However, it does mean that you are benefiting from a system that others do not benefit from and that, to be of help to those individuals, you need to be able to see these inequities and work to make these benefits more accessible for all. For instance, this kind of exploration helped me (LR) to realize that my parents' educational status made it easier for me to navigate higher education contexts, which helped me to pursue doctoral study and to be successful in that context. That didn't mean I didn't also work hard to get my degree, but there were a lot of parts of it that came more easily to me than it would to others just because of my family's background and things I was exposed to. Examining and understanding this makes it easier for me to leverage my privilege to advocate for students. It helps me be aware that I may not always recognize the structural barriers students are facing and that I can't assume they've had access to the same resources and opportunities that I have. This helps me refrain from imposing the myth of meritocracy on others and helps me to actively address these barriers in my mentoring.

Exploring our areas of privilege doesn't mean that we ignore the areas in which we face marginalization and challenges. Nor does it mean that we discount the challenges or barriers we face when we have relative privilege compared to some. But, as Oluo (2018) notes, we can easily focus on our areas of disadvantage to avoid the pain of recognizing that we also receive benefits that others do not. So, for this exercise, take some time to focus specifically on these areas of relative privilege and consider what that privilege keeps you from noticing, recognizing, and addressing. And then choose one thing you're going to do in order to increase your awareness in one of those areas: you could decide to read articles or books written by people who identify with marginalized statuses in those areas, or watch documentaries or movies in that area, or listen to podcasts focused on those aspects of identity.*

*Anneliese Singh's (2019) *The Racial Healing Handbook,* provides extensive experiential and educational guidance in exploring racial privilege (as well as aspects of intersectional identities), which can also be a model for exploring other areas of privilege such as citizenship, absence of disability, and education.

After validation, acceptance, and compassion have helped to counter some of the detrimental impact of being told not to feel a certain way, therapists may turn to exploring ways to help clients decenter from the internalized thoughts that naturally arise from the experiences they've had and the messages they've been receiving (see Box 10.5 for a brief overview of research on the mental health impact of internalization of discrimination experiences). As Graham, Sorenson, and Hayes-Skelton (2013) suggest in their thoughtful discussion of culturally competent CBT, trying to target thoughts about the likelihood of discrimination occurring is invalidating because these thoughts aren't unrealistic and present a risk. Instead, they recommend targeting the internalization of these thoughts (e.g., "I'm less competent because English is not my first language"; "I'm not a *real* man because of my sexual orientation"; "This disability prevents me from contributing at work in a meaningful way"). In ABBT, we can help clients decenter from these thoughts—that is, see that these thoughts, just like other thoughts we've explored in therapy, are occurring due to socialization and are not indicators of truth. Remembering the role of learning history in producing painful thoughts can help to reduce fusion with these thoughts and provide some increased flexibility from which to make behavioral choices.

In terms of selecting actions, we can help clients to make choices within the real constraints they're facing. This may include intentionally choosing to stay in a situation where a client is the target of microaggressions because some aspect of the situation is consistent with their values; providing feedback to the aggressor or telling someone else with power in the situation about it; or choosing to leave the situation. Values-based actions may also include intentionally leaving certain contexts to preserve resources and engage in self-care. And, for some clients, values-based actions will include identifying ways to challenge injustices and inequities either individually or communally. Exploring different options can help clients to reclaim a sense of their agency and power, even in the midst of contexts in which their power is also constrained.

BOX 10.5. A CLOSER LOOK:
The Mental Health Impact of Internalized Discrimination and Stigma

Research across different marginalized identities has consistently demonstrated that one mechanism through which discrimination is associated with negative mental health effects (e.g., anxiety, depression, lowered reports of self-esteem) is the internalization of devaluing experiences and messages. This phenomenon has been referred to as internalized racism, internalized heterosexism, internalized transphobia, or internalized stigma. Studies have found that, among individuals with physical disabilities, reports of internalized stigma fully mediate the negative association between reports of personal discrimination and self-esteem (Molero, Recio, Garcia-Ael, & Pérez-Garin, 2019). Similarly, internalized heterosexism appears to mediate the association between heterosexist discrimination and psychological distress among LGB individuals (Szymanski & Mikorski, 2016) and concealment of sexual orientation and psychological distress among LGB older adults (Hoy-Ellis, 2016). Among transgender and gender-nonconforming youth, higher levels of internalized transphobia were associated with diagnoses of GAD and major depressive disorder (Chodzen, Hidalgo, Chen, & Garofalo, 2019). Reports of internalized racism have also been shown to mediate the association between racist experiences and symptoms of anxiety in a sample of Black participants (Graham, West, Martinez, & Roemer, 2016). In contrast, internalized inferiority moderated the association between racial discrimination and mental distress among Asian and Pacific Islanders, such that at higher levels of internalized inferiority, the association between racial discrimination and mental distress was stronger (Garcia, David, & Mapaye, 2019). One recommendation drawn from this body of research is that these internalizations should be targeted in therapy (e.g., Carlson, Endlsey, Motley, Shawahin, & Williams, 2018; Graham-LoPresti, Abdullah, Calloway, & West, 2017). The finding that decentering moderates the relation between internalized heterosexism and psychological distress (Puckett, Mereish, Levitt, Horne, & Hayes-Skelton, 2018) provides some empirical basis for considering decentering and other acceptance-based strategies as one method for targeting these internalized critical beliefs. Acknowledging the external basis for these beliefs is one strategy that can be used to facilitate this decentering. Self-compassion may also be a particularly beneficial strategy for targeting these internalized beliefs (Graham-LoPresti et al., 2017).

Physical Challenges

Physical challenges can be part of clients' lives in a number of different ways. Some clients are born with challenges that they face throughout their lives, and some challenges emerge and have a time-limited, intermittent, or exacerbating course. Clients may acquire physical challenges related to biological factors, while others will experience changes in their abilities due to accidents or illnesses. All of us will find that our physical abilities alter at times in our lives and that some abilities we have when we are younger will naturally change as we age. These challenges all occur in a social context in which we often receive messages that celebrate physical ability and discount or disparage physical challenges, messages that can easily be internalized and that can contribute to distress and restricted engagement in valued action.

Sometimes a shift in health status or physical functioning will naturally lead a person to reconsider and redefine what they value. The recognition that life is fragile and health and physical well-being can't be taken for granted sometimes prompts people to clarify what matters most to them and therefore to more readily engage in these valued actions. Physical changes can also require a change in how long-held values are enacted. Clients who are used to acting consistently with values in ways that are dependent on certain physical abilities may need to consider other options. For example, Regina regularly demonstrated interest in, and care for, her grandchildren by taking them to the playground. As arthritis began to limit her mobility, she found playing board games and doing puzzles to be a more feasible alternative. Therapy can help clients to recognize and acknowledge challenges related to changes in physical ability, validate their new reality and the natural emotional responses to these changes, cultivate self-compassion, and then identify new or modified actions that are still consistent with these values-based actions.[2]

Financial Constraints

Within the United States and globally, income inequity is far too prevalent and, in addition to creating significant stress for many of our clients, this inequity can present barriers that make it more difficult to pursue valued actions. For example, financial constraints can occur at many levels; many people are unable to acquire basic necessities in daily life; some have to make difficult choices about where they can afford to live, whether a member of the family can leave work and primarily serve in a caretaker role for children or aging adults, and when they may be able to retire, while others may be limited in their abilities to pursue enrichment and leisure experiences. Providing for families or for individual needs may necessitate working so many hours that limited time is available to devote to other life domains. Further, economic need may make it more challenging to find a way to pursue one's personal work-related values in the context of a necessary job. Many leisure activities and/or enriching activities (e.g., higher education, further job training, learning arts/music/languages) are associated with significant costs or time away from paid work, making them less accessible to some individuals. Living in a society that emphasizes consumption can be particularly

---

[2]Clients may benefit from reading Toni Bernhard's books, *How to Be Sick* (2010) or *How to Live Well with Chronic Pain and Illness* (2015) or Ezra Bayda and Elizabeth Hamilton's *Aging for Beginners* (2018) for guidance in adjusting to the realities of changes in health status and abilities.

challenging for parents and guardians. For example, Gina works extra hours so she can purchase new clothes and supplies for her children, yet she feels guilty for missing school events and not being home in the afternoons to help with homework. Finally, pervasive and harmful societal messages that equate economic status with self-worth can add muddy emotions of shame and guilt in the context of financial struggles. As we noted earlier, therapists themselves have often been socialized to unconsciously or consciously hold many problematic biases (such as judgments about how people spend their limited funds). We must therefore work to recognize these reactions and act in affirming, validating ways despite this insidious socialization.

Recognizing the impact of financial constraints can help therapists to acknowledge clients' lived experience, respond empathically, and validate the existence of real external barriers to certain values-based actions. This therapist response can help clients decenter from thoughts that financial struggles reflect some internal weakness or pathological, defining characteristic. Practicing decentering and self-compassion again and again can help clients to begin to disentangle from the pervasive, pernicious messages connected to economic status. This process should include recognition that this is an ongoing practice because these messages are so embedded and insidious. From this place of compassion and understanding, therapists can then help clients to identify values-based actions to take that recognize this context. As we have emphasized throughout this chapter, this process often involves modifying an action (e.g., spending an hour with a loved one rather than the entire day), meeting multiple values with the same action (e.g., taking a walk with a friend as a form of exercise and a way to connect), or identifying alternative actions (taking one's children to different museums using library passes over school vacation week instead of going away on a trip), as well as recognizing that we can value something even if we aren't acting consistent with that value at a particular moment in time.

Racism, Discrimination, and Marginalization

People with marginalized identities can experience:

- Overt harm and discrimination such as physical and verbal assaults.
- Microaggressions or subtler communications: intentional or unintentional invalidations and insults that make a person feel inferior or excluded based on identity, such as assuming an Asian American was born outside the United States or denying that discrimination exists in our society.
- Systemic discrimination, including reduced access to job or educational opportunities, more frequent arrests, harsher sentencing, or harsher disciplinary practices in school.

One impact of these experiences is economic inequity, leading to the challenges we have described. However, these experiences create barriers beyond economics.

As noted earlier, these experiences naturally elicit a range of emotional responses. Often others don't acknowledge that discrimination and injustice are taking place, which can lead to intense, muddy emotions and confusion. Chronic invalidation can lead individuals to question, judge, or criticize their own natural, human responses to these injustices. Also, the chronic, widespread nature of discrimination means these clear emotions can be triggered by a broad array of reminders, including news stories about instances of discrimination and hate crimes. When we acknowledge these realities with clients, we need to draw a clear distinction between acceptance and resignation. Although we acknowledge the breadth and depth of discrimination and encourage clients to accept the clear emotions that emerge in response to it, we do not suggest that discrimination and marginalization are acceptable. Instead, acknowledgment and acceptance of the external and emotional realities can help our clients to have compassion for the impact of these experiences, particularly when others deny them. Mindfulness and decentering may help when clients feel entangled with, and defined by, hurtful statements by others. Observing thoughts for what they are can help clients recognize when the hurtful acts of others are leading them to have negative thoughts about themselves, which can help them disentangle further, rather than believing these thoughts. In turn, this process can help with identifying values-based actions to take within these contexts, while acknowledging real barriers.

Although widespread discrimination presents legitimate barriers in people's lives, groups that have experienced discrimination have a long history of coming together, identifying what matters to them, and acting on these values despite substantial obstacles. As Sobczak and West (2013) note, recognizing that feelings of powerlessness are an understandable *response* to discrimination, rather than *evidence* of actual powerlessness, can help people focus on clarifying and choosing actions in the face of harm and injustice. For some, values-based actions may include investing time and energy in directly addressing these injustices. People may also find that pursuing values in other domains, such as in family or community, can enhance their sense of purpose and meaning in the face of persistent barriers and injustices.

BOX 10.6. WHEN TIME IS LIMITED: Working with Contextual Inequities and External Barriers to Values-Based Actions

In therapeutic contexts where sessions are limited, it might be helpful to direct clients who are struggling to balance values across domains and those who find the constraints of time to be challenging to read Chapter 13 in *WLLM* (Orsillo & Roemer, 2016) to supplement in-session work. Given the complexities associated with external barriers to valued actions, and the pervasive role systemic discrimination and marginalization play in society, it can be challenging to effectively address these concerns when time in therapy is limited. In their desire to help clients make changes even in the context of their constraints, therapists might underestimate the importance of acknowledgment and validation. In our experience, it is critical that therapists sufficiently attend and validate clients' lived experience, and make room for a range of painful responses, before shifting into problem solving. In very limited therapeutic contexts, sometimes even just offering the possibility of hope in finding ways to live meaningfully in unfair and unjust contexts after devoting session time to validation and acknowledgment can be therapeutic.

To summarize, therapists should:

- Validate the reality of, and pain associated with, external constraints.
- Explicitly acknowledge systemic, institutional, and personal inequities and injustices.
- Provide opportunity to express grief and disappointment, or at least acknowledge that this will be a necessary part of the process.
- Identify the importance of self-compassion to counter internalization and provide resources for cultivation of these responses.
- Help the client to identify actions that can be taken despite constraints.
  - Explore adaptations to accommodate barriers (e.g., reduce time of action, find another context for actions, develop new actions).
  - Identify opportunities for choice that can be empowering.

How Do You Spend Your Time?

This exercise can be helpful when you're trying to consider where to direct your time and energy. Using the first circle below, draw lines to create pie pieces that represent how much of your time you'd like to devote to different parts of your life and write in that activity. There's no one right way to do this. One person may have a tiny slice devoted to spending time with family, while someone else might choose to make that piece half of their pie. One person may have a large chunk of pie devoted to engaging in creative pursuits, while another person doesn't have that represented at all in their pie. Be sure to include the things that matter to you, as well as other activities that take up your time.

(continued)

Note. Adapted with permission from *Worry Less, Live More* by Susan M. Orsillo and Lizabeth Roemer. Copyright © 2016 The Guilford Press.

Next, create another pie that represents how you're currently spending your time. This pie will have some slices devoted to your daily responsibilities—like cutting the grass or cleaning the house—and others will be devoted to activities that are more likely to be consistent with your values, like being outside in nature or caring for your children.

Now compare the two pies and ask yourself the following questions:

Are there changes you want to make in terms of how you're spending your time? If so, what are they?

_____

_____

_____

_____

(continued)

If there are responsibilities that take up a lot of time, are there ways to attend to them in a way that is values consistent (e.g., could you do them with a family member or appreciate the time alone, or do them mindfully, or pair them with something else meaningful)?

_____

_____

_____

_____

Are there slices of things that you "have to do" that actually reflect things you do in an attempt to control the uncontrollable (e.g., "I have to do more than my share of work, so I never let anyone down," or "I need to have a perfectly manicured lawn so that my neighbors don't judge me")? If so, list them here.

_____

_____

_____

_____

Can any changes be made to those slices?

_____

_____

_____

_____

Are there things you do to "relax" that don't actually replenish your energy (e.g., watching TV, drinking alcohol, gaming) that you could reduce or replace with more nourishing activities?

_____

_____

_____

_____

CHAPTER 11

Evaluating Progress, Relapse Prevention, and Ending Treatment

In this chapter, we discuss ways to monitor the progress of therapy, strategies for addressing lack of progress, methods of preparing clients for challenges they may face after therapy ends (i.e., relapse prevention), and our approach to ending therapy. The application of each of these approaches will vary a great deal depending on clients' presenting problems and the context in which they are being seen (e.g., when sessions are limited for external reasons). Thus, rather than prescribing specific steps to be followed, we share some options and articulate why we make certain choices so that clinicians can adapt our suggestions to meet the specific contexts in which they are working. We have addressed a number of barriers related to specific aspects of treatment throughout the book, so we focus here on additional considerations rather than repeat that material.

What you will learn

- How to incorporate ongoing assessment into therapy.
- How to evaluate progress and address lack of progress.
- Strategies to promote relapse prevention throughout treatment and during termination.
- Issues to consider as therapy ends.

CONTINUAL ASSESSMENT OF PROGRESS

We agree with Persons (2008) that ongoing assessment is an important part of an idiographic, responsive approach to administering and adjusting therapy that helps to enhance outcomes. The form of this assessment will vary depending on your setting, but we encourage the use of brief methods of monitoring key symptoms and processes at each session, as well as the administration of a somewhat more comprehensive assessment at specified intervals across treatment (e.g., a midtreatment review) or if therapy isn't progressing as expected. In our clinical trials, we asked clients to arrive 5–10 minutes early to complete very brief weekly assessments of symptoms, their relationship to their symptoms, and their functioning. We used the single-item assessments we developed specifically to assess the targets of treatment (see Client Form 11.1, *Weekly Assessment,* for an example used with a client with GAD that you can adapt for your purposes). We also used the Outcome Rating Scale,[1] which assesses functioning in personal, interpersonal, social, and overall areas with single items. In addition, we administered a more standard symptom measure such as the Depression Anxiety Stress Scales (described in Chapter 2) in order to assess symptom change more reliably. At longer intervals we might include other full measures described in Chapter 2 in order to get a sense of change over time.

Although we use these assessments partly for research purposes, we also find them clinically important for several reasons. These assessments provide an additional form of monitoring in that clients are asked to reflect on their symptom level and specific aspects of the treatment (e.g., acceptance, mindfulness, engagement in valued action) at least on a weekly basis. This type of reflection is especially helpful for clients who initially have difficulties with daily monitoring and who might not otherwise notice fluctuations across these domains. Completing these ratings allows clients to see changes as they emerge and to notice connections between changes in processes (e.g., increases in their values-based actions) and symptoms (e.g., enhanced mood). Finally, regular, ongoing assessment provides therapists with information about how processes and symptoms are changing over time (or not) for clients, which can inform clinical decisions.

Clinicians may also choose assessments based on what they're observing in therapy. For example, if it seems like a client doesn't understand all or parts of the model, or is particularly skeptical about strategies, an assessment like Client Form 11.2, *Treatment Progress Exploration,* may be helpful to clarify what the client has taken away from therapy. Therapists can also complete this form from their own perspective. In other words, therapists can rate how well they feel the different aspects of the model fit their client's presenting concerns, how explicitly they believe they have presented pieces of the model to their client, and their perceptions of how well the client understands and is responsive to the model. This type of dual assessment can help gauge the extent to which the therapist and client are on the same page and highlight aspects of the treatment plan that may need to be revisited. Similarly, it may be beneficial to assess the therapeutic relationship to determine if an impaired alliance should be addressed. The Session Rating Scale[2] provides a brief assessment of the therapeutic relationship that can be used weekly, while the Working Alliance Inventory[3] provides a somewhat lengthier, heavily researched assessment of bond and agreement on tasks and goals.

---

[1]Available for free to individual practitioners: *https://scott-d-miller-ph-d.myshopify.com/collections/ performance-metrics/products/performance-metrics-licenses-for-the-ors-and-srs.*

[2]Available for free to individual practitioners: *https://scott-d-miller-ph-d.myshopify.com/collections/ performance-metrics/products/performance-metrics-licenses-for-the-ors-and-srs.*

[3]Information on obtaining the Working Alliance Inventory is available at *https://wai.profhorvath.com.*

Evaluating the Course of Change and Addressing Lack of Progress

While assessing the course of change is an essential part of responsive practice, evaluating that course is complicated. Sometimes clients may show a steady or sudden decline in symptoms or problematic behaviors, or a reliable increase in engagement in their lives, indicating the likely effectiveness of their treatment plan. However, often the course of change is nonlinear and requires careful consideration. One evidence-based model of therapeutic change (Hayes, Yaskinski, Barnes, & Bockting, 2015) uses dynamic systems theory to describe how clients who present with chronic challenges might move from a fixed, stable system, in which problematic behaviors are habitual and predictable, into a new pattern (ideally) in which new behaviors and responses will become habitual and predictable. They suggest that once clients' initial system is destabilized, they may go through a period of time in which behavior and responses are more variable and unpredictable, which can even include a worsening of symptoms, before the new system fully stabilizes. Preparing clients for this possibility is an essential part of treatment-informed consent.

Sometimes we illustrate the ways in which the process of changing well-worn habits through therapy can be somewhat destabilizing and nonlinear by asking clients to consider what it's like to switch to our nondominant hand for everyday tasks. Using an example I (LR) learned from Tom Borkovec, we ask a client who always uses their right hand to open doors to imagine switching to using their left hand. We suggest that the process of change is likely to look something like this: First, we keep using our right hand, but after we go through doors we remember we were supposed to try something different and we vow to remember next time. This part of the process might go on for a while! Then we may approach doors, paying close attention to which hand we are using and we force ourselves to use our left hand. We are likely to have a period of time where we find ourselves fumbling around doors, taking a while to get through them, because we know we don't want to follow our established instincts, but we don't yet have new instincts to follow. Our behavior in that moment may look chaotic and ineffective. Eventually, we will use our left hand regularly, but it may require a good bit of our attention. Gradually, if we are consistent with our practice, this new behavior will become a new habit and we will be able easily to open doors again, although, at times of stress or when we are depleted, we may revert to the previous overlearned habit.

The *path up the mountain* metaphor from ACT can also be used as a way to describe the nonlinear course of progress in therapy, particularly with clients who have experience hiking. Switchbacks are twists and turns that are intentionally introduced into trails at points where the incline is steep, such that trying to stay on a direct path to the top of a mountain would be too challenging. Even though following the switchback on a trail can seem like backtracking in the moment and can leave even the most seasoned hiker feeling discouraged, the circuitous path is actually the most reliable route. Similarly, clients may feel discouraged when symptoms increase or their responses are less predictable, but the changes may reflect the nonlinear process of behavioral change.

Given that ABBT encourages clients to turn toward previously suppressed painful internal experiences and reduce behavioral avoidance by engaging more fully in their lives, we expect that clients may exhibit increased symptoms or distress. This increase in symptoms, if accompanied by decreases in behavioral or experiential avoidance, may very well indicate improvement rather than decline. For some clients, practicing mindfulness, focusing on the breath or bodily sensations, initially leads to a noticeable decrease in symptoms. In these cases, it's important to be attuned to challenges that can arise later when practicing mindfulness in more challenging domains, as they elicit an increase in symptoms.

Clinicians need to interpret shifts in symptoms within the context of the goals of treatment so that they can accurately prepare clients at the start of treatment and respond to client concerns that may arise over the course of treatment if symptoms seem to be worsening. Although we expect the path through ABBT to be nonlinear and for symptoms to sometimes increase before they improve, clinicians need to carefully assess indicators of progress to determine if some change to the treatment plan is needed. We assess the following factors to determine whether treatment is unfolding as expected or whether alterations should be made to enhance outcomes.

Understanding of the Model and Its Relevance

As we've described throughout the book, clients' understanding of the ABBT model can enhance their motivation to engage emotionally in sessions, complete in-between-sessions activities, and flexibly apply principles in their lives. When we sense that a client may not fully understand the model or how it fits their experience, we might assess this using Client Form 11.2, *Treatment Progress Exploration*, so that we can get a sense of where the disconnect may lie and address it directly. In other contexts where there are limits to outside assessment time, we may just verbally assess the client's understanding during a session so that we can fill in any holes or address misunderstandings.

Engagement in Treatment

We pay careful attention to whether clients are using self-monitoring, engaging in mindfulness practice, and attending to values-based action as each of these elements is introduced. When clients are not engaging in treatment, we explore with them what might be getting in the way, address these external and internal obstacles (as described in Chapters 4–7, 9, and 10), and evaluate the impact of these alterations. Throughout this work, we maintain a focus on our conceptualization so that if clients face obstacles with one set of strategies, we can flexibly choose alternative methods that serve the same intended function.

One modification we sometimes make to treatment, particularly with clients who are extremely disengaged, is to move more rapidly to encouraging values-based action even before fully introducing other elements of treatment. Jade came to treatment to address her chronic excessive anxiety and worry, which was interfering with her life so much that she was currently unemployed. She was 30–40 minutes late to her first three sessions. When her therapist asked what was interfering with Jade's ability to get to session, Jade responded with a stream of apparently external obstacles (e.g., she had to return several phone calls, she had job-related letters to send, she ran into a neighbor as she was leaving, she hit unexpected traffic on the way). When her therapist asked what would happen if Jade left for therapy before completing her planned tasks, Jade described the intense anxiety she experienced when she left something unfinished, revealing a previously unidentified internal obstacle. Jade's therapist highlighted the way that Jade's motivation to reduce her anxiety and worry were leading her to take a series of actions (staying later to work on her applications, stopping to talk to a neighbor) that were inconsistent with her stated value of attending to the anxiety that she felt was interrupting her life. While each choice made perfect sense at the time, given the sense of completion and relief Jade felt after attending to these responsibilities, the long-term effect was that Jade was not able to fully engage in therapy to make the types of changes she was hoping to make. The therapist asked Jade if, even though it would involve experiencing distress while leaving these situations, Jade might want to commit to leaving early for session and walking away from whatever was in progress in order to act in accord with this stated value. The therapist was careful to clearly validate Jade's distress and the difficulty of making this kind of radical change so early in treatment. This approach both helped Jade to prioritize therapy and work toward effecting the changes she hoped to make and to gain experience choosing a values-based action despite her internal state, which helped illustrate the concepts of ABBT that her therapist subsequently presented.

Patterns of Change Consistent with Conceptualization

Clients vary tremendously in the rate and scale of the changes they make in therapy. We don't necessarily expect change to be apparent until clients have been practicing skills for a few weeks, although some clients do benefit some from simply viewing their symptoms from an ABBT perspective and/or bringing awareness to their internal experiences. Other clients, particularly those who have been restricting their lives significantly, may experience more discomfort as they begin to engage more fully; yet this is an indicator of progress. Similarly, some clients begin to make behavioral changes right away, while others may become much more aware of their internal experiences but continue to feel somewhat stuck behaviorally at first. Clients in this latter category may not start making behavioral changes until they have more fully cultivated mindfulness in their lives and clarified their values.

Based on these observations, we carefully observe clients' course of their symptoms, their relationship to their symptoms, and their behavioral responses during the first several weeks they are practicing and applying the principles of therapy in their lives. As long as these are in some type of flux that is consistent with our conceptualization (e.g., increased distress might coincide with increased behavioral engagement if disengagement has been a form of experiential avoidance), then we consider these changes evidence of therapeutic effect. If, after several weeks, there is no evidence of movement in these domains, then we consider what might be interfering with therapeutic change, as we describe more fully below.

For instance, Edgar came to treatment reporting chronic dysphoria and social isolation. He had a history of moving from job to job. When asked about his current relationships, Edgar described playing a passive role in most relationships, often choosing actions designed to meet others' needs rather than his own. Edgar described significant anxiety at the thought of sharing his own opinion with friends, his partner, or coworkers. He also had a difficult time completing his values writing assignments, saying that he didn't have a clear sense of what was important to him. Edgar and his therapist developed a shared conceptualization tying Edgar's difficulty expressing personal preferences and his habit of choosing to please others rather than himself to his developmental history with affectively intense and demanding parents whom he learned to appease. The treatment plan focused on helping Edgar cultivate mindful-ness of his experiences, enhancing values exploration assignments to help Edgar gain a better sense of his own desires, and encouraging him to practice stating his needs and preferences in various contexts. Although Edgar engaged in therapy-related activities, he did not experience the predicted change in mood or life satisfaction. The therapist suggested that Edgar specifically apply his mindfulness skills during interpersonal sit-uations to monitor his internal experiences carefully so that the information gathered could be used to potentially modify the conceptualization and treatment plan.

Edgar's mindful monitoring revealed some additional information. Based on the initial conceptualization, the therapist predicted Edgar would feel anxious when expressing his needs for fear this wouldn't please others. Although the emphasis of these assignments was on helping Edgar to live consistently with his values, and not on how others responded to his assertiveness, the therapist did predict that a positive response from others would reinforce Edgar's assertive behavior. Instead, when Edgar received an accepting or validating response from someone, his anxiety both escalated in the moment (which was expected) and continued to linger for several days (which was not expected) and was frequently accompanied by feelings of sadness and even anger. For example, Edgar talked with his temporary employer, Frank, about his dis-satisfaction with his current responsibilities. Frank responded positively and offered Edgar a more challenging position that could become permanent. Edgar noticed that he first felt excited and pleased, but more careful monitoring revealed that he also had feelings of anger and dread. A similar mixed response emerged when Edgar's part-ner responded positively to Edgar's suggestion that they try to spend time together on the weekends. Edgar also noticed that he sometimes asserted his needs in a some-what aggressive way. For instance, when a group of coworkers invited him to lunch, he abruptly refused, stating that he couldn't understand how his coworkers could take a true lunch break given how much work he was assigned. This information suggested that the initial conceptualization was incomplete. Upon further reflection, Edgar real-ized that he used his passivity as a means of distancing himself from others. Therefore, when his assertions brought praise or closeness, he actually felt more distressed, and his somewhat aggressive style became another way for him to distance himself from others. Edgar and his therapist concluded that he was fearful and unwilling to be vul-nerable in his relationships. Thus, even though he had started expressing his prefer-ences in relationships, because he was not willing to open up to his own vulnerabilities, Edgar remained stuck in his pattern of avoidance.

Based on this slightly altered conceptualization, Edgar and his therapist collabo-rated on making some changes to Edgar's treatment plan. A shift in the type of values work was made such that rather than looking for and acting on opportunities to be assertive in his relationships, Edgar devoted more time to values articulation and clari-fication in the relationship domain. The treatment plan also included more activities aimed at helping Edgar to change his relationship with the thoughts, emotions, and sensations associated with vulnerability. Edgar spent time in and outside of therapy considering his unwillingness to deepen his connection to others, noticing the costs of that choice, and practicing acceptance and mindfulness toward his responses (e.g., using the *Inviting a Difficulty In and Working It Through the Body* practice in Appendix B). With time and practice, Edgar chose to strengthen his commitment to pursuing and maintaining intimate relationships, with an emphasis on approaching rather than avoiding interpersonal vulnerability. This choice led to greater fluctuation in his mood (with some temporary increases in sadness, followed by significant decreases), suggesting that he and his therapist had identified and moved through an important stuck point.

Edgar's case brings up something that is important to keep in mind, particularly when encouraging clients to engage in values-based actions. We are careful not to assume that certain behaviors, like being more open in relationships, are values-based, adaptive actions for all clients. Instead, we both listen to our clients' description of the changes they want to make, and we attend to the consequences clients experience when they engage in behavioral change. Adaptive actions should lead to a greater sense of flexibility and choice and an increased sense of agency, while reactive, avoidant, or detrimental actions will result in an increased sense of being stuck. Sometimes a process needs to unfold before the distinction is apparent.

Need for Adjunctive Skills Building or Other Behavioral Strategies

ABBT incorporates both acceptance and change strategies; as described in Chapter 9, the balance between them varies depending on the conceptualization of the specific client and should be addressed in the initial treatment plan. However, sometimes the need for adjunctive behavioral treatment or skill building does not become apparent until clients begin engaging in values-based actions and skills deficits in certain areas (e.g., starting a conversation, asserting themselves) become evident. It's not surprising that clients who have had little practice with these highly valued but commonly avoided behaviors would need some additional scaffolding. In these cases, therapists can incorporate skills-building exercises from earlier sessions of ABBT or other behavioral approaches to help clients effectively pursue their desired actions.

Therapist Handout 11.1, *Evaluating and Responding to Potential Obstacles to Treatment Progress*, provides a brief guide to the questions we ask when evaluating progress and addressing any evidence that the therapeutic process is impeded.

RELAPSE PREVENTION

Just as with other cognitive-behavioral treatments, relapse prevention, or strategies aimed at preparing clients to effectively cope with challenges that might arise post-treatment, is a critical element of ABBT and requires careful attention. Even though clients may have made dramatic changes over the course of treatment, it's essential that they continue to practice their skills and revisit core ABBT concepts even after therapy ends, so that they are prepared for the inevitable challenges they will encounter in their daily lives. To maintain the gains they have made, clients need to carry the principles of therapy with them, identify ways to remind themselves of these principles if their memories start to diminish, or reestablish skills that may fade without practice so that they are prepared to move through the apparent setbacks that are an inevitable part of living an engaged life.

Because an acceptance-based approach is often such a radically different way of relating to one's experiences, and experiential escape or avoidance is so often immediately reinforced, in the absence of an intentional plan to continue formal or informal skills practice, clients may lose therapeutic gains and require booster sessions. Also, because ABBT includes multiple components (exercises, concepts, actions in numerous domains), it can be challenging for some clients to develop a coherent model that they remember and follow in the absence of weekly or biweekly sessions. After noticing a slight decline in symptomatic improvement over the follow-up period in the first open-trial investigation we conducted (Roemer & Orsillo, 2007), we increased our emphasis on relapse prevention throughout treatment, particularly in the last several sessions. Our second study (Roemer, Orsillo, & Salters-Pedneault, 2008) revealed changes that were generally maintained over a 9-month follow-up period, which suggested that these alterations were effective. Anecdotally, we have had clients contact us several years posttreatment to comment on how treatment has changed them and to report how these changes have continued over time.

Like other forms of CBT that educate clients about psychological experiences and that teach skills, in a sense the entire course of ABBT is aimed at preparing clients for termination and potential posttreatment lapses. Therapists help clients to adapt treatment so that it makes sense to them, develop new habits that will support the changes being made in therapy, and take ownership of and responsibility for these changes. We give clients a binder to store hard copies of client handouts and writing assignments that are introduced throughout therapy, and we encourage clients to review previously discussed concepts and to refer to and retry past exercises. As treatment progresses, therapists intentionally become less directive, allowing clients to guide the focus of sessions, choose mindfulness and behavioral exercises to work on between sessions, and recognize their active role in therapeutic change and maintenance of this change. As therapists, we consciously step back from a more directive role and point out clients' agency in their change process. Otherwise, clients may attribute any changes to the therapist rather than seeing their own actions and accomplishments. By increasing clients' awareness of the efficacy of their own actions, therapists help clients recognize the impact of their actions and motivate them to continue their efforts toward changes that improve their lives.

Once a decision has been made to terminate therapy, we take several steps to explicitly prevent posttherapy relapse in the remaining sessions. When possible, we taper the last few sessions (i.e., every other week or every third week) so that clients can begin to practice continuing the work of therapy in the absence of a weekly session and address obstacles that arise in a subsequent, planned session. Sometimes clients choose to leave therapy more quickly, and the termination process must be completed in the course of one or two sessions.

Sessions focused on relapse prevention have several goals, including (1) consolidating and reviewing treatment gains, (2) identifying future work to be done independently, (3) predicting lapses (e.g., periods of increased distress and avoidance, decreased practice, apparent setbacks, disconnection from the therapeutic elements of treatment), and (4) developing strategies for addressing lapses (which includes intentionally summarizing skills and practices that were effective during treatment and building in reminders to use those skills and practices posttreatment).

First, we ask clients to complete a between-session treatment review writing assignment (see Client Handout 11.1, *Treatment Review Writing Assignment*, for a model to consider using). This allows clients to reflect on and articulate what they have learned in therapy, consider how they will maintain the gains they have made, identify what else they hope to accomplish, and explore any fears they may have about the end of treatment. In the next session, we review clients' responses to this exercise. It can also be helpful to ask clients to complete a modified treatment review writing assignment when they are considering termination, but a mutual decision has not yet been made. This provides a context in which therapist and client can collaboratively review accomplishments, consider additional goals, and decide whether continued therapy is indicated or whether the goals can be pursued independently. This type of review of gains and work left to be done should be an informal part of therapy throughout. However, we find that a more formal writing and review process can sometimes be additionally beneficial.

Next, we revisit the concept of a lapse and the distinction between lapse and relapse from Chapter 9 to help clients prepare for the inevitable challenges they are likely to face after therapy ends and view them as opportunities to practice skills and reaffirm the commitments. Linehan and colleagues (1999) use the term *dialectical abstinence* to refer to a synthesis of a full commitment to abstaining from a particular behavior, with the recognition that it is likely to reoccur and that this reoccurrence will provide a new learning opportunity that will assist with continued commitment to future abstinence. Similarly, when clients avoid intended values-based actions, this can be seen as an opportunity to identify obstacles and determine strategies for engaging in these actions in the future. And when they drift away from regular mindfulness practice, as with a refocusing on the breath after the attention inevitably wanders from it, clients can simply notice that they didn't act as they would have chosen to, refocus on their commitment to acting a certain way, and proceed accordingly.

When we talk to clients about the likelihood that they will experience lapses after treatment ends and that disappointment, self-criticism, and fear will arise in response to these lapses, we say something like:

> "As you continue through your life, you will face new challenges and new situations. You will inevitably experience times of increased distress when you find it more difficult to continue your mindfulness practice and act consistently with your values. As we have discussed, mindfulness and valued action are processes—we all need to continue to attend to these areas, notice when things are slipping, when our attention has wandered or we've begun to avoid feelings or situations, and gently bring ourselves back. This can be a very difficult and disheartening process. Often, the first response after noticing this kind of lapse is a feeling of disappointment and a thought like 'I'm right back where I started from' or 'I can't do it on my own.' This can easily start a cycle of self-critical reactions, increased distress, and experiential avoidance, which feeds back into the sense of disappointment and self-criticism, continuing the cycle. The longer the cycle, the more challenging it becomes to bring self-compassion to the experience, to lessen self-criticism and reactivity, and to reconnect to the practices that have been helpful.
>
> "I find that knowing this kind of lapse is natural and human helps me more quickly notice the pattern of self-criticism and disappointment and add some self-compassion to my reaction. Sometimes it can still take a long time for me to find a way to stop the cycle. At any moment, I can have the thought, 'Oh, right, this is the part where I feel like I've lost my ability to be mindful and live a valued life.' I can make room for all the doubts and disappointment, as well as my hope that I

can find my way back to the practices that were helpful. I can recommit to doing one thing to begin to bring mindfulness back into my life or find one values-based action to take to begin to set myself back on that path. No matter how many times I wander off the path (and I wander often), I am always just one moment of aware-ness away from stepping back onto it."

We may also revisit the inhibitory learning theory in this discussion (Chapter 9), reminding clients that we don't unlearn our old habitual reactions and behaviors. Rather, we only learn new patterns of responding that we can strengthen with practice. So we can expect old patterns to recur, particularly during times of stress or when our practice has waned. And engaging our newly developed habits again and again will help to restrengthen those responses, leading us to recover from these lapses.

Ironically, clients who rapidly respond to early mindfulness and acceptance prac-tices may be at higher risk for later lapses. When clients experience the relief that can come from practicing mindfulness and learning to relate to internal experiences dif-ferently, they can naturally get attached to that calm and may struggle and return to a pattern of judging and attempting to control feelings of discomfort when mindful-ness practice or life circumstances bring a different response. When these lapses occur while clients are still in therapy, we assure clients that this is an understandable, human lapse, reflecting the habitual and automatic nature of a self-critical reaction and a ten-dency toward avoidance. Clients are encouraged to practice awareness and compassion toward this inevitable response and to recommit to regular mindfulness practice. When these lapses haven't occurred in the latter parts of therapy, we predict that they may do so after therapy ends and we accordingly provide suggestions for responding to them.

We either provide a summary of the main components of treatment or we co-construct a personalized summary of treatment with the client so that they can note the specific concepts, metaphors, principles, handouts, and mindfulness practices that reso-nated with them and be able to refer back to them as reminders.[4] If clients don't already have *WLLM* (Orsillo & Roemer, 2016), we might give them blank copies of Client Forms 9.2 and 9.3, *Clarifying Emotions in the Moment* and *Values-Consistent Action Reflection*, and encourage them to return to these forms when they find they need some more scaf-folding to revisit principles of therapy. We also ensure that clients have a summary sheet of their valued domains to help them remember the areas they have identified as important so that they can bring their attention back to these domains during difficult times. Some of our clients have used physical objects, like stones to put on their desks or books they found particularly inspirational as reminders of their practices. (We include several book recommendations at *http://mindfulwaythroughanxiety.com/resources*, a list that has been supplemented by our clients' suggestions over the years.) Some of our clients have pursued formal practice in organized settings, becoming part of medita-tion groups or sanghas or enrolling in yoga or tai chi classes. Others commit to regular practice in their homes, sometimes setting aside a corner of a room for this practice to mark its importance.

---

[4]We find that metaphors provide clients with a vivid, easily recalled cue of important aspects of treatment. Clients commonly report reminding themselves to "drop the rope" (Chapter 6) or asking, "Who's driving the bus?" (Chapter 9) when they are in an emotionally challenging situation; this can be particularly useful after therapy has ended.

We share the ways that a consistent mindfulness practice may help reduce the risk of escalating lapses by maintaining a habit of awareness. If we haven't already introduced the 3-minute breathing space from Segal and colleagues (2002; see the full script in Appendix B and the audio recording on the Guilford website [see the box at the end of the table of contents]), we introduce it at this point so that clients can have a brief exercise that allows them to gather themselves, focus on their breath, and then expand out with mindful awareness of their full experience. We also might share a handout like Client Handout 11.2, *Mindfulness Practices,* or co-construct a handout together that summarizes mindfulness exercises the client has found helpful, and what they are useful for, so that the client can use this as a reminder after therapy ends. We either provide clients with personalized mindfulness practice recordings or we direct them to websites (like *http://mindfulwaythroughanxiety.com*) that have downloadable recordings. Given our findings that informal practice is particularly important in maintaining gains (Morgan et al., 2014), we also emphasize the importance of bringing mindfulness to daily activities and suggest that clients identify a few regular times to practice informal mindfulness (e.g., when brushing teeth, folding clothes, waiting for the bus) so that it remains part of their daily lives.

We encourage clients to be on the lookout for lapses and opportunities to reengage in practice. We regularly recommend that clients schedule a posttherapy weekly, biweekly, or monthly "check-in" with themselves so that they can bring awareness to their experience, their practice, and their values-based actions. We suggest they particularly check in when they engage in life changes or face new obstacles. We also often find it useful to help clients develop a personalized list of their own signs that a lapse is occurring and it's time to revisit the material of therapy. We list some common indicators that it's time to reengage in therapy in Box 11.1. We recommend that clients contact

---

BOX 11.1. Signs That It's Time to Revisit Mindfulness-, Acceptance-, and Values-Based Actions

- Feeling increasingly anxious/stressed/frazzled.
- Feeling checked out or disconnected, like you are on automatic pilot.
- Having muddied reactions more frequently.
- Feeling constrained in life.
  - Feeling like you don't have freedom or flexibility.
  - Feeling like you spend most of your time doing what you "have" to do.
  - Spending more and more of your free time on activities that don't seem to be enriching your life (aimlessly searching the Internet, watching television programs you don't find entertaining).
  - More frequently passing up valued activities.
  - Avoiding things you may enjoy because they feel like "too much."
- Repeatedly thinking things will get better after this one hurdle is passed.
- Putting off self-care activities and social engagements.

Note. Adapted with permission from *Worry Less, Live More* (2016) by Susan M. Orsillo and Lizabeth Roemer. Copyright © 2016 The Guilford Press.

us for booster sessions if their own methods do not seem to sufficiently reinvoke the aspects of the treatment that helped them in the past. Often, one or two sessions are sufficient, but sometimes a new issue has emerged that requires additional focus in therapy.

ENDING THE THERAPEUTIC RELATIONSHIP

In the course of therapy within an ABBT framework, clients have often engaged in emotionally vulnerable, sometimes frightening, work with the therapist and have expanded their lives in ways that may be novel and unsettling at times. Termination of this strong therapeutic relationship is a significant event that requires attention. Therapists need to be sensitive to individual differences; we are careful neither to overstate the importance of termination for a client who has become less attached to us and is not expressing strong feelings about ending the relationship nor to ignore the significance of termination for a client who has come to rely heavily on us and who will miss us a great deal. Clients often express concerns that, without the support of the therapist, they will lose their newly developed self-compassion or be unable to cope effectively with new challenges. Therapists can validate these fears (it is impossible to know that one can continue this work alone until one has the opportunity to try, so it is natural to fear this kind of change), while also pointing to the ways clients have already been doing this work alone and helping them develop ways to remember the work of the therapy.

Sometimes, clients express a desire to continue the therapeutic relationship as friends. Again, it is important to validate this desire. We ask clients to bring many of the same qualities to the therapeutic relationship that they would to any other intimate relationship, such as openness, honesty, vulnerability, and commitment. Furthermore, acceptance-based behavioral therapists aim to be genuine and unguarded, allowing strong emotions that come up in therapy and self-disclosing in therapeutically useful ways. Given the potential intensity and closeness of the relationship and the ways it can mirror other intimate relationships, it is natural for clients to feel strange about ending the relationship without any conflict or external impetus. It can be useful for therapists to highlight the ways that the therapeutic relationship is different from a friendship, underscoring how these differences are aimed at maximizing the benefits clients may receive from therapy. Clients also may benefit from hearing the therapist's confidence that clients have the skills and abilities necessary to negotiate life's challenges and the rationale that termination will allow clients to experience and recognize their strengths more fully.

In our own practice, we have worked with clients for whom the relationship with the therapist is the most intimate connection they have ever experienced. Many of our particularly isolated clients endorse a value of developing intimate connections and use therapy as a context in which to begin practicing values-consistent behaviors. With clients like these, it is particularly important to expand their social network and support valued actions within those new relationships before therapy ends.

When therapy focuses on interpersonal challenges, these themes are likely to arise in the context of the therapeutic relationship and may be particularly salient as the end of therapy nears. Therapists can share these observations and check in with clients to see if they notice a similar connection. For instance, a client who has avoided making a connection to people in their life due to a fear of being abandoned may find termination particularly evocative. Observing this can provide a context for the distress that is emerging, letting the client see the benefits of opening up to the therapeutic relationship, even though it is ending. This provides experiential evidence for the meaningfulness of pursuing this value, even when doing so also brings fear and sadness, which can be a particularly powerful learning experience. As always, these observations about similarities between the therapeutic relationship and outside relationships need to be presented as hypotheses. Some clients may be unable to see these connections, or the therapist may be inaccurate in these observations. Therapists should gently share their observations, allowing the client to refute them and simply encouraging continued awareness.

Clients often choose to give the therapist some kind of token farewell gift, such as a book on mindfulness, a stone to serve as a mindfulness reminder, or a poem reflecting a therapeutic theme. Although some theoretical perspectives discourage the acceptance of any gift and underscore the importance of processing the meaning of such a gesture with clients, we typically accept these gifts (as long as they are not too extravagant) as a token of gratitude for clients' experiences in therapy.

We honor the end of the therapeutic relationship by expressing our perceptions of the progress clients have made and our appreciation of the effort exerted. We note that we have learned from clients much as they have learned from us. During the final session, we pay particular attention to whether clients seem to be avoiding any negative emotions that arise in the context of saying good-bye and gently bring their attention to these emotions, encouraging an open experience of whatever arises. It is very rare for individuals to have an opportunity to be fully present to a shared termination of an interpersonal relationship; we do our best to take advantage of this opportunity to say an open, emotionally present good-bye.

CHALLENGES THAT ARISE DURING TERMINATION

How to Determine When It Is Time to End Therapy

As discussed earlier, assessment of progress is ongoing throughout therapy so that the therapist and client are both attending to the client's progress. Unlike the case in some traditional approaches to treatment, symptom reduction is not necessarily the central indication that treatment goals have been met. The collaborative treatment plan, which should be continually refined as therapy progresses if new goals emerge or old goals are fine-tuned, will typically contain specific behavioral targets that relate to clients' values-based actions in specific domains, as well as to clients' ways of responding to their own distress (i.e., with openness, curiosity, and acceptance rather than fear, avoidance, and judgment). These are both process goals; clients will not achieve a steady state of mindful, accepting responses while pursuing values-based actions. Therefore, rather than assessing whether a client has achieved a certain state, we assess the degree to which a client has acquired the skills to pursue these process goals on their own.

Often, the valued directions a client has targeted involve long-term life changes, which require time to unfold after years of living a more constrained life. More proximal actions can be taken on the path in these directions, but long-term outcomes may not be observed in the course of therapy. For instance, a client who values work that makes a difference in people's lives might take steps in exploring different career options, start attending to other people more in their current work, and begin some volunteer work over the course of therapy, but might not yet have come to a final career decision when treatment ends. Thus, treatment completion is typically indicated more by some consistent pattern of successful values-based action in multiple domains than by work in these areas feeling complete for the client. As the client begins to exhibit a systematic pattern of approach behavior in intended directions, confronting obstacles relatively independently (with support from the therapist), the therapist should begin to consider termination of therapy so that the client can experience the ability to live their life this way independent of therapy. Concurrent with these behavioral changes, therapists should assess the client's ability to consistently return to mindful, accepting awareness, regardless of the frequency of mindless, judgmental responses, which are inevitable. The ability to return to acceptance and self-compassion is the indicator of treatment success.

Clients may also reach a plateau where they have made significant changes, exhibiting increased skills in acceptance and values-based action, but may still have other areas to explore and that work has stagnated. Therapists and clients may collaboratively choose to take a break from therapy at this point, allowing changes to consolidate and the pattern of values-based action to solidify before beginning to address additional issues. Apparently unresolved issues may resolve in the course of living a mindful, valued life, or subsequent sessions may be needed. Sometimes a scheduled break from therapy can help determine which of these is the case.

Often, when therapists and clients review progress, they come to an agreement regarding the choice to continue or terminate therapy. As noted above, a writing assignment may help clients reflect on progress and their current state, if the decision is not sufficiently clear. Weekly assessments of experiential avoidance, symptoms, and behavioral actions should be reviewed to assess changes and current status to contribute to this decision.

Ending Therapy When the Client Does Not Feel Ready

Sometimes clients do not feel ready to end therapy even though they have made significant gains. They may not recognize the gains that have been made, or they may be afraid that they cannot maintain these gains in the absence of the therapist. Reviewing progress and changes in assessment over time can help illustrate the gains that have occurred. Sometimes a longer series of tapered sessions can be helpful in showing clients what it is like not to have therapy weekly and allowing them to notice their own ability to cope with challenges without the stress of leaving therapy altogether. However, some clients may never feel completely ready to leave therapy. This unwillingness may be another example of experiential avoidance, with clients not wanting to experience the anxiety of losing the safety net of weekly therapy. Framing it this way to clients can be helpful, and they often see that terminating therapy is another values-based action that may not feel comfortable but that they can nonetheless choose.

Sometimes clients continue to hold on to unrealistic goals for therapy, such as being symptom-free. In these cases, reviewing the model of treatment and data that show symptoms often persist intermittently after efficacious treatment (although disorders do not continue) can help clients see that they will not experience a symptom-free life.

Ending Therapy When the Client Has Not Responded to Treatment

Sometimes clients are simply not responding to the treatment approach, and an alternative form of therapy is indicated. In these cases, reviewing whatever gains have been made, as well as the obstacles that seem to have occurred, will still be beneficial. If the ABBT therapist is not able to offer the type of treatment that is indicated, a referral should be made to someone who practices from that perspective. Sometimes clients are interested in ABBT, but they do not feel they are a good fit with therapists who have a particular interpersonal style or cultural identity, and so these clients may ask for a referral to a different provider. Although these therapy challenges can elicit uncomfortable thoughts and feelings in therapists (such as "I am not good enough" or "Why doesn't she like me?"), mindfulness and acceptance skills can help facilitate responses consistent with one's values as a therapist. When these situations arise, clients should be praised for recognizing that the therapy was not a good fit and for being willing to discuss their concerns openly and encouraged to pursue an approach or therapist who may be a better fit. The therapist can review different approaches to treatment at this point and either quell client concerns or help the client select a new therapist.

Sometimes clients are not willing or able to make the kinds of changes that are part of therapy. For example, a client may not be experiencing sufficient distress to motivate them to do the challenging work of therapy, or life circumstances may arise that preclude their current engagement in therapy. Clients are sometimes aware of their own avoidance and the changes they want to make to live a more fulfilling life but are simply unwilling to do so. (In our own work, we find it helpful to think about changes in our lives that we as therapists are aware we could make to improve our lives but that we are not currently working on.) When a client is not willing or able to fully engage in therapy for any of these reasons, the therapist can help the client realize and articulate this rather than allow them to continue to attend sessions without active engagement. Keeping clients in therapy when progress is at a standstill can lead them to believe that therapy is not helpful and may inhibit them from seeking services in the future. Clients can be encouraged to return to therapy when they are willing and able to commit to the work, or sometimes alternative, less demanding approaches can be suggested (such as self-help or Internet approaches if transportation or cost is interfering). In all of these cases, therapists should first work with clients to identify the obstacles to their engagement in therapy, altering treatment so as to optimize their engagement and making sure that clients share therapists' conceptualization and approach. Often, what appears to be disengagement is really the absence of a collaborative treatment plan. Other times, a client is truly not interested in therapy and is pursuing it due to someone else's wishes or a sense that it "should" be done. This is not a good use of the client's time; helping them to realize this and to make a valued choice regarding engagement in therapy can be the most therapeutic choice.

Ending Therapy When External Factors Require It

Sometimes therapy ends for external reasons (e.g., financial constraints, agency limits, a move, new life events). In these cases, reviewing progress, predicting lapses, and putting structures and practices in place to maintain the work of therapy remain important, particularly the emphasis on maintaining the work. Although clients may not have solidified gains yet, therapists can help them recognize the progress they have made and map out the steps they want to follow to maintain and increase these gains. The suggestion to set aside time for weekly reflection and commitment to practice is particularly important in these cases, as it will help clients maintain focus on their progress and implement aspects of therapy on their own. Clients may also benefit from self-help (e.g., *WLLM*; Orsillo & Roemer, 2016) or digital interventions that can provide structure and continue to present the same principles. Termination sessions can focus on identifying these additional resources and providing the client with handouts or co-constructed lists of the personalized aspects of therapy that they can integrate with these resources. Mindfulness recordings or other contexts for mindfulness-based practices can also be beneficial in these cases.

BOX 11.2. WHEN TIME IS LIMITED:
Relapse Prevention

In therapeutic contexts where sessions are limited, it can be easy to overlook relapse prevention. However, helping clients identify ways to keep the principles of treatment in their lives may be particularly important when treatment has been limited. In these contexts, we recommend:

- When appropriate for the client, providing handouts and workbooks (such as *WLLM* [Orsillo & Roemer, 2016]), so that the client can continue psychoeducation and exercises after treatment ends.
- Co-constructing a summary of principles, metaphors, and exercises that clients found useful so they can return to it after treatment ends.
- Psychoeducation about lapse and relapse and a plan for addressing lapses.
- Helping the client develop some new habits/practices that will help with maintaining (and continuing to develop) new learning.
- Recordings of mindfulness practices (such as at *http://mindfulwaythroughanxiety.com*) to help scaffold ongoing formal practice, as well as identification of daily activities during which to practice informal mindfulness.

The following questions are designed to give us a sense of how your week has been in terms of the kinds of things we are focusing on in therapy. There are no right or wrong answers. We just want to get *your* impression of your week.

What percentage of the time did you find yourself worrying over the past week?

0   10   20   30   40   50   60   70   80   90   100

What percentage of the time were you mindful over the past week? By "mindful," we mean aware of your current experience, focused on where you were at that moment and what you were doing, as opposed to what you did earlier or would do later?

0   10   20   30   40   50   60   70   80   90   100

What percentage of the time did you feel accepting of your internal experience (thoughts and feelings) as opposed to trying to push it away?

0   10   20   30   40   50   60   70   80   90   100

What percentage of the time did you feel you were spending on the things that are important to you?

0   10   20   30   40   50   60   70   80   90   100

What percentage of the time did you feel like your thoughts and feelings were getting in the way of what you wanted/needed to be doing?

0   10   20   30   40   50   60   70   80   90   100

CLIENT FORM 11.2. Treatment Progress Exploration

1. Patterns of responding that we learn through our different life events and experiences can be **one of many** factors that contribute to our distress and dissatisfaction. Place a check in front of each of the patterns **your therapist has suggested could** be related to your current distress.

____ Self-criticism in response to painful thoughts, feelings, and physical sensations.

____ Feeling "defined by" one's own painful thoughts, feelings, and physical sensations.

____ Attempts to control or push away certain painful thoughts, feelings, and physical sensations when they arise.

____ Avoiding certain life experiences because they could bring up painful thoughts, feelings, and physical sensations.

____ Trying to control things that are not entirely in your control (like the future or other people's behavior) in order to live a satisfying life.

____ Being unclear about the things you value or the things that could bring meaning to your life.

____ Often not making choices or taking actions based on what is most meaningful to you.

____ Sometimes being distracted by thoughts and feelings that cause you to feel disconnected from whatever is happening in the present moment.

2. Go back through the list in #1 and put a check in front of each of the patterns **you personally think** could be adding to your current distress.

3. Rate the degree to which you agree with each of the following statements on a 0–10 scale (0 = not at all true; 5 = somewhat true; 10 = extremely true).

____ Overall, I think the ABBT model does a good job explaining my distress.

____ Even though I think the ABBT model makes sense logically, I am having a **hard time accepting that some parts of it are true** (e.g., that everyone feels anxious when taking a risk, that people often end up more uncomfortable when they try and change how they feel).

____ Logically, I understand the model, but am struggling because I feel that **some parts of the model don't seem fair** (e.g., there are limits to what I can control).

____ I understand the model, but I don't think it is relevant to me.

____ I forget about the model outside of session, especially when I am in a challenging situation.

____ I don't fully understand the model (some parts seem clear to me, others do not).

____ I don't know what the ABBT model is.

____ Even though the model makes sense logically, I feel like other things are more strongly influencing my distress. Please list: _____

_____

____ I feel like the model (and my therapist) overlook important aspects of my experience. List here: _____

_____

(continued)

4. Put a check in front of each of the following treatment strategies your therapist has suggested you might try to decrease your overall distress and/or improve your life satisfaction.

____ Noticing that we all experience a full range of emotions and that all of our emotions, even the painful ones, serve a function.

____ Noticing that certain ways of responding to painful thoughts, emotions, and physical sensations can make them more distressing and long-lasting.

____ Learning to distinguish "clear" and "muddy" emotions.

____ Using some type of monitoring and/or mindfulness practice to become aware of learned habits of responding.

____ Using mindfulness practice as a way of responding differently to painful thoughts, feelings, and physical sensations.

____ Practicing noticing when you feel pulled to control things out of your control.

____ Thinking or writing about the things you value or the things that could bring meaning to your life.

____ Practicing making choices or taking actions based on what is most meaningful to you rather than responding out of habit.

____ Noticing when you are distracted and bringing your attention to the present moment.

____ Cultivating self-compassion when you are feeling critical and judgmental.

____ Using mindfulness practice as a way of becoming more intentional about the choices you make.

5. Go back through the list in #4 and rate the extent to which you **think** each of these strategies could be helpful if you learned how to apply them in your life on a 0–10 scale (*0 = not at all helpful*; *5 = somewhat helpful*; *10 = extremely helpful*). Mark a strategy N/A if you don't know anything about the strategy or don't understand it.

CLIENT HANDOUT 11.1. Treatment Review Writing Assignment

Set aside 20 minutes during which you can privately and comfortably do this writing assignment. In your writing, we want you to really let go and explore your very deepest emotions and thoughts about the topics listed below.

Write about any or all of the following topics. If you choose to write on only one of the topics, that would be fine. You may write about them in any order you wish. If you cannot think about what to write next, just write the same thing over and over until something new comes to you. Be sure to write for the entire 20 minutes. Please do not spend any time worrying about spelling, punctuation, or grammar—this writing is intended to be a "stream of consciousness"—that is, you may write whatever comes to mind.

- What have you learned about yourself over the course of treatment?
- What methods have you learned that have been helpful to you?
- What changes have you made (if any) that are important to you?
- What methods do you need to continue to practice most once treatment ends?
- What new commitments do you want to make with regard to values-based action?
- What concerns do you have (if any) about treatment ending?

Practice	Helpfulness
Breath	Basic portable practice.
Breathing Space	When racing from one activity to another or to check in and get centered.
Mindfulness of Emotions	When experiencing muddy or intense reactions.
Thoughts on Clouds, Leaves, or Movie Screen	When entangled, fused, or tied in judgments.
Mindfulness of Sounds/Eating Mindfully	When you are bringing expectations to a situation, not necessarily watching as it unfolds.
The Guest House/Inviting a Difficulty In	When you are struggling with willingness.
The Mountain Meditation	When you need help connecting to inner strength and stability in the midst of change.

When clients don't seem to understand all or part of the model:

- Revisit psychoeducation in Chapters 5–8.
- Correct any misunderstandings the client may have about the model (e.g., one has to feel self-compassionate in order to practice self-compassion).

When clients don't think the model applies to aspects of their experience:

- Consider that you may not fully understand the client's experience and ask for input on why the model is insufficient; broaden your assessment, and work with the client to develop a shared conceptualization, using Therapist Forms 3.1 and 3.2.
- Consider contextual factors that you may not have validated or addressed sufficiently; review Chapter 10 for guidance.
- Use information the client provided during the assessment or in treatment to date to place the model in context (e.g., suggesting to a client who doesn't think their struggle with worry or anxiety interferes with values-based actions, "It's like that time you told me that you were so worried that your partner was going to break up with you, that you shut down in a way that was different from how you want to act in that relationship").
- Ask the client if they're willing to bring mindful observation to their behavior and the consequences of behavior in order to get more direct information about the potential relevancy of the model.
- Place any potentially challenging piece of the model aside and ask the client if it could be revisited in the future.

When clients seem disengaged from treatment:

- Assess and address concrete obstacles to engagement in between session activities through problem solving and adjusting activities while maintaining intended function.
- Address any ruptures in the working alliance (see Chapter 4).
- Make sure you are clearly connecting any recommended treatment strategies or practices to the client's goals for treatment and your shared case conceptualization.
- Assess and address obstacles to engagement like nonattendance, possibly through values-based action.

When clients are struggling and/or their symptoms worsened:

- Determine whether their struggle is consistent with your case conceptualization.
  - If so, explain the nonlinear course of change to your client and continue to monitor progress for any unexpected changes.
  - If not,
    - Collaborate with your client in revisiting your conceptualization.
    - Ask your client to practice broadening their awareness and bringing mindfulness to their experiences to see if additional information can be gained to identify potential stuck points.
    - Use in-session mindfulness exercises to explore how application of skills is unfolding for the client, with particular attention to criticism and judgments that arise.
    - Assess whether the client is choosing actions that maintain avoidance rather than engagement.
    - Adaptive actions should lead to a greater sense of flexibility and choice and an increased sense of agency, while reactive, avoidant, or detrimental actions will result in an increased sense of being stuck.
  - Explore whether the client needs additional practice with ABBT skills (revisit Part II) or adjunctive treatment.

APPENDIX A

Measures That Can Be Used to Assess ABBT Model-Specific Processes

Construct	Measure	No. of items	Sample Items	Comments
Measures that assess problematic relationship with internal experiences				
Difficulty identifying and describing emotions	Twenty-Item Toronto Alexithymia Scale[a]	21	I am often confused about what emotion I am feeling. It is difficult for me to reveal my innermost feelings, even to close friends.	Can calculate scores for three factors: difficulty describing feelings, difficulty identifying feelings, and externally oriented thinking.
Fear of physiological arousal-related sensations	Anxiety Sensitivity Index3[b]	16	It scares me when my heart beats rapidly. When I cannot keep my mind on a task, I worry that I might be going crazy.	Can calculate scores for three factors: physical, cognitive, and social concerns.
Fear of emotions	Affective Control Scale[c]	42	Depression is scary to me—I am afraid that I could get depressed and never recover. When I get really excited about something, I worry that my enthusiasm will get out of hand.	Can calculate scores for four factors: fear of anxiety, depression, anger, and positive affect.
Decentering or the ability to observe internal experiences as temporary, objective events	Experiences Questionnaire[d]	20	I can separate myself from my thoughts and feelings. I can observe unpleasant feelings without being drawn into them.	
Cognitive fusion or the extent to which contents of the mind seem true and defining	Cognitive Fusion Questionnaire[e]	7	I tend to get very entangled in my thoughts. I get so caught up in my thoughts that I am unable to do the things that I most want to do.	

283

Construct	Measure	No. of items	Sample Items	Comments
Beliefs about the power of negative, intrusive thoughts	Thought-Action Fusion Scale[f]	19	If I think of a relative/friend being in a car accident, this increases the risk he/she will have a car accident. If I wish harm on someone, it is almost as bad as doing harm.	Items measure the belief that thinking about an unacceptable or disturbing event will increase its probability and the belief that having an unacceptable thought is almost the same as carrying out an unacceptable action.
Difficulty with the idea that future events are unknown and unpredictable	Intolerance of Uncertainty Scale—Short Form (IUS-12)[g]	27	The smallest doubt can stop me from acting. My mind can't be relaxed if I don't know what will happen tomorrow.	Can calculate scores for four factors: uncertainty is stressful and upsetting, uncertainty leads to the inability to act, uncertain events are negative and should be avoided, and being uncertain is unfair.
Self-compassion	Self-Compassion Scale[h]	26	I'm kind to myself when I'm experiencing suffering. I try to see my failings as part of the human condition.	Items measure self-kindness, self-judgment, common humanity, isolation, mindfulness, and overidentification. A shorter version of the scale is also available.

Measures that assess both problematic relationship with internal experiences and experiential avoidance

Construct	Measure	No. of items	Sample Items	Comments
Mindfulness	Philadelphia Mindfulness Scale[i]	20	I am aware of what thoughts are passing through my mind. I try to put my problems out of mind.	Can calculate scores for awareness and acceptance.
Mindfulness in everyday life	Five Facet Mindfulness Questionnaire[j]	39	I notice the smells and aromas of things. When I have distressing thoughts or images, I am able just to notice them without reacting.	Includes skills of observing, describing, acting with awareness, nonjudging, and nonreactivity.

Construct	Measure	Items	Example items	Notes
Emotion Regulation	Difficulties in Emotion Regulation Scale[k]	36	When I'm upset, I become embarrassed for feeling that way.	Can calculate scores for acceptance of emotions, ability to engage in goal-directed behavior when distressed, impulsivity when distressed, access to strategies for regulation, awareness of emotions, and clarity of emotions.

Measures that assess experiential avoidance

Construct	Measure	Items	Example items	Notes
Tendency to suppress thoughts	White Bear Suppression Inventory[l]	15	I always try to put problems out of mind. There are things I prefer not to think about.	Very widely used in research.
Strategies used to try and control unpleasant and unwanted thoughts	Thought Control Questionnaire[m]	30	I punish myself for thinking the thought. I call to mind positive images instead.	Can calculate scores for five factors: distraction, social control, worry, punishment, and reappraisal.
Experiential avoidance	Brief Experiential Avoidance Questionnaire[n]	15	I work hard to keep out upsetting feelings. The key to a good life is never feeling any pain.	Can calculate scores for behavioral avoidance, distress aversion, procrastination, distraction and suppression, repression, and denial.
Acceptance/ experiential avoidance/ psychological inflexibility	Acceptance and Action Questionnaire –II[o]	10	Worries get in the way of my success. Emotions cause problems in my life.	There are multiple versions of this measure. Some are specific to particular populations (e.g., chronic pain, alcohol misuse).

Construct	Measure	No. of items	Sample Items	Comments
			Measures that assess values	
Values importance and consistency	Valued Living Questionnaire[p]	20	Parenting Recreation/fun	Can calculate an importance and a consistency score.
Values attainment and persistence	Bull's-Eye Values Survey[q]	Varies	Relationships Personal growth	Respondents generate values within four domains and place a mark on a target at a distance from the center (i.e., bull's eye) that shows how closely they are living in accordance with their values. They also describe obstacles and rate the extent to which they interfere. Finally, they generate values-consistent actions.

[a]Bagby, Parker, and Taylor (1994). Available at *www.gtaylorpsychiatry.org/tas.htm*.

[b]Taylor et al. (2007). Available at *www.idspublishing.com/docs08/ASI%20Order%20Form.pdf*.

[c]Williams, Chambless, and Ahrens (1997). Available at *https://web.sas.upenn.edu/dchamb/questionnaires*.

[d]Items available in Fresco, Moore, et al. (2007).

[e]Items available in Gillanders et al. (2014).

[f]Items available in Shafran et al. (1996).

[g]Carleton, Norton, and Asmundson (2007). Items available at *www.midss.org/content/intolerance-uncertainty-scale-short-form-ius-12*.

[h]Neff (2003). Available at *https://self-compassion.org/wp-content/uploads/2015/06/Self_Compassion_Scale_for_researchers.pdf*.

[i]Items available in Cardaciotto et al., (2008); the scale is also available by contacting LeeAnn Cardaciotto, Department of Psychology, La Salle University, Box 268, 1900 West Olney Avenue, Philadelphia, PA 19141; email: *cardaciotto@lasalle.edu*.

[j]Baer el al. (2006). Available at *http://ruthbaer.com/academics/FFMQ.pdf*.

[k]Items available in Gratz and Roemer (2004). Also available at *http://cairncenter.com/forms/difficultiesinemotionalregulation_scale.pdf*.

[l]Items available in Wegner and Zanakos (1994) and at *https://scholar.harvard.edu/dwegner/publications/chronic-thought-suppression*.

[m]Wells and Davies (1994). Available at *www.clintools.com/victims/resources/assessment/affect/tcq.pdf*.

[n]Available at Gámez et al. (2014).

[o]Bond et al. (2011). Available at *http://ruthbaer.com/academics/AAQ-II.pdf*.

[p]Wilson et al. (2010). Available at *www.div12.org/wp-content/uploads/2015/06/Valued-Living-Questionnaire.pdf*.

[q]Items cited in Lundgren et al. (2012).

APPENDIX B

Mindfulness Exercises

MINDFULNESS OF BREATH

"Noticing the way you are sitting in the chair. . . . Noticing where your body is touching the chair. . . . Now beginning to bring your attention to your breath. . . . Noticing where you feel your breath in your body . . . it may be in your throat, your nostrils, your chest, or your belly . . . allowing your awareness to settle in this place. . . . Paying attention to the sensations you experience . . . each time your mind wanders, bringing it back to this place where you feel your breath in your body. . . . "

MINDFULNESS OF CLOUDS AND SKY

"Close your eyes . . . first focusing on your breathing, just noticing your breath as you take it in, it travels through your body and then back out of your body. Noticing how your body feels. . . . Now picturing yourself lying someplace outside where you can see the sky. You can picture any place that feels comfortable and vivid to you—lying on a raft in a pond, on a blanket in a field, on the deck of a house, on the roof of a car, anyplace where you have a clear full view of the sky. Now imagining yourself, comfortably lying, your body sinking into whatever you're lying on, as you gaze at the sky. Noticing the sky, and the clouds that hang in the sky, moving across it. Seeing how the clouds are part of the sky, but they are not the whole sky. The sky exists behind the clouds. Imagining that your thoughts and feelings are the clouds in the sky, while your mind is the sky itself. Seeing your thoughts and feelings gently drifting across the sky . . . as you notice thoughts and feelings, placing them in the clouds and noticing them, as they pass across the sky. . . . Noticing yourself as you become distracted, or immersed in the clouds, losing sight of the sky . . . noticing how the clouds can be very light and wispy, or dark and menacing . . . noticing how even when the clouds cover the sky, the sky exists behind them. . . . Noticing moments when your thoughts and feelings feel separate from you . . . and moments when they feel the same as you . . . picturing the sky behind the clouds and the clouds drifting across the sky . . . practicing putting your thoughts and feelings on to the clouds . . . noticing the different shapes they take . . . the different consistency of the clouds they are on . . . when you find yourself on the clouds, slowly shifting your attention back to the sky behind the clouds and practicing putting your thoughts and emotions on the clouds. . . . [Leave the client time to do the exercise in silence, then gently guide awareness back to the room, present sensations, sitting in a chair, and invite client to open eyes when ready.]"

INVITING A DIFFICULTY IN AND WORKING IT THROUGH THE BODY[1]

"Now, once you are focusing on some troubling thought or situation—some worry or intense feeling—allow yourself to take some time to tune into any physical sensations in the body that the difficulty evokes. See[ing] if you are able to notice and approach any sensations that are arising in your body, becoming mindful of those physical sensations, deliberately, [but gently] directing your focus of attention to the region of the body where the sensations are the strongest in the gesture of an embrace, a welcoming. This gesture might include breathing into that part of the body on the in-breath and breathing out from that region on the out-breath, exploring the sensations, watching their intensity shift up and down from one moment to the next.

"[. . .]Seeing if you can bring to this attention an even deeper attitude of compassion and openness to whatever sensations, [thoughts, or emotions] you are experiencing, however unpleasant, by saying to yourself from time to time, 'It's okay. Whatever it is, it's already here. Let me open to it.' Then just stay with the awareness of these [internal] sensations, breathing with them, accepting them, letting them be, allowing them to be just as they are. It may be helpful to repeat, 'It's here right now. Whatever it is, it's already here. Let me open to it.' Soften[ing] and open[ing] to the sensations you become aware of, letting go of any tensing and bracing. Remember that by saying, 'It's already here' or 'It's okay,' you are not judging the original situation or saying that everything's fine, but simply helping your awareness, right now, to remain open to the sensations in the body. If you like, you can also experiment with holding in awareness both the sensations of the body and the feeling of the breath moving in and out, as you breathe with the sensations moment by moment.

"And when you notice that the bodily sensations are no longer pulling your attention to the same degree, simply return 100% to the breath and continue with that as the primary object of attention."

3-MINUTE BREATHING SPACE

"Now, closing your eyes, if that feels comfortable for you, the first step is being aware . . . of what is going through your mind; what thoughts are around? Here, again, as best you can, just noting the thoughts as mental events. . . . So we note them, and then noting the feelings that are around at the moment . . . in particular, turning toward any sense of discomfort or unpleasant feelings. So rather than trying to push them away or shutting them out, just acknowledging them, perhaps saying, 'Ah, there you are, that's how it is right now.' And similarly with sensations in the body . . . Are there sensations of tension, of holding, or whatever? And again, awareness of them, simply noting them. Okay, that's how it is right now.

"So, [we've] got a sense of what is going on right now. We've stepped out of automatic pilot. The second step is to collect our awareness by focusing on a single object—the movements of the breath. So . . . focusing attention in the movements of the abdomen, the rise and fall of the breath . . . spending a minute or so focusing on the movement of the abdominal wall . . . moment by moment, breath by breath, as best we can. So that you know when the breath is moving in, and you know when the breath is moving out. Just binding your awareness to the pattern of movement down there . . . gathering yourself, using the anchor of the breath to really be in the present.

[1] Adapted with permission from *The Mindful Way through Depression* by Mark Williams, John Teasdale, Zindel V. Segal, and Jon Kabat-Zinn. Copyright © 2007 The Guilford Press.

"And now as a third step, having gathered ourselves to some extent, we allow our awareness to expand. As well as being aware of the breath, we also include a sense of the body as a whole. So that we get this more spacious awareness. . . . A sense of the body as a whole, including any tightness or sensations related to holding in the shoulders, neck, back, or face . . . following the breath as if your whole body is breathing. Holding it all in this slightly softer . . . more spacious awareness.

"And then, when you are ready, just allowing your eyes to open."[2]

---

[2]Reprinted with permission from *Mindfulness-Based Cognitive Therapy for Depression, Second Edition*, by Zindel Segal, Mark Williams, and John Teasdale. Copyright © 2013 The Guilford Press.

APPENDIX C

A Model of Integration of Topics, Exercises, and Forms across Sessions

Session goals	Psychoeducation topics and handouts	Self-monitoring activities	In-session and out-of-session experiential practices	In-session and out-of-session values practices
Assessment: Develop preliminary understanding of client's presenting concerns, history, and current context (Chapter 2) Begin to build therapy relationship (Chapter 4)	Handouts/readings on the ABBT model to be read at home (Chapter 1) Chapter 1 in *WLLM* may be given to be read at home			Assess cost of presenting concerns on values
Treatment planning: Develop shared case conceptualization and treatment plan (Chapter 3)	ABBT Model and Rationale for Treatment (Chapters 1 and 5) Client Handout 5.1, *Fear Is Learned* Client Handout 5.2, *What Are Fear and Anxiety Made Up Of?*	Client Form 5.1, *Monitoring Your Fear and Anxiety*	Imaginal recall of fear/anxiety to notice elements of response in session (Chapter 5) *Mindfulness of breath* practiced at end of session (Appendix B)	Review of cost of struggle on values using information from assessment in session
Introduce mindfulness practice	Overview of formal and informal mindfulness, connect mindfulness practice to presenting problems (Chapter 6) Client Handout 6.1, *What Is Mindfulness?* Client Handout 6.2, *Mindfulness Skills*	Monitor at-home mindfulness practice (formal and informal)	*Mindfulness of breath* (Appendix B) *Raisin practice* (Chapter 6) *Progressive muscle relaxation* adapted (Chapter 6)	Client Form 8.1, *Values Writing Exercise I*

Explicit efforts aimed at helping client to change client's relationship with internal experiences Thoughts and worries	Overview of how minds work (Chapter 5) Chapter 2 in WLLM may be given to read at home Client Handout 5.6, *Common Reasons We Turn Our Attention to the Future (Worry) and Past (Rumination)* Client Handout 5.7, *Am I Problem Solving, Worrying, or Ruminating?*	Client Form 5.4, *Worry or Problem Solving?* Continue monitoring at-home mindfulness practice (formal and informal)	*Mindfulness of sounds* (Chapter 6) Work through examples of problem solving, rumination, and worrying Exploration of experience with formal and informal mindfulness practice	Consideration of how worry and rumination reduce the quality of engagement in valued activities Hidden costs of worry-driven activities is time away from valued activities
Explicit efforts aimed at helping client to change client's relationship with internal experiences Emotions and physical sensations	Function of emotion Concept of clear and muddy emotions (Chapter 5) Client Handout 5.3, *Clear Emotions* Client Handout 5.4, *Differentiating Clear and Muddy Emotions*	Client Form 5.2, *Monitoring Emotions* Continue monitoring at-home mindfulness practice (formal and informal)	*Mindfulness of emotion* (Chapter 6) Metaphors and stories from Chapter 5 (e.g., Sam suppressing his sadness; Peggy's anger at the neighbors)	Cost of control efforts tied to *Values I* review
Factors that contribute to muddy emotions	Muddy emotions and control efforts (Chapter 5) Client Handout 5.5, *Factors That Contribute to Muddy Emotions* Chapter 4 in WLLM may be given to read at home	Client Form 5.3, *Clarifying Emotions Reflections* Continue monitoring at-home mindfulness practice (formal and informal)	*Mindfulness of clouds and sky* (Appendix B) *White Bear*; adapted polygraph exercise; love story (Chapter 5) Discuss challenges that arise when practicing mindfulness (Chapter 6)	Client Form 8.2, *Values Writing Exercise II*

Session goals	Psychoeducation topics and handouts	Self-monitoring activities	In-session and out-of-session experiential practices	In-session and out-of-session values practices
Values articulation and clarification	Overview of values, distinguishing from goals, and rationale for focus (see Chapter 8) Chapter 9 in *WLLM* may be given to read at home Misunderstandings associated with self-compassion (Chapter 7) Client Handout 8.1, *Intentional Responses That Differ from Emotion-Driven Reactions*	Continued use of Client Form 5.3, *Clarifying Emotions Reflection* Continue monitoring at-home mindfulness practice (formal and informal)	*Inviting a difficulty in and working it through the body* (Appendix B) *Skiing* and *falling in love* metaphors (Chapter 8) *Choosing an ice cream flavor* metaphor (Chapter 8)	Client Form 8.3, *Values versus Goals* Define one or two values in each domain (Chapter 8)
Continue values clarification/Introduce commitment and willingness	Identifying and working through values stuck points (Chapter 8) Chapter 10 in *WLLM* may be given to read at home Commitment as a process, not an outcome (Chapter 9) The defining characteristics of willingness (Chapter 9)	Client Form 8.4, *Monitoring Opportunities for Valued Action* Continue monitoring at-home mindfulness practice (formal and informal)	*The Guest House* (Chapter 6) *Aim your arrow* metaphor (Chapter 9) Choose metaphors—some options include *gardening, passengers on the bus, swamp, the party* (Chapter 9)	Client Form 9.1, *Values Writing Exercise III*

Phase II Sessions Depending on client multiple sessions that could be focused on one or more topic Planning and implementing values-based actions Working through obstacles to values-based actions Working with painful emotions as they arise in daily life	Review and elaboration of previously covered topics, if needed Addressing the barriers of limited time, relationships, physical, societal, systemic barriers, and inequities as relevant (Chapter 10)	Client Form 9.2, *Clarifying Emotions in the Moment* Continue monitoring at-home mindfulness practice (formal and informal)	*3-minute breathing space* (Appendix B) Client's choice of practice	Client Form 9.3, *Values-Consistent Actions Reflection* If needed, Client Form 10.1, *How Do You Spend Your Time?*
Preparing for Termination/ Relapse Prevention	Lapse versus relapse (Chapters 9 and 11) Plan to retain skills posttreatment (Chapter 11) Client Handout 11.1, *Treatment Review Writing Assignment*	Client Form 9.1 *Clarifying Emotions in the Moment* Plan for ongoing check-ins/signs of relapse (Chapter 11) Client Handout 11.2, *Mindfulness Practices*	*Mountain meditation* (Chapter 6)	Client Form 9.2 *Values-Consistent Actions Reflection*

References

A-Tjak, J. G. L., Davis, M. L., Nexhmedin, M., Powers, M. B., Smits, J. A. J., & Emmelkamp, P. M. G. (2015). A meta-analysis of the efficacy of acceptance and commitment therapy for clinically relevant mental and physical health problems. *Psychotherapy and Psychosomatics, 84,* 30–36.

Addis, M., & Martell, C. R. (2004). *Overcoming depression one step at a time: The behavioral activation approach to getting your life back.* Oakland, CA: New Harbinger.

Amodio, D. M., Devine, P. G., & Harmon-Jones, E. (2007). A dynamic model of guilt: Implications for motivation and self-regulation in the context of prejudice. *Psychological Science, 18,* 524–530.

Antony, M. M., Orsillo, S. M., & Roemer, L. (Eds.). (2001). *Practitioner's guide to empirically based measures of anxiety.* Dordrecht, the Netherlands: Kluwer Academic.

Antony, M. M., & Roemer, L. (2011). *Behavior therapy.* Washington, DC: American Psychological Association Press.

Arch, J. J., & Craske, M. G. (2008). Acceptance and commitment therapy and cognitive behavioral therapy for anxiety disorders: Different treatments, similar mechanisms? *Clinical Psychology: Science and Practice, 15,* 263–279.

Arch, J. J., Eifert, G. H., Davies, C., Vilardaga, J. C. P., Rose, R. D., & Craske, M. G. (2012). Randomized clinical trial of cognitive behavioral therapy (CBT) versus acceptance and commitment therapy (ACT) for mixed anxiety disorders. *Journal of Consulting and Clinical Psychology, 80*(5), 750–765.

Baer, R. A., Smith, G. T., Hopkins, J., Krietemeyer, J., & Toney, L. (2006). Using self-report assessment methods to explore facets of mindfulness. *Assessment, 13,* 27–45.

Bagby, R. M., Parker, J. D., & Taylor, G. J. (1994). The twenty-item Toronto Alexithymia Scale—I. Item selection and cross-validation of the factor structure. *Journal of Psychosomatic Research, 38,* 23–32.

Bailey, T. H., & Phillips, L. J. (2016). The influence of motivation and adaptation on students' subjective well-being, meaning in life and academic performance. *Higher Education Research and Development, 35,* 201–216.

Barlow, D. H. (1991). Disorders of emotion. *Psychological Inquiry, 2,* 58–71.

Barlow, D. H. (Ed.). (2014). *Clinical handbook of psychological disorders: A step-by-step treatment manual* (5th ed.). New York: Guilford Press.

Barlow, D. H., Farchione, T. J., Sauer-Zavala, S., Latin, H. M., Ellard, K. K., Bullis, J. R., . . .

Cassiello-Robbins, C. (2017). *Unified protocol for transdiagnostic treatment of emotional disorders: Therapist guide.* New York: Oxford University Press.

Barnard, L. K., & Curry, J. F. (2011). Self-compassion: Conceptualizations, correlates, and interventions. *Review of General Psychology, 15*(4), 289–303.

Bayda, E., wth Hamilton, E. (2018). *Aging for beginners.* Somerville, MA: Wisdom.

Benish, S. G., Quintana, S., & Wampold, B. E. (2011). Culturally adapted psychotherapy and the legitimacy of myth: A direct-comparison meta–analysis. *Journal of Counseling Psychology, 58,* 279–289.

Bernhard, T. (2010). *How to be sick: A Buddhist-inspired guide for the chronically ill and their caregivers.* Somerville, MA: Wisdom.

Bernhard, T. (2013). *How to wake up: A Buddhist-inspired guide to navigating joy and sorrow.* Somerville, MA: Wisdom.

Bernhard, T. (2015). *How to live well with chronic pain and illness: A mindful guide.* Somerville, MA: Wisdom.

Bernstein, D. A., Borkovec, T. D., & Hazlett-Stevens, H. (2000). *New directions in progressive relaxation training: A guidebook for helping professionals.* Westport, CT: Praeger.

Bishop, S. R., Lau, M., Shapiro, S., Carlson, L., Anderson, N. D., Carmody, J., . . . Devins, G. (2004). Mindfulness: A proposed operational definition. *Clinical Psychology: Science and Practice, 11,* 230–241.

Bond, F. W., Hayes, S. C., Baer, R. A., Carpenter, K. M., Guenole, N., Orcutt, H. K., . . . Zettle, R. D. (2011). Preliminary psychometric properties of the Acceptance and Action Questionnaire–II: A revised measure of psychological inflexibility and experiential avoidance. *Behavior Therapy, 42,* 676–688.

Borkovec, T. D., Alcaine, O. M., & Behar, E. (2004). Avoidance theory of worry and generalized anxiety disorder. In R. G. Heimberg, C. L. Turk, & D. S. Mennin (Eds.), *Generalized anxiety disorder: Advances in research and practice* (pp. 77–108). New York: Guilford Press.

Borkovec, T. D., & Sharpless, B. (2004). Generalized anxiety disorder: Bringing cognitive-behavioral therapy into the valued present. In S. C. Hayes, V. M. Follette, & M. M. Linehan (Eds.), *Mindfulness and acceptance: Expanding the cognitive-behavioral tradition* (pp. 209–242). New York: Guilford Press.

Bouton, M. E. (1988). Context and ambiguity in the extinction of emotional learning: Implications for exposure therapy. *Behaviour Research and Therapy, 26,* 137–149.

Bouton, M. E., & King, D. A. (1983). Contextual control of the extinction of conditioned fear: Tests for the associative value of the context. *Journal of Experimental Psychology: Animal Behavior Processes, 9,* 248–265.

Bowen, S., Chawla, N., Collins, S. E., Witkiewitz, K., Hsu, S., Grow, J., . . . Marlatt, G. A. (2009). Mindfulness-based relapse prevention for substance use disorders: A pilot efficacy trial. *Substance Abuse, 30*(4), 295–305.

Brach, T. (2003). *Radical acceptance: Embracing your life with the heart of a Buddha.* New York: Bantam Dell.

Breines, J. G., & Chen, S. (2012). Self-compassion increases self-improvement motivation. *Personality and Social Psychology Bulletin, 38*(9), 1133–1143.

Bronfenbrenner, U. (1979). *The ecology of human development: Experiments by nature and design.* Cambridge, MA: Harvard University Press

Cacioppo, J. T., & Hawkley, L. C. (2009). Perceived social isolation and cognition. *Trends in Cognitive Sciences, 13,* 447–454.

Cacioppo, J. T., Hughes, M. E., Waite, L. J., Hawkley, L. C., & Thisted, R. A. (2006). Loneliness as a specific risk factor for depressive symptoms: Cross-sectional and longitudinal analyses. *Psychology and Aging, 21,* 140–151.

Calloway, A., Hayes-Skelton, S. A., Roemer, L., & Orsillo, S. (2017, April). *Working alliance over time across an acceptance-based behavioral therapy and applied relaxation for clients with generalized anxiety disorder.* Paper presented at the annual meeting of the Anxiety and Depression Association of America, San Francisco, CA.

Cardaciotto, L., Herbert, J. D., Forman, E. M., Moitra, E., & Farrow, V. (2008). The assessment of present-moment awareness and acceptance: The Philadelphia Mindfulness Scale. *Assessment, 15,* 204–223.

Carleton, R. N., Norton, M. A., & Asmundson, G. J. G. (2007). Fearing the unknown: A short version of the Intolerance of Uncertainty Scale. *Journal of Anxiety Disorders, 21,* 105–117.

Carlson, M., Endlsey, M., Motley, D., Shawahin, L. N., & Williams, M. T. (2018). Addressing the impact of racism on veterans of color: A race-based stress and trauma intervention. *Psychology of Violence, 8,* 748–762.

Catterson, A. D., Eldesouky, L., & John, O. P. (2017). An experience sampling approach to emotion regulation: Situational suppression use and social hierarchy. *Journal of Research in Personality, 69,* 33–43.

Chervonsky, E., & Hunt, C. (2017). Suppression and expression of emotion in social and interpersonal outcomes: A meta-analysis. *Emotion, 17,* 669–683.

Cheung, W.-Y., Maio, G. R., Rees, K. J., Kamble, S., & Mane, S. (2016). Cultural differences in values as self-guides. *Personality and Social Psychology Bulletin, 42,* 769–781.

Chishima, Y., Mizuno, M., Sugawara, D., & Miyagawa, Y. (2018). The influence of self-compassion on cognitive appraisals and coping with stressful events. *Mindfulness, 9,* 1907–1915.

Chodron, P. (2001). *The places that scare you: A guide to fearlessness in difficult times.* Boston: Shambhala.

Chodron, P. (2007). *Practicing peace in times of war.* Boston: Shambhala.

Chodzen, G., Hidalgo, M. A., Chen, D., & Garofalo, R. (2019). Minority stress factors associated with depression and anxiety among transgender and gender-nonconforming youth. *Journal of Adolescent Health, 64*(4), 467–471.

Cohen, G. L., Garcia, J., Apfel, N., & Master, A. (2006). Reducing the racial achievement gap: A social-psychological intervention. *Science, 313,* 1307–1310.

Cohen, G. L., Garcia, J., Purdie-Vaughns, V., Apfel, N., & Brzustoski, P. (2009). Raising minority performance with a values-affirmation intervention: A two-year follow-up. *Science, 324,* 400–403.

Craske, M. G. (2010). *Cognitive-behavioral therapy.* Washington, DC: American Psychological Association.

Craske, M. G., & Barlow, D. H. (2014). Panic disorder and agoraphobia. In D. H. Barlow (Ed.), *Clinical handbook of psychological disorders: A step-by-step treatment manual* (5th ed., pp. 1–61). New York: Guilford Press.

Craske, M. G., Treanor, M., Conway, C. C., Zbozinek, T., & Vervliet, B. (2014). Maximizing exposure therapy: An inhibitory learning approach. *Behaviour Research and Therapy, 58,* 10–23.

Crenshaw, K. (1991). Mapping the margins: Intersectionality, identity politics, and violence against women of color. *Stanford Law Review, 43*(6), 1241–1299.

Creswell, J. D., Welch, W. T., Taylor, S. E., Sherman, D. K., Gruenewald, T. L., & Mann, T. (2005). Affirmation of personal values buffers neuroendocrine and psychological stress responses. *Psychological Science, 16,* 846–851.

Curry, S., Marlatt, G. A., & Gordon, J. R. (1987). Abstinence violation effect: Validation of an attributional construct with smoking cessation. *Journal of Consulting and Clinical Psychology, 55*(2), 145–149.

Danitz, S. B., & Orsillo, S. M. (2014). The mindful way through the semester: An investigation of the effectiveness of an acceptance-based behavioral therapy program on psychological wellness in first-year students. *Behavior Modification, 38,* 549–566.

Danitz, S. B., Suvak, M., & Orsillo, S. M. (2016). The mindful way through the semester: Evaluating the impact of integrating an acceptance-based behavioral program into a first-fear experience course for undergraduates. *Behavior Therapy, 47,* 487–499.

Davey, G. C., Tallis, F., & Capuzzo, N. (1996). Beliefs about the consequences of worrying. *Cognitive Therapy and Research, 20,* 499–520.

Deci, E. L., & Ryan, R. M. (1985). The general causality orientations scale: Self-determination in personality. *Journal of Research in Personality, 19,* 109–134.

Derogatis, L. R. (2000). *Brief Symptom Inventory (BSI)–18: Administration, scoring and procedures manual.* Minneapolis, MN: NCS Pearson.

Epton, T., Harris, P. R., Kane, R., van Koningsbruggen, G. M., & Sheeran, P. (2015). The impact of self-affirmation on health-behavior change: A meta-analysis. *Health Psychology, 34,* 187–196.

Erskine, J. A. K., Georgiou, G. J., & Kvavilashvili, L. (2010). I suppress, therefore I smoke: Effects of thought suppression on smoking behavior. *Psychological Science, 21,* 1225–1230.

Eustis, E. H., Hayes-Skelton, S. A., Orsillo, S. M., & Roemer, L. (2018). Surviving and thriving during stress: A randomized clinical trial comparing a brief web-based therapist assisted acceptance-based behavioral intervention versus waitlist control for college students. *Behavior Therapy, 49,* 889–903.

Eustis, E. H., Hayes-Skelton, S. A., Roemer, L., & Orsillo, S. M. (2016). Reductions in experiential avoidance as a mediator of change in symptom outcome and quality of life in acceptance-based behavior therapy and applied relaxation for generalized anxiety disorder. *Behaviour Research and Therapy, 87,* 188–195.

Eustis, E. H., Morgan, L. P., Orsillo, S. M., Hayes-Skelton, S. A., & Roemer, L. (2017, April). *Examining the relations among facets of mindfulness, acceptance, and outcomes in acceptance-based behavior therapy and applied relaxation for generalized anxiety disorder.* Poster presented at the annual conference of the Anxiety and Depression Association of America, San Francisco, CA.

Eustis, E. H., Williston, S. K., Morgan, L. P., Graham, J. R., Hayes-Skelton, S. A., & Roemer, L. (2017). Development, acceptability, and effectiveness of an acceptance-based behavioral stress/anxiety management workshop for university students. *Cognitive and Behavioral Practice, 24,* 174–186.

Ferssizidis, P., Adams, L. M., Kashdan, T. B., Plummer, C., Mishra, A., & Ciarrochi, J. (2010). Motivation for and commitment to social values: The roles of age and gender. *Motivation and Emotion, 34,* 354–362.

Foa, E. B., & Kozak, M. J. (1986). Emotional processing of fear: Exposure to corrective information. *Psychological Bulletin, 99,* 20–35.

Freeston, M. H., Rhéaume, J., Letarte, H., Dugas, M. J., & Ladouceur, R. (1994). Why do people worry? *Personality and Individual Differences, 17,* 791–802.

Fresco, D. M., Moore, M. T., van Dulmen, M. H., Segal, Z. V., Ma, S. H., Teasdale, J. D., & Williams, J. M. G. (2007). Initial psychometric properties of the Experiences Questionnaire: Validation of a self-report measure of decentering. *Behavior Therapy, 38,* 234–246.

Fresco, D. M., Segal, Z. V., Buis, T., & Kennedy, S. (2007). Relations of posttreatment decentering and cognitive reactivity to relapse in major depression. *Journal of Consulting and Clinical Psychology, 76*(3), 447–455.

Fuchs, C. H., West, L. M., Graham, J. R., Kalill, K. S., Morgan, L. P., Hayes-Skelton, S. A., . . . Roemer, L. (2016). Reactions to an acceptance-based behavior therapy for GAD: Giving voice to the experiences of clients from marginalized backgrounds. *Cognitive and Behavioral Practice, 23*(4), 473–484.

Fulton, P. R. (2013). Mindfulness as clinical training. In C. K. Germer, R. D. Siegel, & P. R. Fulton (Eds.), *Mindfulness and psychotherapy* (2nd ed., pp. 59–75). New York: Guilford Press.

Gámez, W., Chmielewski, M., Kotov, R., Ruggero, C., Suzuki, N., & Watson, D. (2014). The Brief Experiential Avoidance Questionnaire: Development and initial validation. *Psychological Assessment, 26,* 35–45.

Garcia, G. M., David, E. J. R., & Mapaye, J. C. (2019). Internalized racial oppression as a moderator of the relationship between experiences of racial discrimination and mental distress among Asians and Pacific Islanders. *Asian American Journal of Psychology, 10*(2), 103–112.

Garland, E. L., Brown, S. M., & Howard, M. O. (2016). Thought suppression as a mediator of the association between depressed mood and prescription opioid craving among chronic pain patients. *Journal of Behavioral Medicine, 39,* 128–138.

Germer, C. K. (2005). Anxiety disorders: Befriending fear. In C. K. Germer, R. D. Siegel, & P. R. Fulton (Eds.), *Mindfulness and psychotherapy* (pp. 152–172). New York: Guilford Press.

Germer, C. K. (2009). *The mindful path to self-compassion: Freeing yourself from destructive thoughts and emotions.* New York: Guilford Press.

Germer, C. K., Segal, R. D., & Fulton, P. R. (Eds.). (2013). *Mindfulness and psychotherapy* (2nd ed.). New York: Guilford Press.

Gilbert, P. (2009). *The compassionate mind.* Oakland, CA: New Harbinger.

Gillanders, D. T., Bolderston, H., Bond, F. W., Dempster, M., Flaxman, P. E., Campbell, L., . . . Masley, S. (2014). The development and initial validation of the Cognitive Fusion Questionnaire. *Behavior Therapy, 45,* 83–101.

Goldberg, S. B., Tucker, R. P., Greene, P. A., Davidson, R. J., Wampold, B. E., Kearney, D. J., & Simpson, T. L. (2018). Mindfulness-based intervention for psychiatric disorders: A systematic review and meta-analysis. *Clinical Psychology Review, 59,* 52–60.

Graham, J. R., Sorenson, S., & Hayes-Skelton, S. A. (2013). Enhancing the cultural sensitivity of cognitive behavioral interventions for anxiety in diverse populations. *The Behavior Therapist, 36,* 101–107.

Graham, J. R., West, L. M., Martinez, J., & Roemer, L. (2016). The mediating role of internalized racism in the relationship between racist experiences and anxiety symptoms in a Black American sample. *Cultural Diversity and Ethnic Minority Psychology, 22,* 369–376.

Graham, J. R., West, L., & Roemer, L. (2013). The experience of racism and anxiety symptoms in an African American sample: Moderating effects of trait mindfulness. *Mindfulness, 4,* 332–341.

Graham, J. R., West, L. M., & Roemer, L. (2015). A preliminary exploration of the moderating role of valued living in the relationships between racist experiences and anxious and depressive symptoms. *Journal of Contextual Behavioral Science, 4,* 48–55.

Graham-LoPresti, J. R., Abdullah, T., Calloway, A., & West, L. M. (2017). How Black Americans can cope with anxiety and racism. Retrieved from *www.anxiety.org/black-americans-how-to-cope-with-anxiety-and-racism.*

Gratz, K. L., & Roemer, L. (2004). Multidimensional assessment of emotion regulation and dysregulation: Development, factor structure, and initial validation of the difficulties in emotion regulation scale. *Journal of Psychopathology and Behavioral Assessment, 26,* 41–54.

Greenberg, L. S., & Safran, J. D. (1987). *Emotion in psychotherapy.* New York: Guilford Press.

Grilo, C. M., & Shiffman, S. (1994). Longitudinal investigation of the abstinence violation effect in binge eaters. *Journal of Consulting and Clinical Psychology, 62*(3), 611–619.

Griner, D., & Smith, T. B. (2006). Culturally adapted mental health intervention: A meta-analytic review. *Psychotherapy: Theory, Research, Practice, Training, 43*(4), 531–548.

Gross, J. J. (Ed.). (2014). *Handbook of emotion regulation* (2nd ed.). New York: Guilford Press.

Gross, J. J., & Levenson, R. W. (1997). Hiding feelings: The acute effects of inhibiting negative and positive emotion. *Journal of Abnormal Psychology, 106,* 95–103.

Hall, G. C. N., Hong, J. J., Zane, N. W. S., & Meyer, O. L. (2011). Culturally competent treatment for Asian Americans: The relevance of mindfulness- and acceptance-based psychotherapies. *Clinical Psychology: Science and Practice, 18,* 215–231.

Hall, G. C. N., Ibaraki, A. Y., Huang, E. R., Marti, C. N., & Stice, E. (2016). A meta-analysis of cultural adaptations of psychological interventions. *Behavior Therapy, 47,* 993–1014.

Harrell, S. P. (2018). Soulfulness as an orientation to contemplative practice: Culture, liberation, and mindful awareness. *Journal of Contemplative Inquiry, 5*(1), 9–40.

Harris-Perry, M. (2017, July). How Squadcare saved my life. Retrieved from *www.elle.com/culture/career-politics/news/a46797/squad-care-melissa-harris-perry.*

Hawkley, L. C., & Cacioppo, J. T. (2007). Aging and loneliness: Downhill quickly? *Current Directions in Psychological Science, 16*(4), 187–191.

Hayes, A. M., Laurenceau, J. P., Feldman, G., Strauss, J. L., & Cardaciotto, L. (2007). Change is not always linear: The study of nonlinear and discontinuous patterns of change in psychotherapy. *Clinical Psychology Review, 27*, 715–723.

Hayes, A. M., Yasinski, C., Barnes, J. B., & Bockting, C. L. (2015). Network destabilization and transition in depression: New methods for studying the dynamics of therapeutic change. *Clinical Psychology Review, 41*, 27–39.

Hayes, S. A., Orsillo, S. M., & Roemer, L. (2010). Changes in proposed mechanisms of action during an acceptance-based behavior therapy for generalized anxiety disorder. *Behaviour Research and Therapy, 48*, 238–245.

Hayes, S. C. (2016). Acceptance and commitment therapy, relational frame theory, and the third wave of behavioral and cognitive therapies. *Behavior Therapy, 47*, 869–885.

Hayes, S. C., Barnes-Holmes, D., & Roche, B. (2001). *Relational frame theory: A post-Skinnerian account of human language and cognition.* New York: Kluwer Academic/Plenum.

Hayes, S. C., Batten, S. V., Gifford, E. V., Wilson, K. G., Afari, N., & McCurry, S. M. (1999). *Acceptance and commitment therapy: An individual psychotherapy manual for the treatment of experiential avoidance.* Reno, NV: Context Press.

Hayes, S. C., & Shenk, C. (2004). Operationalizing mindfulness without unnecessary attachments. *Clinical Psychology: Science and Practice, 11*, 249–254.

Hayes, S. C., Strosahl, K. D., & Wilson, K. G. (1999). *Acceptance and commitment therapy: An experiential approach to behavior change.* New York: Guilford Press.

Hayes, S. C., Strosahl, K. D., & Wilson, K. G. (2012). *Acceptance and commitment therapy: The process and practice of mindful change* (2nd ed.). New York: Guilford Press.

Hayes, S. C., Villatte, M., Levin, M., & Hildebrandt, M. (2011). Open, aware, and active: Contextual approaches as an emerging trend in the behavioral and cognitive therapies. *Annual Review of Clinical Psychology, 7*, 141–168.

Hayes, S. C., Wilson, K. G., Gifford, E. V., Follette, V. M., & Strosahl, K. (1996). Experiential avoidance and behavioral disorders: A functional dimensional approach to diagnosis and treatment. *Journal of Consulting and Clinical Psychology, 64*, 1152–1168.

Hayes-Skelton, S. A., Calloway, A., Roemer, L., & Orsillo, S. M. (2015). Decentering as a potential common mechanism across two therapies for generalized anxiety disorder. *Journal of Consulting and Clinical Psychology, 83*, 395–404.

Hayes-Skelton, S. A., Roemer, L., & Orsillo, S. M. (2013). A randomized clinical trial comparing an acceptance-based behavior therapy to applied relaxation for generalized anxiety disorder. *Journal of Consulting and Clinical Psychology, 81*(5), 761–773.

Hayes-Skelton, S. A., Roemer, L., Orsillo, S. M., & Borkovec, T. D. (2013). A contemporary view of applied relaxation for generalized anxiety disorder. *Cognitive Behavioural Therapy, 42*, 292–302.

Hays, P. A. (1995). Multicultural applications of cognitive-behavior therapy. *Professional Psychology: Research and Practice, 26*, 309–315.

Hays, P. A. (2016). *Addressing cultural complexities in practice: Assessment, diagnosis and therapy* (3rd ed.). Washington, DC: American Psychological Association.

Hebert, E. A., Dugas, M. J., Tulloch, T. G., & Holowka, D. W. (2014). Positive beliefs about worry: A psychometric evaluation of the Why Worry–II. *Personality and Individual Differences, 56*, 3–8.

Hofmann, S. G., & Asmundson, G. J. G. (2017). *The science of cognitive behavioral therapy.* Cambridge, MA: Elsevier.

Holt-Lunstad, J., Smith, T. B., & Layton, J. B. (2010). Social relationships and mortality risk: A meta-analytic review. *PLOS Medicine, 7*(7), 1–20.

Hoy-Ellis, C. P. (2016). Concealing concealment: The mediating role of internalized heterosexism in psychological distress among lesbian, gay, and bisexual older adults. *Journal of Homosexuality, 63*(4), 487–506.

Huntley, C. D., & Fisher, P. L. (2016). Examining the role of positive and negative metacognitive beliefs in depression. *Scandinavian Journal of Psychology, 57*(5), 446–452.

Huron, D. (2018). On the functions of sadness and grief. In H. Lench (Ed.), *The function of emotions* (pp. 59–91). Cham, Switzerland: Springer International.

Iijima, Y., & Tanno, Y. (2013). The moderating role of positive beliefs about worry in the relationship between stressful events and worry. *Personality and Individual Differences, 55,* 1003–1006.

Jacobson, E. (1934). *You must relax.* New York: McGraw-Hill.

Jones, K. D. (2010). The unstructured clinical interview. *Journal of Counseling and Development, 88,* 220–226.

Jordan, J. V. (2010). *Relational–cultural therapy.* Washington, DC: American Psychological Association.

Kabat-Zinn, J. (1994). *Wherever you go there you are: Mindfulness meditation in everyday life.* New York: Hyperion.

Kabat-Zinn, J. (2005). *Coming to our senses: Healing ourselves and the world through mindfulness.* New York: Hyperion.

Kanter, J. W., Santiago-Rivera, A. L., Rusch, L. C., Busch, A. M., & West, P. (2010). Initial outcomes of a culturally adapted behavioral activation for Latinas diagnosed with depression at a community clinic. *Behavior Modification, 34,* 120–144.

Kaplan, J. S. (2010). *Urban mindful: Cultivating peace, presence, and purpose in the middle of it all.* Oakland, CA: New Harbinger.

Kazantzis, N., Dattilio, F. M., & Dobson, K. S. (2017). *The therapeutic relationship in cognitive-behavioral therapy: A clinician's guide.* New York: Guilford Press.

Khoury, B., Lecomte, T., Fortin, G., Masse, M., Therien, P., Bouchard, V., . . . Hofmann, S. G. (2013). Mindfulness-based therapy: A comprehensive meta-analysis. *Clinical Psychology Review, 33,* 763–771.

King, L., & Polaschek, D. (2003). The abstinence violation effect: Investigating lapse and relapse phenomena using the relapse prevention model with domestically violent men. *New Zealand Journal of Psychology, 32*(2), 67–75.

King, R. (2018). *Mindful of race: Transforming racism from the inside out.* Louisville, CO: Sounds True.

Kircanski, K., Lieberman, M. D., & Craske, M. G. (2012). Feelings into words: Contributions of language to exposure therapy. *Psychological Science, 23,* 1086–1091.

Kircanski, K., Thompson, R. J., Sorenson, J. E., Sherdell, L., & Gotlib, I. H. (2015). Rumination and worry in daily life: Examining the naturalistic validity of theoretical constructs. *Clinical Psychological Science, 3*(6), 926–939.

Klein, A. A. (2007). Suppression-induced hyperaccessibility of thoughts in abstinent alcoholics: A preliminary investigation. *Behaviour Research and Therapy, 45,* 169–177.

Koerner, K. (2011). *Using dialectical behavior therapy: A practical guide.* New York: Guilford Press.

Kolts, R. L. (2016). *CFT made simple.* Oakland, CA: New Harbinger.

Kubiak, T., Zahn, D., Siewert, K., Jonas, C., & Weber, H. (2014). Positive beliefs about rumination are associated with ruminative thinking and affect in daily life: Evidence for a metacognitive view on depression. *Behavioural and Cognitive Psychotherapy, 42,* 568–576.

La Roche, M. J., D'Angelo, E., Gualdron, L., & Leavell, J. (2006). Culturally sensitive guided imagery for allocentric Latinos: A pilot study. *Psychotherapy: Theory, Research, Practice, Training, 43*(4), 555–560.

Ladouceur, R., Blais, F., Freeston, M. H., & Dugas, M. J. (1998). Problem solving and problem orientation in generalized anxiety disorder. *Journal of Anxiety Disorders, 12,* 139–152.

Laugesen, N., Dugas, M. J., & Bukowski, W. M. (2003). Understanding adolescent worry: The application of a cognitive model. *Journal of Abnormal Child Psychology, 31*(1), 55–64.

Le, B. M., & Impett, E. A. (2016). The costs of suppressing negative emotions and amplifying positive emotions during parental caregiving. *Personality and Social Psychology Bulletin, 42*(3), 323–336.

LeDoux, J. (1998). *The emotional brain: The mysterious underpinnings of everyday life.* New York: Simon & Schuster.

Lejuez, C. W., Hopko, D. R., Acierno, R., Daughters, S. B., & Pagoto, S. L. (2011). Ten year revision of the Brief Behavioral Activation Treatment for Depression: Revised treatment manual. *Behavior Modification, 35,* 111–161.

Linehan, M. M. (1993). *Cognitive-behavioral treatment of borderline personality disorder.* New York: Guilford Press.

Linehan, M. M. (1997). Validation and psychotherapy. In A. C. Bohart & L. S. Greenberg (Eds.), *Empathy reconsidered* (pp. 353–392). Washington, DC: American Psychological Association.

Linehan, M. M. (2015). *DBT skills training manual* (2nd ed.). New York: Guilford Press.

Linehan, M. M., Schmidt, H., Dimeff, L. A., Craft, J. C., Kanter, J., & Comtois, K. A. (1999). Dialectical behavior therapy for patients with borderline personality disorder and drug-dependence. *American Journal on Addictions, 8,* 279–292.

Lovibond, P. F., & Lovibond, S. H. (1995). The structure of negative emotional states: Comparison of the Depression Anxiety Stress Scales (DASS) with the Beck Depression and Anxiety Inventories. *Behaviour Research and Therapy, 33,* 335–343.

Lundgren, T., Luoma, J. B., Dahl, J., Strosahl, K., & Melin, L. (2012). The Bull's-Eye Values Survey: A psychometric evaluation. *Cognitive and Behavioral Practice, 19,* 518–526.

Lyubomirsky, S., Tucker, K. L., Caldwell, N. D., & Berg, K. (1999). Why ruminators are poor problem solvers: Clues from the phenomenology of dysphoric rumination. *Journal of Personality and Social Psychology, 77*(5), 1041–1060.

Magee, J. C., Harden, K. P., & Teachman, B. A. (2012). Psychopathology and thought suppression: A quantitative review. *Clinical Psychology Review, 32,* 189–201.

Magee, R. V. (2016). Teaching mindfulness with mindfulness of race and other forms of diversity. In D. McCown, D. Reibel, & M. S. Micozzi (Eds.), *Resources for teaching mindfulness: An international handbook* (pp. 225–246). Cham, Switzerland: Springer International.

Markus, H. R., & Kitayama, S. (1991). Culture and the self: Implications for cognition, emotion, and motivation. *Psychological Review, 98,* 224–253.

Marlatt, G. A., & Gordon, J. R. (1980). Determinants of relapse: Implications for the maintenance of behavior change. In P. O. Davidson & S. M. Davidson (Eds.), *Behavioral medicine: Changing health lifestyles* (pp. 410–452). New York: Brunner/Mazel.

Marlatt, G. A., & Gordon, J. R. (Eds.). (1985). *Relapse prevention: Maintenance strategies in the treatment of addictive behaviors.* New York: Guilford Press.

Martell, C. R., Addis, M. E., & Jacobson, N. S. (2001). *Depression in context: Strategies for guided action.* New York: Norton.

Martell, C. R., Dimidjian, S., & Herman-Dunn, R. (2010). *Behavioral activation for depression: A clinician's guide.* New York: Guilford Press.

Martinez, J. H., & Roemer, L. (2019, November). A brief mindfulness- and acceptance-based intervention for coping with race-related stress. In J. H. Martinez (Chair), *Mindfulness- and acceptance-based approaches for addressing racism-related stress.* Symposium presented at the annual meeting of the Association for Behavioral and Cognitive Therapies, Atlanta, GA.

Matsumoto, N., & Mochizuki, S. (2018). Why do people overthink?: A longitudinal investigation of a meta-cognitive model and uncontrollability of rumination. *Behavioural and Cognitive Psychotherapy, 46,* 504–509.

Mattick, R. P., & Clarke, J. C. (1998). Development and validation of measures of social phobia scrutiny fear and social interaction anxiety. *Behaviour Research and Therapy, 36,* 455–470.

McBee, L. (2008). *Mindfulness-based elder care: A CAM model for frail elders and their caregivers.* New York: Springer.

McQueen, A., & Klein, W. M. (2006). Experimental manipulations of self-affirmation: A systematic review. *Self and Identity, 5,* 289–354.

Mennin, D. S., & Fresco, D. M. (2014). Emotion regulation therapy. In J. J. Gross (Ed.), *Handbook of emotion regulation* (2nd ed., pp. 469–490). New York: Guilford Press.

Michelson, S. E., Lee, J. K., Orsillo, S. M., & Roemer, L. (2011). The role of values-consistent behavior in generalized anxiety disorder. *Depression and Anxiety, 28*(5), 358–366.

Miller, A. N., & Orsillo, S. M. (2020). Values, acceptance, and belongingess in graduate school: Perspectives from underrepresented minority students. *Journal of Contextual Behavioral Science, 15,* 197–206.

Miller, W. R., & Rollnick, S. (1991). *Motivational interviewing: Preparing people to change addictive behavior.* New York: Guilford Press.

Miller, W. R., & Rollnick, S. (2012). *Motivational interviewing: Helping people change* (3rd ed.). New York: Guilford Press.

Millstein, D. J., Orsillo, S. M., Hayes-Skelton, S. A., & Roemer, L. (2015). Interpersonal problems, mindfulness, and therapy outcome in an acceptance-based behavior therapy for generalized anxiety disorder. *Cognitive Behaviour Therapy, 44*(6), 491–501.

Miyake, A., Kost-Smith, L. E., Finkelstein, N. D., Pollock, S. J., Cohen, G. L., & Ito, T. A. (2010). Reducing the gender achievement gap in college science: A classroom study of values affirmation. *Science, 330,* 1234–1237.

Molero, F., Recio, P., Garcia-Ael, C., & Pérez-Garín, C. (2019). Consequences of perceived personal and group discrimination against people with physical disabilities. *Rehabilitation Psychology, 46,* 212–220.

Moore, T. J., & Mattison, D. R. (2017). Adult utilization of psychiatric drugs and differences by sex, age, and race. *JAMA Internal Medicine, 177,* 274–275.

Morgan, L., Graham, J. R., Hayes-Skelton, S. A., Orsillo, S. M., & Roemer, L. (2014). Relationships between amount of post-intervention of mindfulness practice and follow-up outcome variables in an acceptance-based behavior therapy for generalized anxiety disorder: The importance of informal practice. *Journal of Contextual Behavioral Science, 3,* 173–178.

Murphy, J. T. (2016). *Dancing in the rain: Leading with compassion, vitality, and mindfulness in education.* Cambridge, MA: Harvard Education Press.

Narrow, W. E., Clarke, D. E., Kuramoto, S. J., Kraemer, H. C., Kupfer, D. J., Greiner, L., & Regier, D. A. (2013). DSM-5 field trials in the United States and Canada: Part III. Development and reliability testing of a cross-cutting symptom assessment for DSM-5. *American Journal of Psychiatry, 170*(1), 71–82.

Neff, K. D. (2003). Development and validation of a scale to measure self-compassion. *Self and Identity, 2,* 223–250.

Neff, K. D. (2015). *Self-compassion: The proven power of being kind to yourself.* New York: HarperCollins.

Neff, K., & Germer, C. (2018). *The mindful self-compassion workbook.* New York: Guilford Press.

Newman, M. G., & Llera, S. J. (2011). A novel theory of experiential avoidance in generalized anxiety disorder: A review and synthesis of research supporting a contrast avoidance model of worry. *Clinical Psychology Review, 31*(3), 371–382.

Nezu, A. M., Ronan, G. F., Meadows, E. A., & McClure, K. S. (Eds.). (2000). *Practitioner's guide to empirically-based measures of depression.* Berlin, Germany: Springer Science + Business Media.

Nikčević, A. V., Marino, C., Caselli, G., & Spada, M. M. (2017). The importance of thinking styles in predicting binge eating. *Eating Behaviors, 26,* 40–44.

Nolen-Hoeksema, S. (1991). Responses to depression and their effects on the duration of depressed mood. *Journal of Abnormal Psychology, 100,* 569–582.

Norcross, J. C. (2011). *Psychotherapy relationships that work: Evidence-based responsiveness* (2nd ed.). New York: Oxford University Press.

Okun, B. F., & Suyemoto, K. L. (2013). *Conceptualization and treatment planning for effective helping.* Belmont, CA: Brooks/Cole.

Oluo, I. (2018). *So you want to talk about race.* New York: Seal Press.

Orsillo, S. M., Danitz, S. B., & Roemer, L. (2016). Mindfulness- and acceptance-based cognitive and behavioral therapies. In A. M. Nezu & C. M. Nezu (Eds.), *The Oxford handbook of cognitive and behavioral therapies* (pp. 172–199). New York: Oxford University Press.

Orsillo, S. M., & Roemer, L. (2016). *Worry less, live more: The mindful way through anxiety workbook.* New York: Guilford Press.

Orsillo, S. M., Roemer, L., Lerner, J. B., & Tull, M. T. (2004). Acceptance, mindfulness, and cognitive-behavioral therapy: Comparisons, contrasts, and application to anxiety. In S. C. Hayes, V. M. Follette, & M. M. Linehan (Eds.), *Mindfulness and acceptance: Expanding the cognitive-behavioral tradition* (pp. 66–95). New York: Guilford Press.

Papageorgiou, C., & Wells, A. (2009). A prospective test of the clinical metacognitive model of rumination and depression. *International Journal of Cognitive Therapy, 2*(2), 123–131.

Parsons, C. E., Crane, C., Parsons, L. J., Fjorback, L. O., & Kuyken, W. (2017). Home practice in mindfulness-based cognitive therapy and mindfulness-based stress reduction: A systematic review and meta-analysis of participants' mindfulness practice and its association with outcomes. *Behaviour Research and Therapy, 95*, 29–41.

Pennebaker, J. W. (1997). Writing about emotional experiences as a therapeutic process. *Psychological Science, 8*, 162–166.

Pennebaker, J. W., & Smyth, J. (2016). *Opening up by writing it down: The healing power of expressive writing* (3rd ed.). New York: Guilford Press.

Penney, A. M., Mazmanian, D., & Rudanycz, C. (2013). Comparing positive and negative beliefs about worry in predicting generalized anxiety disorder symptoms. *Canadian Journal of Behavioural Science, 45*, 34–41.

Persons, J. B. (2008). *The case formulation approach to cognitive-behavior therapy.* New York: Guilford Press.

Pratt, L. A., Brody, D. J., & Gu, Q. (2017). *Antidepressant use in persons aged 12 and over: United States, 2011–2014* (National Center for Health Statistics Data Brief, No. 283). Hyattsville, MD: National Center for Health Statistics.

Puckett, J. A., Mereish, E. H., Levitt, H. M., Horne, S. G., & Hayes-Skelton, S. A. (2018). Internalized heterosexism and psychological distress: The moderating effects of decentering. *Stigma and Health, 3*(1), 9–15.

Purdon, C., Rowa, K., & Antony, M. M. (2005). Thought suppression and its effects on thought frequency, appraisal and mood state in individuals with obsessive–compulsive disorder. *Behaviour Research and Therapy, 43*, 93–108.

Quillian, L., Pager, D., Hexel, O., & Midtbøen, A. H. (2017). Meta-analysis of field experiments shows no change in racial discrimination in hiring over time. *Proceedings of the National Academy of Sciences of the USA, 114*(41), 10870–10875.

Rescorla, R. A. (1996). Preservation of Pavlovian associations through extinction. *Quarterly Journal of Experimental Psychology B: Comparative and Physiological Psychology, 49*(3), 245–258.

Rescorla, R. A., & Wagner, A. R. (1972). A theory of Pavlovian conditioning: Variations in the effectiveness of reinforcement and nonreinforcement. *Classical Conditioning II: Current Research and Theory, 2*, 64–99.

Robins, C. J., Schmidt, H., III, & Linehan, M. M. (2004). Dialectical behavior therapy: Synthesizing radical acceptance with skillful means. In S. C. Hayes, V. M. Follette, & M. M. Linehan (Eds.), *Mindfulness and acceptance: Expanding the cognitive-behavioral tradition* (pp. 30–44). New York: Guilford Press.

Roemer, L., Arbid, N., Martinez, J. H., & Orsillo, S. M. (2017). Mindfulness-based cognitive behavioral therapies. In S. Hofmann & G. Asmundson (Eds.), *The science of cognitive behavioral therapy: From theory to therapy* (pp. 175–197). New York: Elsevier.

Roemer, L., & Borkovec, T. D. (1994). Effects of suppressing thoughts about emotional material. *Journal of Abnormal Psychology, 103*, 467–474.

Roemer, L., & Orsillo, S. M. (2002). Expanding our conceptualization of and treatment for generalized anxiety disorder: Integrating mindfulness/acceptance-based approaches with existing cognitive-behavioral models. *Clinical Psychology: Science and Practice, 9,* 54–68.

Roemer, L., & Orsillo, S. M. (2007). An open trial of an acceptance-based behavior therapy for generalized anxiety disorder. *Behavior Therapy, 38,* 72–85.

Roemer, L., & Orsillo, S. M. (2014). An acceptance-based behavioral therapy for generalized anxiety disorder. In D. H. Barlow (Ed.), *Clinical handbook of psychological disorders: A step-by-step treatment manual* (5th ed., pp. 206–236). New York: Guilford Press.

Roemer, L., Orsillo, S. M., & Salters-Pedneault, K. (2008). Efficacy of an acceptance-based behavior therapy for generalized anxiety disorder: Evaluation in a randomized controlled trial. *Journal of Consulting and Clinical Psychology, 76*(6), 1083–1089.

Rogers, C. R. (1961). *On becoming a person: A therapist's view of psychotherapy.* Boston: Houghton Mifflin.

Rush, A. J., First, M. B., & Blacker, J. (Eds.). (2008). *Handbook of psychiatric measures* (2nd ed.). Arlington, VA: American Psychiatric Publishing.

Ryan, R. M., & Deci, E. L. (2000). Intrinsic and extrinsic motivations: Classic definitions and new directions. *Contemporary Educational Psychology, 25,* 54–67.

Safran, J. D., Muran, J. C., & Eubanks-Carter, C. (2011). Repairing alliance ruptures. *Psychotherapy, 48*(1), 80–87.

Safran, J. D., & Segal, Z. V. (1990). *Interpersonal process in cognitive therapy.* New York: Basic Books.

Sagon, A. L., Danitz, S. B., Suvak, M. K., & Orsillo, S. M. (2018). The mindful way through the semester: Evaluating the feasibility of delivering an acceptance-based behavioral program online. *Journal of Contextual Behavioral Science, 9,* 36–44.

Santor, D. A. (2017). Registry of scales and measures: Psychological tests, scales, questionnaires, and checklists. Retrieved from *www.scalesandmeasures.net.*

Segal, Z. V., Anderson, A. K., Gulamani, T., Dinh Williams, L. A., Desormeau, P., Ferguson, A., . . . Farb, N. A. (2019). Practice of therapy acquired regulatory skills and depressive relapse/recurrence prophylaxis following cognitive therapy or mindfulness based cognitive therapy. *Journal of Consulting and Clinical Psychology, 87*(2), 161–170.

Segal, Z. V., Williams, J. M. G., & Teasdale, J. D. (2002). *Mindfulness-based cognitive therapy for depression: A new approach to preventing relapse.* New York: Guilford Press.

Segal, Z. V., Williams, J. M. G., & Teasdale, J. D. (2013). *Mindfulness-based cognitive therapy for depression* (2nd ed.). New York: Guilford Press.

Seidman, A. J., Wade, N. G., Lannin, D. G., Heath, P. J., Brenner, R. E., & Vogel, D. L. (2018). Self-affirming values to increase student veterans' intentions to seek counseling. *Journal of Counseling Psychology, 65,* 653.

Serowik, K. L., Roemer, L., Suvak, M., Liverant, G., & Orsillo, S. M. (in press). A randomized controlled trial evaluating *Worry Less, Live More: The Mindful Way through Anxiety Workbook.*

Shafran, R., Thordarson, D. S., & Rachman, S. (1996). Thought–action fusion in obsessive compulsive disorder. *Journal of Anxiety Disorders, 10,* 379–391.

Shapiro, S. L., Carlson, L. E., Astin, J. A., & Freedman, B. (2006). Mechanisms of mindfulness. *Journal of Clinical Psychology, 62,* 373–386.

Sheldon, K. M., & Elliot, A. J. (1999). Goal striving, need satisfaction, and longitudinal well-being: The self-concordance model. *Journal of Personality and Social Psychology, 76,* 482–497.

Sheldon, K. M., & Kasser, T. (2001). Getting older, getting better?: Personal strivings and psychological maturity across the life span. *Developmental Psychology, 37,* 491–501.

Sherman, D. K., & Cohen, J. L. (2006). The psychology of self-defense: Self-affirmation theory. In M. P. Zanna (Ed.), *Advances in experimental social psychology* (pp. 183–242). San Diego, CA: Academic Press.

Shipherd, J. C., & Beck, J. G. (2005). The role of thought suppression in posttraumatic stress disorder. *Behavior Therapy, 36,* 277–287.

Singh, A. (2019). *The racial healing handbook: Practical activities to help you challenge privilege, confront systemic racism, and engage in collective healing.* Oakland, CA: New Harbinger.

Smith, T. B., Domenech Rodriguez, M. M., & Bernal, G. (2011). Culture. In J. C. Norcross (Ed.), *Psychotherapy relationships that work: Evidence-based responsiveness* (2nd ed., pp. 316–335). New York: Oxford University Press.

Sobczak, L. R., & West, L. M. (2013). Clinical considerations in using mindfulness and acceptance-based behavioral approaches with diverse populations: Addressing challenges in service delivery in diverse community settings. *Cognitive and Behavioral Practice, 20,* 13–22.

Sommers-Flanagan, J., & Sommers-Flanagan, R. (2016). *Clinical interviewing* (6th ed.). Hoboken, NJ: Wiley.

Spears, C. A., Houchins, S. C., Bamatter, W. P., Barrueco, S., Hoover, D. S., & Perskaudas, R. (2017). Perceptions of mindfulness in a low-income, primarily African American treatment-seeking sample. *Mindfulness, 8*(6), 1532–1543.

Steele, C. M., & Aronson, J. (1995). Stereotype threat and the intellectual test performance of African Americans. *Journal of Personality and Social Psychology, 69,* 797–811.

Stoddard, J. A., & Afari, N. (2014). *The big book of ACT metaphor: A practitioner's guide to experiential exercises and metaphors in acceptance and commitment therapy.* Oakland, CA: New Harbinger.

Sue, D. W., & Sue, D. (2016). *Counseling the culturally diverse: Theory and practice* (7th ed.). New York: Wiley.

Szabó, M., & Lovibond, P. F. (2002). The cognitive content of naturally occurring worry episodes. *Cognitive Therapy and Research, 26*(2), 167–177.

Szymanski, D. M., & Mikorski, R. (2016). External and internalized heterosexism, meaning in life, and psychological distress. *Psychology of Sexual Orientation and Gender Diversity, 3*(3), 265–274.

Taylor, S., Zvolensky, M. J., Cox, B. J., Deacon, B., Heimberg, R. G., Ledley, D. R., . . . Cardenas, S. J. (2007). Robust dimensions of anxiety sensitivity: Development and initial validation of the Anxiety Sensitivity Index–3. *Psychological Assessment, 19,* 176–188.

Tirch, D. (2012). *The compassionate-mind guide to overcoming anxiety: Using compassion-focused therapy to calm worry, panic, and fear.* Oakland, CA: New Harbinger.

Tolin, D. F. (2016). *Doing CBT: A comprehensive guide to working with behaviors, thoughts, and emotions.* New York: Guilford Press.

Tsai, M., Kohlenberg, R. J., Kanter, J. W., Kohlenberg, B., Follette, W. C., & Callaghan G. M. (Eds). (2009). *A guide to functional analytic psychotherapy: Awareness, courage, love, and behaviorism.* New York: Springer.

Tsai, W., Nguyen, D. J., Weiss, B., Ngo, V., & Lau, A. S. (2017). Cultural differences in the reciprocal relations between emotion suppression coping, depressive symptoms and interpersonal functioning among adolescents. *Journal of Abnormal Child Psychology, 45*(4), 657–669.

Vettese, L. C., Toneatto, T., Stea, J. N., Nguyen, L., & Wang, J. J. (2009). Do mindfulness meditation participants do their homework? And does it make a difference?: A review of the empirical evidence. *Journal of Cognitive Psychotherapy, 23*(3), 198–225.

Wadsworth, L. P., Morgan, L. P. K., Hayes-Skelton, S. A., Roemer, L., & Suyemoto, K. L. (2016). Way to boost your research rigor through increasing your cultural competence. *The Behavior Therapist, 39,* 76–92.

Ward, T., Hudson, S. M., & Marshall, W. L. (1994). The abstinence violation effect in child molesters. *Behaviour Research and Therapy, 32*(4), 431–437.

Watkins, E., & Moulds, M. (2005). Positive beliefs about rumination in depression—a replication and extension. *Personality and Individual Differences, 39,* 73–82.

Watson-Singleton, N. N., Black, A. R., & Spivey, B. N. (2019). Recommendations for a culturally responsive mindfulness-based intervention for African Americans. *Complementary Therapies in Clinical Practice, 34,* 132–138.

Wegner, D. M. (1989). *White bears and other unwanted thoughts: Suppression, obsession, and the psychology of mental control.* London: Penguin Press.

Wegner, D. M., & Schneider, D. J. (2003). The white bear story. *Psychological Inquiry, 14*(3–4), 326–329.

Wegner, D. M., Schneider, D. J., Carter, S. R., & White, T. L. (1987). Paradoxical effects of thought suppression. *Journal of Personality and Social Psychology, 53,* 5–13.

Wegner, D. M., & Zanakos, S. (1994). Chronic thought suppression. *Journal of Personality, 62,* 615–640.

Wells, A., & Davies, M. I. (1994). The Thought Control Questionnaire: A measure of individual differences in the control of unwanted thoughts. *Behaviour Research and Therapy, 32,* 871–878.

West, L., Graham, J. R., & Roemer, L. (2013). Functioning in the face of racism: Preliminary findings on the buffering role of values clarification in a Black American sample. *Journal of Contextual Behavioral Science, 2,* 1–8.

Williams, J. M. G., Teasdale, J. D., Segal, Z. V., & Kabat-Zinn, J. (2007). *The mindful way through depression: Freeing yourself from chronic unhappiness.* New York: Guilford Press.

Williams, K. E., Chambless, D. L., & Ahrens, A. H. (1997). Are emotions frightening?: An extension of the fear of fear concept. *Behaviour Research and Therapy, 35,* 239–248.

Wilson, K. G., & Murrell, A. R. (2004). Values work in acceptance and commitment therapy: Setting a course for behavioral treatment. In S. C. Hayes, V. M. Follette, & M. M. Linehan (Eds.), *Mindfulness and acceptance: Expanding the cognitive-behavioral tradition* (pp. 120–151). New York: Guilford Press.

Wilson, K. G., Sandoz, E. K., Kitchens, J., & Roberts, M. (2010). The Valued Living Questionnaire: Defining and measuring valued action within a behavioral framework. *Psychological Record, 60,* 249–272.

Witkiewitz, K., & Marlatt, G. A. (2004). Relapse prevention for alcohol and drug problems: That was Zen, this is Tao. *American Psychologist, 59*(4), 224–235.

Woods-Giscombé, C. L., & Gaylord, S. A. (2014). The cultural relevance of mindfulness meditation as a health intervention for African Americans: Implications for reducing stress-related health disparities. *Journal of Holistic Nursing, 32*(3), 147–160.

Yang, L. (2017). *Awakening together: The spiritual practice of inclusivity and community.* Somerville, MA: Wisdom.

Yogis, J. (2009). *Saltwater Buddha: A surfer's quest to find zen on the sea.* Somerville, MA: Wisdom.

Zuckerman, E. L. (2012). *Clinician's thesaurus: The guide to conducting interviews and writing psychological reports* (7th ed.). New York: Guilford Press.

Index

Note. *f, t, b,* or *n* following a page number indicates a figure, table, box, or note.

Experiential avoidance *(cont.)*
reducing, 22–23
working with, 197
Experiential awareness, 11–13
Experiential practices, role of, 22
Exposure therapy, 225b–226b
External barriers; *see* Contextual inequities/
external barriers

F

Fear
client handouts on, 127–129, 216b
functions of, 103
message, elicitors, actions, 130
monitoring, form for, 122
Feelings, unreciprocated, 248
Financial constraints, 253–254
Fusion, 10–11

G

Gardening metaphor, 228b
Generalized anxiety disorder (GAD),
mindfulness practices and, 147
Goals, *versus* values, form for distinguishing,
193f, 205
Guilt, message, elicitors, actions, 130

H

Habitual responses, benefits and costs of, 8
Hopelessness, working with, 197

I

Identity; *see also* Cultural identity
importance of, 20, 20n6
marginalized, psychological "armor" and,
116
Indecision, working with, 196–197
Inhibitory learning theory (ILT), 225b–226b,
269
Inner experiences
assessing, 46–47
contextual triggers of, assessing, 46–47

Instruction, as source of learning, 8
Integrating goals of ABBT, 213–237, 214–217
and actions in difficult situations, 230–232
early sessions
selecting strategies for, 214–216, 214f, 216b
teaching model and skill development,
214–217, 214f, 216b
later sessions, applying ABBT components,
223–229
learning goals, 213
with limited time, 232b
model for, across sessions, 290–293
second phase, commitments to valued
actions, 217–223, 230b
Internal experiences
altering client's relationship with, 21–23,
80–87, 83b, 89b
by encouraging decentering/defusion,
84–87
by enhancing acceptance/willingness,
87–89
by promoting values-based actions, 89–90
using validation, 81–84, 83b
assessing, 26–28, 28t
assessing relationship with, 27–28
client history and, 41, 42t
control efforts and, 111–113
cultivating compassionate relationship
with, 21
emotional reactions to, 11–12
experiential awareness and, 11–13
fusion and entanglement with, 10–11
increasing acceptance of/willingness to
have, 22–23
judgment of, 9–10
learned qualities of relating to, 8–9
measures assessing relationship with,
283–285
problematic relationship with, 9–13
reducing discomfort of, 217
relationship with, 5, 6
assessing, 47
and stuck points in values writing, 190–196,
191b
Interviews
for assessing engagement in meaningful
activities, 31–33
for assessing experiential avoidance, 29–30
for assessing internal experiences, 26–28, 28t
"Inviting difficulty in" practice, 247–248

List of Audio Tracks

Title	Length
Mindfulness of Breath	3 minutes
Mindfulness of Sounds	5 minutes
Mindfulness of Physical Sensations	3 minutes
Mindfulness-Based Progressive Muscle Relaxation: Instructions	11 minutes
Progressive Muscle Relaxation, 16 Muscle Group Exercise	37 minutes
Progressive Muscle Relaxation, 7 Muscle Group Exercise	19 minutes
Progressive Muscle Relaxation, 4 Muscle Group Exercise	13 minutes
Mindfulness of Emotions	5 minutes
Mindfulness of Emotions and Physical Sensations	6 minutes
Mindfulness of Clouds and Sky	7 minutes
Mountain Meditation	8 minutes
Inviting a Difficulty In and Working It through the Body	6 minutes
Your Personal Experience with Self-Compassion	4 minutes
Mindful Observation of Self-Critical Thoughts	4 minutes

TERMS OF USE